MW01487483

The Addict

The True Path to Inner Peace and Self-Mastery

By Ronnie Landis

"The Addiction Free Lifestyle is superb writing, bringing a depth of clarity and direction to this topic. I appreciate Ronnie's wealth of knowledge and experience that he brings into this to see beyond surface level illusions and to dive deep into how to acknowledge what is really happening. He brings the pathway to change the game with it, if you choose."

-Marci Lock

Copyright

Disclaimer

This book is meant to narrate one man's subjective journey while learning about how to use the power of his mind for a happy and healthy life. The information provided by the author, website, or this company is not a substitute for a face-to-face consultation with your physician and should not be construed as individual medical advice. If a condition persists, please contact your physician. This book is provided for personal and informational purposes only. This book is not to be construed as any attempt to either prescribe or practice medicine. Neither is the book to be understood as putting forth any cure for any type of acute or chronic health problem.

You should always consult with a competent, fully licensed medical professional when making any decision regarding your health. Ronnie Landis and the owners of the Website will use reasonable efforts to include up-to-date and accurate information on our Internet site, but make no representations, warranties, or assurances as to the accuracy, currency, or completeness of the information provided. The owners of this book and our corresponding internet site shall not be liable for any damages or injury resulting from your access to, or inability to access this book, our Internet site, or from your reliance upon any information provided. All rights reserved. No part of this publication may be reproduced, transmitted, transcribed, stored in a retrieval system, or translated into any language, in any form, by any means, without the written permission of the author.

Ronnie Landis
www.hhphealth.com

Table of Contents

Warning: Before You Read This Book

WAIT!

Stop before you read this book!

I can't let you dive into this book without a warning...

...So, give me just two minutes before you start reading (although I know you're really excited.)

Look, if you're anything like me, which I imagine you are to have picked up this book in the first place, self-mastery is a huge deal to you.

Due to the sobering nature of what you're about to read in this book, you're going to likely experience a wide range of emotions... and not all of them feel good, at first.

You see, because of what you're about to read, you're going to want to make some immediate changes to your lifestyle.

On one hand, you're right where you need to be. The goal of this book is to inspire positive change.

On the other hand, making immediate changes to your lifestyle can and most likely will beget some discomfort.

Over the past several decades that you've been alive, you've been conditioned to believe in a "normal" based on social mores, laws, regulations, family domestication, and beliefs.

You may find that habits you never considered to be detrimental are, in fact, holding you back from the success, self-actualization, or peace of mind that you want and deserve.

When people read this book, they are immediately confronted by the truth of their habits, patterns, self-destructive tendencies, and underlining addictions.

You will likely be motivated to make abrupt changes all at once.

However, I want to encourage you to take your time with this process and focus on changing one thing at a time.

It can be overwhelming to feel that we must do everything all at once, and much more difficult to try to do it all on our own.

But you don't have to do this alone.

Please join me at **www.AFLSupport.com** where we have a community of Addiction-Free Lifestyle participants, leaders, mentors, and teachers eager to support you on your journey... no matter what step you're at.

I can't wait to get to know you and some of the people you love most in our Addiction-Free Lifestyle Tribe at **www.AFLSupport.com.**

Freedom from addiction is freedom to be truly, deeply happy.

Let's walk this road together.

With respect and admiration,

Ronnie Landis

Foreword

As an author I am often asked to write testimonials for the books of others. To be quite honest, this is something of a dilemma, for I personally don't think it is right to speak of a book unless one has read the whole of it first, which obviously is quite a commitment in one's precious time and energy. Having said this, I am very glad I agreed to take a look at this book when Ronnie asked me if I would consider writing the Foreword. It is a truly important book. Ronnie has taken on a subject patrolled by armies of experts the world over, so I salute his bravery before he even began!

But this book is not really another book about addiction. It isn't even a book about how to break addiction. It goes much further than this. Ronnie grounds his reader in a simple, controversial but undeniable truth - that we all are addicts in one form or another. To live without addiction presupposes a high level of awareness and even spiritual development. As I read through these pages, I began to realize subtle places in my own life where addictive tendencies still linger, like stubborn lichens clinging to the rocks on mountaintops.

The fact is that addiction is one of the fundamental universal human shadows. No one is immune from addiction in one form or another. As the Buddhists have testified for eons, it is our clinging addictive human tendencies that keep bringing us back to the earth realm. To really understand addiction, therefore, is to understand the very basis of what keeps us from awakening to our highest crest of self-realization. This makes addiction the ultimate spiritual journey, for only when we can live what Ronnie terms 'The Addiction Free Lifestyle' will we have fully awakened.

This is, however, not only a book for spiritual types. It is for everyone. Writing in his clear, flowing and friendly prose, Ronnie speaks from his heart to our heart. He also speaks from the heart of his suffering, and you get the feeling he truly empathizes with our addictions, whatever they may be. He also gives us hope where many feels there is no hope:

This can begin to become a bit of a rude awakening for us when we realize that we have been carrying out seemingly benign behaviors, day after day, month after month, year after year, maybe even decade after decade and unable (or unwilling) to see the accumulative effect they have had on our lives. It can feel like we have dug ourselves so deep due to our willful unconsciousness that the road back to self-confidence, self-esteem, and self-respect feels too far gone and hopeless. This feeling is completely normal and is a sign of hope in of itself because the pain that arises from this realization is a glimmer of consciousness pouring in.

There are a hell of a lot of great insights in this book. There is fascinating science, but it isn't long-winded or boring. There are forays into the various areas where addiction is most commonly found - diet, technology, sex and a deeply relevant focus on the addictive power of social media. However, as you read the whole book you soon begin to realize that it doesn't really matter so much *what* you are addicted to, just that it is there because there is a hole in your soul, and the addiction is your way of wishing it wasn't there. This is the insight around which Ronnie builds his approach - that the key is not to simply lock addiction down through an act of will, but to understand its roots in our physical body, our emotional body, our mind and deepest of all, in our soul. And from this profound understanding, our action flows effortlessly and our addictions are permanently dismantled, rather than simply transferred from one area of our life to another.

I don't wish to distract you the reader from beginning this journey with Ronnie with too many more words. All I wish to say is that from my perspective, Ronnie knows this territory and his insights and advice can truly help you if you are courageous enough to read the book and then apply it to your own addictive patterns. Addiction is memory stored in the cells of the body and is usually rooted in childhood. Addiction is also loosened or tightened through the mind. And perhaps above all, Ronnie's greatest insight: Addiction thrives where relationships wither. We have to open our hearts up to life again and to others - this is perhaps the greatest step of all.

I wholeheartedly encourage you to read and re-read this book and then work with it. Let it be a breakthrough book for you - one of those rare events that swings a whole life in a new direction. If you've made it this far, then I wish you well on your journey and I commend you into the hands of this most excellent guide, a man with humility and integrity with a message of practical hope that can reshape your life from this moment forth. Go to it. Dive in and contemplate these words and insights. Resonate these lessons deep in your cells and you will come to understand the power of Grace to transform a life of suffering into a life of freedom...

Richard Rudd

Author & Founder of The Gene Keys

Introduction

This book is a summation of all the years of research and personal investigation into the fields of human development from the perspective of what holds us back the most from accessing and embodying our greatest potential in life. In the Westernized socialized world, the idea of personal development is heavily focused upon doing more, becoming more, accumulating more, and adding layer upon layer as to block out the inadequacies or short comings that do not reflect excellence. Although there is great merit in the tenets of work ethic, motivation, setting and getting goals, and all the rest, that is only one part of the equation and all too often the singular focus on personal growth can leave us feeling a bit empty once we discover that no amount of worldly success can fulfill an empty void or in the phraseology of Dr. Gabor Mate, author of **In the Realm of Hungry Ghosts**, it does not satisfy the hungry ghosts that we try to feed from these pursuits.

It is becoming soberingly clear and obvious that at the root of all psychological and emotional distresses worldwide has less to do with a chemical imbalance (although this is a big factor and we will discuss this in detail), it has much more to do with a crisis of meaning and what we are making our lives mean. You see, we as human beings are brilliant and highly imaginative meaning making machines. We can make any situation mean virtually anything we want based on our perspectives, our adopted belief systems, and however negative or positive our frame of mind tends to be on a regular basis. In other words, we are making it all up as we go along and the meaningfulness in our lives is directly proportionate to the meaning we give to our lives. We can look out into the world for meaning all we want and derive conclusions about what is true or what is false based on circumstances (which most people tend to do) but ultimately that is all something of a holographic illusion and changes in appearance based on the changes that occur within ourselves.

What I have found for myself and thousands of clients I have worked with over the last 15 years or so is that the gold we seek is buried deep inside ourselves. What that means is that the things we want to achieve outside of us have much less to do with an external phenomenon and much more with an internal feeling we are trying to gain access to. For simplicity's sake, let's call this internal sensation an emotion or a consistent state of feeling that we are searching for. So, if this is the case and I attest that it always has been, then that begs the question which is do I need to do more or add more on in order to gain it or do I do less and strip away more in order to find it?

Once we begin asking this kind of question the mysteries of life begin to open themselves up to us in a way that was once previously blocked from our awareness and simply cannot be found outside of us in the wide world out there. There is a paradox built into this kind of inquiry for sure and that will be unpacked as we continue through this book but let's address the elephant in the room as to get a crystal-clear understanding of what stops us all from, not only accessing the states of feeling we wish to experience daily but also what sabotages us from experiencing all of life and our personal potential at its peak.

It would be all too easy to say that the biggest challenge people seem to face in life (and in their health) is one form or another of self-sabotage. In fact, what exactly does that mean; to sabotage oneself? Does that even make sense logically? This will definitely make a lot more sense as we navigate these concepts deeper in the coming pages but for now just consider that there is an inner tension that exists within just about every human walking the planet. Something of an inner conflict and for some a full-blown inner civil war that has left a feeling of disconnection or dislocation from what we can call someone's true authentic self and their 'not self' or simply their inauthentic self. Well then, what is this inauthentic self? Good question! It is what some refer to as the ego yet that is a grossly oversimplified term and has influenced a culture of spiritual oriented minds to think the ego is somehow bad or wrong, which is absolutely false and could not be further from the truth.

The ego, as it were, is simply a mental identity structure that contains its own set of values, morals, ethics, and ways of seeing the world. This can be an extremely useful tool, or it can also become a detrimental hinderance depending on how it is trained. Similar to a dog. It can be free flowing, develop new skills, fluid and full of life or it can also be angry, calcified, incapable of learning new things, and sickly. It all depends on how it is trained, treated, and exercised.

So, back to the tension between the authentic and inauthentic self. The inauthentic self is essentially a repository of personality programming that has been accumulated over our lives and has been switched on autopilot whereas the authentic self is who you actually are, underneath the cultural programming, reactive patterning, belief systems, ingrained habits, familial ties, and behavior tendencies. It is the true authentic spark of divinity that represents what is absolutely unique about you and cannot be replicated, duplicated, or emulated by another being on the planet, like your fingerprint or snowflake but far, far more unique and special than even that. It is the mark of your soul and so long as we live from that space within us, we are living outside of the personality program and so long as we are disconnected from that we are trapped in the personality programming. Make sense?

This then begs the question; what keeps us from living in that space of our own uniqueness. This of course becomes the most important question and the inquiry into this is far more of a deconstructive process than it is constructive. What I mean by this is we begin to deconstruct the personality programming or conditioning rather than continuing to build upon its hollow foundation. Once we have thoroughly delayered the faulty foundation of conditioning, we can then begin installing new patterns, informational programs (beneficial belief systems), and productive routines that allow our true self to flourish within the structured habitat of a lifestyle that supports our dreams and produces vigorous health, happiness, fulfillment, and harmonious relationships. Consider it a detoxification process for the ego identity that was based entirely on external circumstances and worldly achievements rather than being content and satisfied internally, regardless of what is happening around us.

> *"Everything can be taken from a man but one thing: the last of the human freedoms — to choose one's attitude in any given set of circumstances, to choose one's own way."*
>
> *Viktor Frankl, Man's Search for Meaning*

My Personal Journey with Addiction & Self Sabotage

The overall purpose of this book is twofold. On one level it is to provide a valuable resource for those who struggle with any form of addiction and self-defeating patterns. This much is likely obvious to the reader. This is a manual for addressing the underlining roots of addiction, how to overcome internal conflict, and transcend these limitations so that one may begin living the life they truly deserve. The other purpose is for me to also unpack and unwind my own internal conflicts that have arisen throughout my life as a way to liberate myself from my own limiting patterns. I, like you, and all of us are very much human and have experienced a life of intensity, trauma, struggle, and challenges just as much as I have also been able to overcome myself time and time again. In fact, I would say that the underlining theme of my own life has been overcoming my limitations, powering through life circumstances, developing a greater sense of faith in the unknown, and persisting relentlessly towards my dreams in the face of total uncertainty and unpredictability.

So, in essence, we are both going on a journey here and what makes me uniquely qualified to be the tour guide is that every single thing I communicate is coming from deep personal experience. I am a very seasoned researcher, holistic health educator, and transformational coach but it is not as if that happened overnight or simply due to serendipity. It has been a long road full of insurmountable obstacles, many dark nights of the soul, and in many instances having to reconcile shattered dreams on the riverbank of reality. The greatest attribute I have received through my own life journey is the realization that there are no victims in life, and I certainly have never felt like I was a victim. I am simply a soul in this human avatar called a body and have done my best, despite self-sabotage tendencies, to rise up to the occasion and claim victory in the face of prior defeat. I have maintained the attitude of a winner and champion through my adult life, and this is the single saving grace that has allowed me to make it through the journey and that is what I wish to impart to you as well, among many other highly valuable pieces of wisdom.

Over the last decade of being a global health and nutrition educator I have given hundreds of lectures on topics such as raw foods, super foods, herbalism, detoxification, disease recovery and prevention, and the mind-body connection. Throughout the years it became clearer to me that there were two distinct types of people I would come across in my work; those who heal and those who simply do not. I have worked with countless individuals with a range of conditions from all forms of cancer, heart conditions, diabetes, digestive gut problems, autoimmune issues, neurological dysfunctions (MS, Parkinson's, etc.), and others. I began to see that there were some people that took all of my advice, implemented the changes, and were on a fast track towards recovery. I also noticed, and more times than not, others would get the same advice but struggled to stay consistent in implementing it and seemed to be on a constant up and down spiral which ultimately led to them never truly healing.

Over the years I became far more interested in the psychology of health than merely just the physiology itself. I realized that consciousness has a huge part to play in all forms of healing whether physical, psychological, emotional, and/or spiritual. In fact, I would go so far to say that 90% of "diet" is psychological in nature due to the simple fact that in order to make necessary changes one must be compliant to the changes first. Compliance is key and if our default belief systems/stories do not support the changes we are attempting to make than those changes have no anchor and ultimately fall off, sometimes in extreme ways where someone yo-yos to the other extreme and becomes worse off than they were before. As one can imagine, this was very perplexing for me and this began my deeper exploration in the nature of psychotherapy, past life regressions, metaphysics, trauma and wound clearing, plant medicines, as well as other unique aspects of the human condition.

What I would like to share with you now is that through this deeper exploration into the human condition I began to unearth my own traumas that had been deeply layered in my psyche as well as in my neuromuscular system, and it was not as if I knew exactly how to address them when they arose. I was in the position of the teacher and coach, but when I came across someone who mirrored an internal conflict/tension point, I began to sense the tension within my own operating system and found myself unwinding long held trauma's that had always been there but were undetectable up to that point. This is really where my deeper spiritual initiation began because as I began to explore and unpack my own inner tension, I began to witness certain behavioral patterns in my life that were out of alignment with who I knew I was; out of alignment with who others knew me as. As I began to become more aware of this it felt unsettling to say the least, and I did not exactly know what to do with it, other than just keep moving forward and assume it would all take care of itself.

Every chapter in this book is specifically chosen based on two factors. One is the understanding that these are the very real challenges that virtually everyone in society either experiences directly or is directly affected by, in one way or another. The second factor is that I have personally experienced each one of these challenges and have personally "suffered" through my own ignorance and willingness to perpetuate addictive tendencies all while fully experiencing the pain it has caused in my life and my psyche. The world is our mirror and what we see on the hologram outside of us is an exact reflection of what is residing within our own unconscious minds. Consciousness is primary but the unconscious is always seeking to become conscious, and will use the props, the stages, and actors in our lives to bring forth aspects of ourselves to the surface.

When I think about the most dominant and obvious addictions (we will further define that word just a bit later) there are a number of things that come to mind. The most obvious in our culture is recreational street drugs, pharmaceutical drugs, prescription medications, alcohol, tobacco, and some others. These lead the list in most people's minds. Lesser acknowledged addictions begin to include pornography, coffee/caffeine, processed foods, internet scrolling and digital devices including our computers, phones, tablets, television, and video games. Underneath all of that we can begin to look at addictive patterning such as workaholism, compulsions around sexuality, moodiness, which can be an addiction associated with lower emotional states, codependency in relationships, social approval from friends, partners, co-workers, or society as a whole, and on and on the list goes.

I have to a greater or lesser degree experienced all of these which gives me a lot of depth and width to discuss in greater detail moving forward. I have experienced the hyper-stimuli rush from online pornography which was always followed up by the crashing wave of shame and guilt after ejaculation. I remember getting so worked up and aroused during the engagement only to find myself quickly cleaning up, zipping up my pants, and walking away as if I was leaving a crime scene. That may seem a bit overdramatic, but when you understand what pornography really is and what happens to the male brain during watching it, and how it feels to be looped in a downward sexualized cycle such as that, then it becomes easier to understand why it feels so awkward and uncomfortable of a thing to participate in. That is only one example of many that virtually all men can relate to, and most women have been affected by through their sexual partners or society as a whole.

I have also experienced the neuro-chemical dependency of stimulants, particularly caffeine in the form of the world's favorite and most accepted drug of choice, coffee. At first glance this does not appear to be anything out of the ordinary but when we consider that historically a civilization's substance of choice in maintaining itself is the same substance it used to build itself it becomes clear that our society has been running on what I call 'caffeinated consciousness'. I know first-hand the dangerous allure this seemingly innocent substance has on people's brains, nervous system, adrenal-thyroid glands, mood imbalances, etc. I was a closet coffee drinker for many years and in no time at all I was making excuses for why coffee was a "super food". But in reality, it was all marketing nonsense and had devastating health consequences. I felt like I needed coffee in the morning in order to feel "normal" but by the time it became a compulsive habit my new normal was far below optimal where coffee allowed me to function at 60% capacity at best but once I completely removed it for good, I was able to function at 100% capacity and that became my new normal, without the coffee bean drug to slow me down.

Internet addiction is another one most of us can relate to in our day and age. I became obsessed with scouring the net for all bits of information and research to compile into my brain. As useful as this tool has been (and I am thankful for it) it also became a double edge sword. Social media platforms are designed in the same way mainstream media outlets are designed; to extract energy through the onlooker's attention i.e., their consciousness. Attention is the new currency in our technological world and our energy is precious and finite which is why the internet scrolling culture has become increasingly disturbed, disassociated from reality, failing in developing true relationships, is susceptible to all kinds of propaganda, false teachings, and corporate marketing programs among other things such as easy access to things such as pornography, the dark web, misinformation, and all the rest. I know this one all too well and it

19

was a blessing when I began to pull back from the virtual reality simulation of the internet (and social media) and began writing this book, which I had on me to do list for months, but it was not until I pulled out of the matrix of the social media that I actually got on with the process of writing.

I know all too well how deep the rabbit hole of addiction goes and how subtle the onset of an additive compulsive tendency begins. It seems innocent and even playful at first but remember in all the great mythological and spiritual stories that seduction and lure are the gateways to compromising our highest virtues and settling for the leftovers of those who work their butts off, do not compromise their virtues, and steadily discipline themselves towards the realization of a worthy ideal. The habituation of self-defeating patterns is what robs us of our dreams, our goals, our relationships, our health and vitality, our longevity, our quality of life, our financial stability, and our deeper sense of meaning and purpose. When I began discipling myself to refrain from giving into the temporary gratification of compulsive patterns and relaxed into the tension in my body from the space in between (instead of trying to fill it right away) I began to experience more inner freedom which resulted in more energy, more cognitive focus, more self-respect, more confidence, more money, more impact in the world, and more of a connection with my creator, whom I call God.

So, with all of this laid out, we are now ready to embark upon our journey together traversing through the layers of the addiction onion, peeling back one at a time, deeply investigating them with a microscope, seeing aspects of ourselves that may not have seen the light of truth, and starting the journey back to wholeness, health, sanity, and maturation as we soon understand that all addictive tendencies are rooted in the avoidance of becoming a fully integrated adult, whether we are man or woman, it really is all the same. In one way or another, when an addictive pattern is taking place, we are simultaneously in an avoidance pattern from ourselves, our true authentic selves, that is.

And this meeting with destiny can no longer be postponed. We have an appointment to get too!

Section 1

The Foundations of Addiction & Recovery

You have been properly introduced to the basic premise of this book and it's now time for us to embark upon the journey together. The topic of addiction is a very interesting and uniquely nuanced one amongst all other themes surrounding health and personal growth. So much of the information on addiction alludes to some of these nuances and basic principles, but I found it challenging to find any single source that truly pulled everything together in a truly holistic way. Don't get me wrong, there are great works on the subject available by many incredible experts in the field of study, and yet I found that there were missing elements in all that I came across. In fact, to be bluntly honest, I found more times than not that there were gaping holes yearning to be filled and that is what sparked the motivation to begin this project.

In this section we are going to deeply explore the foundation of addiction and how it manifests itself from all angles. We are not leaving any stone unturned or any relative sub-topic unaccounted for. There are both subtle and not so subtle aspects of the addiction equation and from what I can see there is not a tremendous amount of clarity or holistic understanding as to the more subtle components of this topic. They say that necessity is the mother of all invention and innovation in the world. I certainly felt the pulse of necessity when I began contemplating about writing this book, how I wanted to structure it, and the underlining theme that would carry it all together from start to finish.

The first phase of this journey will be to explore the subtle nature of addiction and what that all means. From there we will take a close look at the biochemical and epigenetic factors relating to addiction and how the cycle of addictive tendencies creates a biological dependency over time. This is extremely important and essential to inner stand for success. Following that we will drop into a transformational session on the power of living with purpose, mastering the art of goal setting, and most importantly, developing a beautiful vision for your life. That in itself has the power to break the proverbial chains of any addiction and set you free to be and do exactly what you desire.

Let's Dive In…

The Subtle Nature of Addiction

"It does not matter how slowly you go as long as you do not stop."

Confucius

"My recovery must come first so that everything I love in life doesn't have to come last."

Unknown

As we discuss the topic of addiction, it's important that we go beyond the chosen habits themselves and quickly pierce through the foggy veil where the root of the problem exists. It is very common in much of our societies efforts to overcome addiction to focus mostly, if not entirely on the so-called addiction itself without addressing the cause of it and why it continues to persist for so many people. We must understand the subtle nature of this phenomenon in order to see it for what it really is, or we will continue to chase our tail in a perpetual cycle of seeking to be healed yet never truly healing at all.

The journey from addiction to recovery is simply a personal path towards inner freedom, self-sovereignty, and personal empowerment. To the degree that we feel the absence of freedom, sovereignty, and empowerment we will find ourselves susceptible to compulsive habit patterns that tend to temporarily fill in these inner voids but always leave us emptier than we were before and cause a kind of craving sensation that reinforces the cycle of addiction. In essence, this is truly a journey of healing those areas within ourselves where we feel empty, broken, wounded, unloved, dissatisfied, judged, and providing the necessary medicine that allows for healing to happen. The medicine will take many different forms such as organic whole foods, clean structured water, restorative sleep, exercise and movement practices, stilling the mind through meditation and breath work, trauma release work, healthy relationships, among other positive life affirming practices.

On one level this must seem fairly obvious and straight forward. On another level it may feel a bit overwhelming, daunting, or perhaps it feels like a Herculean effort to establish these habits because there seems to be something within us blocking all the goodness from happening in our lives. This brings up a key question which is if healing is simple, and I know the things to help me heal, then why does it feel so hard to maintain momentum once I get started? This my friend is one of the most important questions to sit with because the answer holds the golden key to all of our challenges when it comes to making the positive changes in all areas of our life that will produce positive results and also why we sometimes find ourselves unconsciously sabotaging the fruits of our labor, time and time again.

The simple answer to this can and will only be found inside what is sometimes referred to as 'wholeness'. You see, the entire process of healing is an internal journey back to wholeness. What exactly does this mean, to be whole? Well, consider something for a moment here. Over the last 150 years or so (perhaps much more) all of us and our ancestors have been brought up within what could easily be described as a 'rigged system'. A social system that has been rigged against the average individual from experiencing life in wholeness, health, and prosperity. Throughout all of the socially engineered events that have taken place in our world history we have suffered a type of psychological trauma that has laid deeply below the surface of our conscious mind. This has created a type of psychological fracturing where we have been trained to rely upon our left-brain hemisphere to navigate our personal lives and make sense of the world around us. This is the inception point of the collective trauma we all have inherited from our parents, grandparents, and all those who have come before us.

The left hemisphere of the brain complex is entirely focused on analysis and by overcompensating in this way we have been trained to analyze our lives, our relationships, and our world through the filter of a binary linear mechanism and filter out all of the magnificent aspects of life that live within the right hemisphere of our brain. This has caused a kind of hyper stress adaptation within our nervous system simply called a 'sympathetic overload'. This means that for most people they are living mostly or almost entirely in a state of stress which physiologically speaking is a sympathetic stress response. This causes us to be reactive instead of responsive and this, my friend, is the reason why breaking old habits becomes so hard.

When our bodies are flooded with the chemical cocktail of stress, blood flow to the right hemisphere of the brain decreases and we are pitted in a physiological state of survival, fear, and carnal desires begin to kick on, sometimes in very intense and overwhelming ways. The chosen habit patterns, i.e., the addictions at hand, are a way to self sooth our nervous system, which is going into a state of red alert. When our minds are thrown out of balance we begin to panic and will sometimes do anything within our immediate ability to regulate our system, which is feed-backing to us that something is drastically out of whack. Sometimes this reaction in the body can be so intense that we feel as if we are dying and at that point all capacity for critical thinking goes out the window and we find ourselves in a state of absolute primal survival, which can only produce further distress and disorientation of the mind.

Begin to sit with this explanation for a moment. Take a deep diaphragmatic inhalation, hold it in the upper chest cavity for 5 seconds, and slowly exhale through the nose for another 5 seconds. Notice the subtle changes to your state of mind as you repeat this process another 5-10 times. Your bodily system begins to go into a state of calm and all of the electrical-chemical reactions in the body begin to self-regulate all on their own. Take it a step further and go into the shower, turn it all the way cold, and let the water pour onto you for 15-30 seconds without getting out. Notice how the body, at first, goes into a reactive state and maybe even panics for a few moments. Notice how you begin to breath excessively as an automatic response to the temporary shock of the cold energy. Then, as you stay in the temporary discomfort, see how your body system starts to regulate itself and normalize to what was previously a very uncomfortable or even unbearable shock.

This is the miracle technology of your human body. It is entirely designed to self-sooth and self-regulate all on its own but we often times avoid temporary discomfort in order to sooth our inner tension with habits that provide immediate pleasure yet tend to rob us our innate capacity for long term healing and wholeness. Which again, is the true path towards inner freedom and there are no loopholes, shortcuts, or bypasses to healing and recovery. There simply is giving our power away

25

to things outside of us which is the epitome of addiction or exercising our innate power within us and releasing the tentacles of self-destructive patterns that do not serve our evolution and growth.

Subtle Death Habits Revealed

As we continue to pull back the layers of this overall conversation, we discover nuances, subtleties, and unique perspectives emerge as what was once unconscious becomes conscious in our awareness. The discovery that behind every addictive tendency resides an energetic cord linked to an aspect of our own inner experience that has been fragmented or misplaced becomes unavoidable in the healing process. Every behavior is linked to a set of motivators that emerge as part of our own personal identity and as we become more conscious of these motivations, we also become more aware of the identities we have assumed for ourselves to navigate the world around us. So then, as we become more aware of the roles, we have been playing out in our lives we can then begin the deconstruction process of shedding outdated identities and begin reconstructing productive and authentic roles for our life moving forward.

When we are operating within a belief construct or false identity it has a way of creating inner tension and distress within our bodily system. This is due to the fact that our nervous system is a highly intelligent, self-organizing technology that acts as a feedback system to communicate with our conscious mind as to whether we are on track with our higher path or slipping off track. Whether we are in alignment with our truth or living a lie based on misaligned habits and identity structures. Consider it as something of a lie detector technology and when we are telling ourselves a lie i.e., living a lie we feel pain and tension. In order to compensate for the tension, as we have explained before, we may use any manner of habits to neutralize the tension and medicate the pain, for the time being. As we tend to discover though, this is only a temporary band aid, at best, and what is really being called for is an intervention of consciousness by way of stilling the reactive mind through our full presence.

Over the last decade of my professional investigations into the wide world of health and human transformation I came across a great book entitled *Breaking the Death Habit* by *Leonard Orr* which describes what I have been calling for years "subtle death habits". Once we become aware that all of us have had and likely still have a combination of tendencies leaning towards affirming life or affirming death, we can earnestly begin the recovery journey. Until we become aware of this, we will likely keep up false appearances, play out inner child traumas, make up all manner of excuses for our short comings, and remain in a state of limbo; between the true self and false self (dharma & karma). As the saying goes, the truth will set us free but first it will hurt like a MF!

So, what constitutes as a subtle death habit, you may ask. Well, it should be fairly obvious once you begin to look at the cause-and-effect equation of things. What habits, patterns, and routines do you carry out in your life that you know are not assisting in the production of health, positivity, and abundance? What tendencies do you lean towards that seem to lower your energy levels, create fogginess of mind, interrupt your sleep patterns, contribute to unhealthy relationships, and for simplicity's sake, lead to a less than preferable experience for yourself and others? All of these, no matter how small or how big should be categorized within the subtle death habit folder. Anything that is being repeated that produces low energy in the body is slowly damaging the body. So, then what do you call that exactly? You certainly cannot label it as life affirming or life supportive.

This can begin to become a bit of a rude awakening for us when we realize that we have been carrying out seemingly benign behaviors, day after day, month after month, year after year, maybe even decade after decade and unable (or unwilling) to see the accumulative effect they have had on our lives. It can feel like we have dug ourselves so deep due to our willful unconsciousness that the road back to self-confidence, self-esteem, and self-respect feels too far gone and hopeless. This feeling is completely normal and is a sign of hope in of itself because the pain that arises from this realization is a glimmer of consciousness pouring in. In this moment we are being totally authentic and truthful about how we feel, and the key word here is FEEL. Prior to this we likely had done all we could to avoid feeling our feelings and using all of these addiction mechanisms to further suppress these pesky emotions below the surface until we were no longer burdened by them.

What we often do not recognize is how truly burdened we have become due to our distractions and how much density/stagnation we have picked up in our bodies simply by using so much energy to compress our feelings. The opposite of compression is expression and in order to overcome depression it requires an expression of energy that had been suppressed. Anything in our lives that contributes to the suppression of energy will ultimately land in the subtle death habit folder because it causes the body to steadily lose life force, which is why we feel weighed down, have a heavy heart, can't sleep at night, carry guilt or shame, and generally do not feel all that great about ourselves while we are engaged in these patterns. The first step towards liberating ourselves is to liberate our bundled-up energy in the form of unexpressed emotions. We will discuss more in the book about specific practices, modalities, and lifestyle upgrades that will help you unlock your energy/life force but also how to access dormant depths of life force that are the literal cause of all bodily and psychological healing itself.

Why We Do What We Do

"The strongest force in the human personality is the need to stay consistent with how we define ourselves. Identity is a set of beliefs and rules that you use to define yourself and that other people use to define you."

Anthony Robbins

When we find ourselves caught in the cycle of self-destructive patterns it can and usually does feel that there is no way out. I know this feeling all too well. I also know the subconscious programming that creates these patterns and locks them in place like a finely tuned loop. It is important to first recognize that our patterning develops a looping cycle within our psychophysiology that hardwires itself based on repetition. On a more scientific level this is why old habits are so hard to break, we are running on a looping cycle and it eventually becomes a software program within our nervous system that begins to run on autopilot. In order to free ourselves from the prior programming we must see it for what it is and then relentlessly interrupt the pattern as it arises.

This is far easier said than done and as I write these words, I can feel the subtle discomfort in my own body from years of prior patterning. You see, all of the information we have absorbed in our lives inside of our physical bodies. Our body is the grand repository of all our life experiences, successes and failures, victories and triumphs, defeats and disappointments, and to the degree that we are conscious of this is the degree that we have control over ourselves. Once we become more aware, then we can install new habits in place of the old. Throughout the book this idea will be further elaborated on and with specific tools to assist the process.

There are two distinct processes I have seen for reprogramming ourselves and they both work in tandem with each other. One approach is to completely overwhelm our old habits with brand new habits and suffocate out the old. I call this subtraction by addition which means we add in new lifestyle habits and eventually it crowds out the old habits as a result. This requires a solid motivation, focus, and will power to begin, maintain, and eventually the momentum of consistency takes over. The challenge with this is that it does not fully address the root cause of these prior habit patterns and all too often we slip back into old habits as a way to remain consistent with who we believe we are (and who we are used to being). So, this is only one step of the equation and without the next step locked in place it tends to be unsustainable for most.

The other part of the transformational formula is what I call upgrading the operating system and belief system adaptation. The operating system I am referring to is your brain, nervous system complex, and overall biological warehouse including the endocrine system, neuromuscular system, cardiovascular system, immune system, hepatic system (liver-gallbladder), and glandular system. It is not necessary to comprehend in great detail how all of these bodily systems work and interact with one another. What is important to understand is that how feel mentally and emotionally is directly correlated with how we feel physically and when our physiology is in what I called a high-performance health state our emotional constitution and cognitive capacity are far more capable of fulfilling the most important functions of self-transformation, belief system adaptation.

Belief system adaptation is a loose term that came to me when I began to see how our beliefs in life can be like a moving target, constantly in motion, and have their own moving goal posts that are subject to change and adjust based on numerous factors. In the world of personal development and goal setting it has become painfully evident that the smallest percentage of people can absorb information, immediately organize their thoughts, and execute their plans without skipping a beat or feeling overwhelmed as a result of this process. Logically it seems clear and cut that if we take in good information about whatever our goals are that all it takes is creating a basic road map and then just taking the actions consistently and we should arrive at the same outcome, right? Wrong! In fact, this is so wrong for many reasons that I cringe when I think about how much time, energy, money, and years have been expended trying to emulate this formula only to come up short time and time again. I also discovered for myself that there were times where I would not follow this exact formula and somehow arrive at the results I was aiming for or even much better.

I do not want to harp too much on my gripes with the self-help or personal growth communities because I have profound respect and admiration for so much of it but what needs to be understood is so much of it over the last 20ish years is more cosmetic than it is addressing the core concerns. It is like rearranging furniture in our home but continuing to ignore the accumulation of dirt in the corner or pass over the mounting ant hill behind the trash can. Once we take a closer inspection as to what is working well for us and also an honest observation as to what is not working for us then we can make the choice to change. And that choice to change does not just happen once. It happens many times, sometimes multiple times in a single day and continuing to make this choice is the most important choice we can make because it gives us the little boost of hope we need to keep going.

So, now returning back to belief adaptation. You see, we go through many phases and cycles in our life journey. Rarely are we ever the same identical person in our early adult developing years as we are in our 30's, 40's, 50's, etc. We are meant to be constantly changing, fluid like water in motion and our ability to adapt to constant change is based on our internal adaptability. For most people this is extremely difficult because they have a set-in personality program based on external factors and we often call this our personal identity or persona. We build up this identity structure (ego complex) through our formative years as a way to navigate our social environment and for most people this identity becomes the foundation that they stand on moving into adulthood. For some people this can actually be very positive because they had a supportive upbringing and were given the love, care, attention they required along with provisions that allowed for greater access to information, opportunities, and activities to explore their innate creativity. For many people they had the privilege of growing up relatively trauma free. And I say the word privilege simply because this is not the case for the vast majority of people.

For many others, including myself, the reality was far less of a smooth ride and many of us have accrued wounding from childhood experiences and even carry micro-PTSD from trauma's that we may not even know happened to us. All of our life experiences encode energetically into the physical bodily system and are stored deeply into our nervous system until we are consciously capable to healthfully process them and move on. As we continue on in life, we develop our own ego identity based on life experience and when there is more of this unprocessed information in the system then all of that contributes to the identity structure itself. This means that who we believe we are and what we believe we are capable of in life is fundamentally influenced by our unhealed traumas and unconscious programs.

"Our childhood affects every aspect of our health."

Dr. Gabor Mate

This is a major discovery in the field of consciousness work and overall healing because these unconscious programs literally dictate, not only our ability to think and feel, but also to take consistent action. It will never be enough to exercise all the will power in the world if we still have painful experiences living inside of our nerves, muscle cells, immune cells, and blood cells that are contradictory to the goals we are pursuing. This approach can and does only lead to physical burn out, emotional depletion, mental exhaustion, and spiritual crisis over enough time. It is a very sad and disheartening thing to watch, especially because I have also been through it myself and I would not wish this upon anyone. This is also the same process with health and fitness goals by the way. You can take tremendous action towards eating better and working out but if you do not address the underlining identity conflict those habits will begin to die off and/or your body will not respond in a way that it logically should, based on the actions you are taking.

So, with this explanation laid out a bit more let's discuss belief system adaptation and how it works. Most people have a pretty locked in place set of beliefs, for all of the reasons we already mentioned. This can actually allow someone to be relatively successful in their lives depending on the nature of their belief system and how it corresponds to the structure of their life. Perhaps you have heard the saying that what got you here will not get you there in reference to advancing to a new level in life, usually related to business but it applies to everything. In order to play a bigger and more rewarding game we have to be willing to let go of what is holding us back and paradoxically that usually means letting go of doing what worked to get us to where we are now. This requires tremendous flexibility and non-attachment. We have to be 100% committed to the results of our vision instead of being tightly held to the routines and habits of our current circumstances.

Belief adaptation is literally adapting our beliefs, like accessible software programs, to meet the vision of our chosen future and to become the kind of person required to live that reality now. The mistake is to adapt our beliefs based on our circumstances, obstacles, and limited perspective of what is truly possible. We can easily minimize our potential simply by looking outside of us for references of what has been done, either by us in the past or by others. The biggest common denominator in our society is mediocrity and if we only adapt ourselves to what we see outside of us we will adopt the identity of mediocrity at best, by choice or by mistake. Either way it is a bad return on investment for the same amount of energy it takes to upgrade our belief systems and chart the course for a more inspiring future.

When we understand and 'inner stand' these two principles, our lives become a lot more interesting, entertaining, and often a lot easier in many ways. There is really no complexity or complication here either. It is simple, straight forward, and can be acted upon at any moment anyone so chooses. And yet so few tend to successfully upgrade their entire operating systems, develop the ability to toggle between relative belief systems by choice, and more to the point, create the life of their hearts desire. A million books have been written about this general topic and me writing one on top of it was not exactly my highest excitement at first but there was a major elephant sitting in the room of this conversation that I felt uniquely qualified to address. And the fact was that I did not see many others addressing it other than a few landmark educators sharing their wisdom in their own way. Let's discuss the elephant we are all looking at and is looking right back at us.

The Existential Crisis of Disconnection

What if I told you that your addiction to specific habits, routines, patterns, and what can only seem like compulsive tendencies i.e., compulsions to do a certain activity (drugs, porn, smoking, unhealthy food, etc.) are not the problem. In fact, they are far from the actual problem itself but are sign posts pointing towards a deeper causation. I've hinted at this truth a few different ways up to this point and now is where we drop into the nitty gritty of our journey together. This will not be easy and certainly will not be comfortable, for the reader and also for the author as well. But it is time to face the truth because the truth is truly what will set us free from our own self-inflicted captivity and we all deserve to live life freely.

Years ago, when I discovered that I may have developed compulsive addictive tendencies that were slowly weakening my resolve, leaking my bodily life force energy, and building up judgement in my mind it was a long journey of delayering the seemingly simple and benign nature of habitual patterning. I figured that I could stop smoking tobacco (organic), eating excessive carbohydrates at night (organic chips, etc.), or refrain from masturbation at any point I chose. The problem I kept coming up against was I kept putting off making the choice to interrupt my prior patterning and choose a new direction. Before I knew it, I had gotten myself into a spider's web of habits that were all robbing me of long-term fulfillment in place for immediate pleasure. The illusion of this pattern was that I was receiving little to no true pleasure from any of it but my resolve to evolve out of it was lessening and I found myself unable to face the deeper truth underneath the surface of my habituation to downward behaviors.

As I pointed out in the paragraphs before when we begin shifting our energy in a positive and productive direction it begins to take energy away from habits that are leading us elsewhere. So, I noticed that my tobacco smoking habit would come in cycles. When I was living my life more mentally such as writing my books, building online businesses, or in states of consistent stress I would use hand rolled cigarettes as a way to sooth the pressure of not being fully in my body. I also noticed that when I would be fully committed to going to the gym every day, working out with heavy weights, and doing high intensity interval training the tobacco habit would completely lift. When I exercised my respiratory capacity, it become obvious that smoking was a detriment and was unbearable because my workouts were so much harder with that habit in my life. So, the clear demarcation in the sand was obvious and the moment of decision was effortless because my goal for physical fitness was greater than my desire to continue smoking.

So, in essence, this is an example of why the habit kept popping back up in my life, the common themes that played out such as being too mentally focused and not as much in my body, and also what it took of me to shift the habit itself by focusing on getting in my body and literally pushing the stagnation the smoking caused out of my lungs. I would not have been able to do it by simply quitting cold turkey but not changing another major aspect of my lifestyle. You see, when we have stagnation in one area of our life it allows for stagnation to creep into another area. This is also how infectious pathogens work. A bacterial infection or fungal infection will find its way into a localized point of the body, let's say the small intestine and over time if it has the right inner environment that is hospital for it to live it will cultivate microorganism colonies and eventually travel systemically throughout the body and set up breeding locals wherever the immune system is not able to track it down.

Consider that underneath the surface theme of addiction we are unpacking that what we are actually dealing with is a psychological pathogen, like a psycho-parasite that operates in every way a physical parasite does and the more room we allow for it to roam the more opportunity it has to take control of the operating system. I will dive

34

deeper in depth into this later in the book but for the sake of this conversation take this concept to heart. There is a good reason we often can feel like we do not have any control over our impulses and feel terribly uncomfortable when the urge arises in our bodily system. We can turn our attention elsewhere, we can talk ourselves out of the moment, and we can force ourselves through will power to do something else but at the end of this power struggle we are still stuck in a tug a war with ourselves. And no matter where we go or what we do we continue to find ourselves right back where we left off. In a power struggle and the tension that is created through this back and forth creates more internal friction which urges us to self sooth the pressure and thus the cycle is put on repeat.

Now, with all of this said, there is a very important idea I want to relay to you in relation to this idea of a psychological pathogen/parasite and how it actually takes foot in our mind. On one hand it is true that all forms of parasites, physical and non-physical, use their host for their own ends and are energy extraction organisms which draw energy from its host into itself which creates a nasty codependent cycle. Throughout the decade of investigation into parasitology and all forms of bodily disease I have a pretty solid comprehension and direct experience on this topic. I would assert anyone with a serious compulsive addiction problem should go onto a parasite cleanse, more on that later in the book. I also want to illuminate something very important for you with this in mind. The only way a pathogen can take hold of someone, in any way at all, is if that person gives permission and consent for it to do so. Wait, What? Let me explain further.

From a purely physical health perspective, if someone has any form of parasite infection it is because either they consumed a food/contaminated liquid that had a parasite and/or usually is the case they have a deep imbalance in their inner-echo system (microbiome-intestinal tract) and their inner terrain has become hospital for pathogens to live and breed in. Under normal healthy conditions a person's body contains a set of buffering systems such as gastric acids (stomach acid), detoxification and elimination organs, and an immune system that self protects against these foreign invasive organisms. If someone's immune system and stomach acid is not optimal due to poor food choices, lack of movement, and other unhealthy habits they are unconsciously giving consent for parasites, fungi, and bacteria to move in because these organisms are actually the clean-up crew that eat up and dispose of the waste products in the body itself.

So, if someone is choosing a particular lifestyle, they are also choosing what all comes along with that chosen lifestyle and that is what I mean by it being permission based. If we carry unhealthy thought patterns it literally creates acidity in our blood stream and reinforces future acidic behaviors due to the law of correspondence. Something of a like nature corresponds equally to that thing. The idea to consider here before we move on is that the process of regaining self-sovereignty and inner freedom is one of taking total responsibility for our actions, our thoughts, our lifestyle choices, and also for our urges which lead to habits we often times demonize and reject instead of embrace and accept as all part of our consent based human experience.

If we have any area within us that is disempowered, rejected, disowned, or simply not optimally functional such as the example with our bodies then that is a target for something of a lower nature to come and fill in the void. Because, make no mistake, all forms of addictive tendencies arise and sustain themselves entirely based on there being an inner void or disconnect from our true nature/Self which then leads us into what is known as an existential crisis, whether we experience it as a crisis or we simply soften the felt experience of disconnection from our soul/source through these compensatory habits.

"In psychology, compensation is a strategy whereby one covers up, consciously or unconsciously, weaknesses, frustrations, desires, or feelings of inadequacy or incompetence in one life area through the gratification or (drive towards) excellence in another area. Compensation can cover up either real or imagined deficiencies and personal or physical inferiority. Positive compensations may help one to overcome one's difficulties. On the other hand, negative compensations do not, which results in a reinforced feeling of inferiority."

Wikipedia-

Compensatory strategies are an idea that we should all become familiar with because all of us, in one way or another, use them in order to make our way through life and ease the tension we experience as a result of being human beings in a very confusing world. The confusion we often feel in of itself is a psychological compensatory strategy because when we are not in a state of mental clarity, we are not able to address the challenges in our lives. When we experience heightened states of stress it creates a disorientation of the mind and scatters our thoughts as a result. Although this phenomenon clearly does not support us in any real productive way, it is one of the ways the overwhelmed and exhausted psyche compensates for lack of any better option at any given moment.

The body can easily go into a state of panic and survival which we call a sympathetic overload and although there may be no immediate threats in our environment the nervous system can go into red alert as if our life is being threatened. In order to down regulate the system, we have buffer programs kick on and compensate for the stress, anxiety, panic, and fear that we may experience because the system is overloaded and must decompress as its top priority. The body system operates on a hierarchy of survival priorities and if it's overwhelmed it will boot up survival software programs in order to release the pressure valve. This also means we are completely incapable of clear, coherent, and critical thinking in those heightened moments of stress. It then becomes a bit more obvious to see how we use other activities such as various drugs, medications, tobacco, cannabis, psychedelics, pornography, masturbation, junk food, overeating, etc. to compensate for the unrest and distress that has accumulated inside of us.

At the point of systematic overwhelm it is crucial to understand that this is the boiling point for the built-up pressure and tension within us. This is not a mild sign that we need to take a quick break, go blow off some steam, work it out in a gym session, or whatever and go back to our habituated way of life. This is a clear-cut sign that this is a wakeup call from our body and more to the point from our soul that we are living in a way that is unsustainable and has to change, otherwise the alarm clock from our nervous system will only get louder and louder. And the way the feedback repository of our body gets our attention tends to be in the form of tension and tension eventually becomes pain and pain eventually becomes emergency care.

So, what we get to inner stand about this entire process is that our discomfort, tension, pain, and existential pressure is like a finger pointing to the moon, to quote the great Bruce Lee, if we only focus on the finger then we will miss all of the heavenly glory. What he was saying in this legendary statement is that if we focus on the finger i.e., the signpost i.e., the symptoms we will find ourselves obsessing over symbols such as the reactionary symptom but fail to recognize the deeper meaning for why the symptom has occurred. This is exactly what the entire industrialized medical model including pharmaceutical medicine, surgical interventions, dentistry, and disease management have all done and it should be self-evident based on the results how that has been working out. We must take our attention from the symptom and redirect it to where the root cause is and from there, we can see what the full scope of possibilities for true healing are, meaning take our attention from the simple finger and turn our gaze towards the heavenly glory of possibilities.

"Knowing oneself comes from attending with compassionate curiosity to what is happening within."

Dr. Gabor Mate

In essence, all addictions are coping mechanism, compensatory responses to sooth the tension we feel inside. Now, let's take this a step deeper into the core of the problem itself which is an inner divide from our true Self and the inauthentic self. The inauthentic self is a compilation of stories, rehearsed patterns, ego-identity programs, and at the root of all of that is a disconnection to self-i.e., our true and authentic self. Dr. Gabor Mate has brilliantly explained that all addictions are really formed from a disconnection that occurred earlier on in our life experience. In this way all addictions are formed in childhood and the form of the addiction itself is not the issue at hand. The issue is the core trauma imbedded in the human being (or the body system) that makes them susceptible to compulsive tendencies i.e., addiction cycles.

When we were children in our formative years, our nervous systems were still developing and, in truth, our brains do not fully develop until around the age of 25. If we had experienced a traumatic event in early childhood, it is likely we did not have the processing power to properly internalize the situation, process it safely, and discharge it form our body like an animal would in nature. There is a phenomenon called neurogenic tremors where an animal experiences the full-bodied stress of being hunted and if it gets away it then begins to shake convulsively for a short duration and once the stress is completely discharged from the body, it then goes on its way. We as humans also carry this innate intelligence but as children, we are rarely educated on how to operate our bodies intelligence and instead of discharging these experiences we store them up in the neuromuscular system as accumulated information. This information in-forms our psychology, our biology, our muscular system, and our nervous system which tends to get overloaded like backed up files on our hard drive or too many tabs open on our desktop browser and slows down the operating system over time.

Because of this we progressively lose touch with the incredible technology that is our body and we become further disconnected from its innate healing capacities. In order to compensate for this our ego develops identities, sub-identities, and 'stories' to explain why we are the way we are which creates the structure for the inauthentic self. The tension below the surface never really goes away though and eventually the well-constructed identity begins to crack, and this is the start of what later can become an existential crisis. I know this all too well because I have experienced many instances of existential crisis. Another phrase that is commonly used in spiritual circles is a dark night of the soul which, in truth, can be more like dark months or even years where the soul is emerging into consciousness, but the structures of our ego protection system is defending itself against the integration of the true Self. More on this later.

So, in order to synthesize this entire train of thought and all of the pieces coming into a synchronized geometry it is easy to say that the root source of all addictions can be found in a fundamental disconnection that occurred at the moment of our most sensitive traumatic experiences. As mentioned, children do not possess the ability to effectively process a traumatic experience and thus it creates a disconnect internally. It is common in classical psychotherapy sessions to lay on a couch and unwind one's thoughts and childhood experiences until they come to the realization of what had happened to them. This can be extremely helpful in part but is still critically lacking in whole because, again, the body keeps the score and simply becoming consciously aware of one's pain points does not extinguish the pain itself. It merely illuminates the mental processes around it and, in some cases, rehashing the same old stories can create a mental looping cycle that only perpetuates further.

We often make the mistake of assuming that what happened to us i.e., our stories about the event, is the cause of our issues or addictions. In truth, that is not factual at all, not even partly factual. Dr. Joe Dispenza has explained that scientific studies have demonstrated that at least 50% of our memories about the past are fabricated, meaning we make up at least half of the details in order to reaffirm how we feel about the situation itself. This is also called cognitive bias where we have a mental bias towards certain pieces of information and all other details that would contradict our bias are filtered out from our conscious awareness. So, what does that mean? It means that if we are unconsciously making up at least 50% of our memories based on how we feel about ourselves then if we feel like a victim all of our memories are going to confirm that we were victimized. Now, this may be true that we experienced being a victim. This is a valid experience to acknowledge but where it gets tricky is when we see through the perceptual lenses of being a victim and the rest of our bodily experience confirms that based entirely on a misperception or misappropriation of our creative imagination.

The only clear-cut path towards healing is to see a situation in its entirety and for what it really is. And what it really is entirely based on how we perceive the situation which then informs our reality, and our reality is entirely based on our felt experience of it, moment by moment by moment. In order to be fully present in the moment requires us to be fully embodied as a way of life. When we experience a disconnection internally due to trauma or wounding it can feel so painful that we want to eject ourselves from the physical body in order to avoid experiencing the pain. Imagine, an entire population of people, in a socialized, artificially constructed, consumer-based world void of true intimacy, connection to nature, and frequently in the beta brain wave state of reaction and survival. Is it any question why addiction of all kinds runs absolutely wild in our world, suicide rates are as high as they ever been, people feel deeply isolated within a hyper virtually connected landscape, and we are the most unhealthy and unfulfilled population of people in recorded history?

The answer for all of our dilemmas in life can be translated into a need for connection. For over ten years in my professional speaking career the number one piece of advice I have given countless audiences and clients is returning back to nature. I remember a client who had stage 3 breast cancer, was completely unfulfilled in her life, and was living in London which was not where she wanted to be. She was stuck in paralysis by analysis meaning she wanted to make bold changes but was stuck in her head. She did not want to go down the allopathic medical route for cancer therapies, which by the way has an extremely low success rate statistically, and she felt trapped by her circumstances. She asked me, what would you do if you were in my situation? So, I told her, if I was in your situation, I would immediately close out all of my lose ends, book a plane flight for Hawaii, go onto a green juice and raw food cleanse, and then once I landed, I would find the nearest waterfall, then, and only then would I make my decision about what to do next in my life. She was in a state of total disarray and there would be no solutions found in that place. What she was suffering from was not solely a physical ailment but in truth, she was under the weight of overwhelm due to a total lack of connection. Connection to the earth, connection to her body, connection to community, and connection to her soul.

This is a perfect opportunity to tie a bow on this topic and let it percolate inside your soul a bit. There is no rush to the finish line, in fact, that is another trap we can fall into which is thinking there is a finish line to healing. It is simply a continual flow of energy moving from one moment to the next and one day into another. So be easy on yourself, release the tendencies to judge or shame yourself for any reason. Being a human is incredible challenging and you are not alone.

Now, let's prepare to move into the next phase of this journey which is understanding what I call the Dopamine Dilemma and how our neurochemistry plays a major role in how we form habits and how we detach from compensatory habits and begin to experience life at its fullest potential!

The Dopamine Dilemma

"Of all the chemical transmitter substances sloshing around in your brain, it appears that dopamine may be the most directly related to the neural correlates of belief. Dopamine, in fact, is critical in association learning and the reward system of the brain that Skinner discovered through his process of operant conditioning, whereby any behavior that is reinforced tends to be repeated. A reinforcement is, by definition, something that is rewarding to the organism; that is to say, makes the brain direct the body to repeat the behavior in order to get another positive reward."

Michael Shermer, Author of The Believing Brain

The subtle nature of addiction, as we've explored, is very nuanced and has deeper elements at play than what appears on the surface. We, as human beings, are a complex mixture of elemental forces, personalities, beliefs, and have a diversity of lifestyle habits and motivations in life. This is why addiction is such a tricky thing to get a handle on, let alone break free from all together. And perhaps the biggest factor in all addictive patterns is exactly what is just beneath the surface itself. Just beneath the epidermal layers of the skin that is. We are also a highly complex chemistry set that is producing, synthesizing, and managing trillions of bio-chemical reactions per second. Of course, we would never know this because the entire system functions independent of our awareness but most certainly it can be slowed down or brought to entire screeching halt by us.

Over recent years it has become much more well understood that our bodies chemistry is playing a massive role in forming and reinforcing habitual patterns. This seems obvious I am sure but how well aware are you about this? And how much are you consciously working to change the chemistry set to positively affect you or otherwise? To assume that the trillions of chemical reactions occurring second by second in our bodies do not have a role in addiction formation or addiction repatterning is naive at best and dangerous at worst. Over the last decade in my work with nutrition, holistic health modalities, and cleansing protocols I can tell you that the biggest lever that makes the most difference comes down to how we take care of our body. The food we eat, the supplements we take, the water we drink, the exposure to sun, the quality of our sleep, and the movement of our bodies will trump any psychotherapy or prescription medication day in and day out.

The most interesting conversation surrounding addiction and habit formation over recent years has been around dopamine. Dopamine is a neuro-hormone called a neurotransmitter which could also be viewed as a chemical messenger in the nervous system. Serotonin, choline, and Gaba are also neurotransmitters of equal importance but dopamine has a special focus in its role with addictive tendencies and up and down withdrawal cycles. Dopamine is commonly known as a pleasure hormone and stimulates chemical sensations of feel-good states of being. In truth, dopamine is so much more than that, but this assertion is also very true; it is part of the pleasure pathway of the brain. This is why activities such as pornography can become so overwhelmingly addictive because the brain is being overloaded with an immense amount of dopaminergic stimulation (hyper-stimuli) and it associates what the eyes are seeing as the source of this intense flooding of pleasure. The brain over time becomes compartmentalized in a way and then becomes reliant on the fantasy to produce heightened sensations of pleasure rather than fully engaging in our own reality. This will be explained in more detail in the chapters **Virtual Simulated Reality** and **Pornography | Sexuality.**

What is critical to consider is that the frequent hyper stimulation of our pleasure sensations in the brain sets us up for dependency to recreate the same experience. The bad news is that every time we go back to the chemical slot machine, we tend to have a lower amount of dopamine and it takes more of it in order to recreate the same experience. This is what it means when people say robbing Peter to pay Paul; we are robbing ourselves of a healthier future in order to sustain an unhealthy habit. In the end, we are literally robbing ourselves of our future in order to produce heightened states of pleasure in this moment. And, of course, underneath this pattern is the desire to avoid the discomfort of the present moment. To avoid the void of the moment and distract from feeling the emptiness of the void. So, we distract ourselves in all kinds of ways and if you have not noticed by now, that tends to leave us off exactly where we started. Exactly where we started but usually worse off than before because now our chemistry set is producing less and less of the hormonal fuel our holistic system requires for optimal function.

There is a very important concept I want to drive into this discussion. Within the nature of addiction cycles there is a very clear back and forth sequence of events that play out. The form of the events is unique to the individual but the nature of them is universal to one another. This is called the pain/pleasure cycle or more to the point seeking pleasure to avoid pain and avoiding pain to seek pleasure. This phrase could define the heartbeat of our consumer driven, hyper sexualized, processed food eating, alcohol partying, workaholic culture in a nutshell. We drive towards habits that will produce pleasure but how many times do we consciously drive towards pain/discomfort? You may ask, well why would I want to focus on things that are pain or uncomfortable? The answer is simple; so, you grow and mature as an adult. Children tend to gravitate mostly towards activities that are entirely pleasurable. In fact, children can easily become addicted to simple pleasure but in their development if they do not eventually learn how to be ok with discomfort than they never fully mature into an independent integrated adult. The key distinction between an adolescent and an adult is one is codependent, and one is interdependent. We live in a society that has far more children in adult bodies than we have fully mature adults. This is why it is easy to say that the vast majority of our population is hiding out with some form of addiction.

At the end of this chapter, I will be walking you through a concise list of habits you can begin practicing and exploring to build back your dopamine receptors naturally. Over the course of our lives and especially our adult lives our hormones and neurotransmitters begin to slowly decline in response to our lifestyle. The harder we push on the body the more hormonal power is required to buffer the acidity, inflammation, toxicity, and pressure placed upon it. Eventually we reach a tipping point and over a very short period of time someone can go from appearing relatively healthy to looking like they have ages 10-20 years. I have witnessed this play out in the extreme cases of cancer, diabetes, and other hormonal dysregulations but make no mistake these conditions do not happen out of nowhere. They incubate and ferment over time until the body's immune system can no long buffer the damage and overnight everything begins to break down. It is rarely a slow gradual process towards disease or dysfunction, it can happen at the drop of a dime but appears to happen over the course of a lifetime which is why we have this phrase "age associated illness".

Knowing how to build back our dopamine receptors and our overall hormonal system (endocrine system) is one of the most important aspects to addiction, physical illness, sports performance, sexual virility, cognitive fitness, and restorative sleep. When we invert an addictive pattern what we are doing is changing the program of seeking pleasure to avoid pain to seeking discomfort to cultivate long lasting pleasure. For example, taking a cold shower in the morning instead of taking the hot shower. The comfort of the hot warm water soothes us and puts us into a sleepy like comfort zone. The cold water slightly shocks the system, forces us to deeply breath, and invigorates the body but is not immediately pleasurable (until you do it a lot). Hot water expands and creates a disordering of hydrogen-oxygen molecules, which also in turn does the same to our energy particles. This is why we could easily go into a slight hypnotic state, particularly in a sulfur hot spring. The cold water concentrates energy and bonds the oxygen-hydrogen molecules together, which again, is exactly what happens in our own body. This is why hot water tends to make us more lethargic the longer we stay in, but cold water energizes the body.

In order to reroute our chemical messaging system, we need to change the input and output sequence. Addiction is when we are habituated to immediate dopamine producing inputs. For example, waking up and reaching for the phone or quickly making a pot a coffee to "get going" in the morning. The coffee is one-part ritual and one-part immediate stimulation. The stimulatory effect drives the sympathetic response and that is where the energy in the morning is being sourced. Checking the phone first thing in the morning engages us with the energy of the world via this virtual interface. It may seem benign, but it really can cause a problem when we get looped into morning rituals that distract from powering on the system organically. When we are seeking outside of ourselves for something to turn us on opposed to turning ourselves on naturally.

Dopamine addiction interrupts the rhythms of our hormonal cycles. When we awake in the morning, our body is not fully online, and to force it to perk up all at once is not ideal. It is a slower process; the rituals in our morning determine the overall energy we have throughout the day. This is also why withdrawal is so uncomfortable. We are chemically withdrawing from immediate stimulation that drives dopamine and serotonin thus making us feel "normal". If we have been normalized to addiction, then we need a brand new normal, and the transition period is where we need to reroute our inputs and outputs. The first 3-7 days tend to be the hardest but if someone can stay steadfast for 7-10 days then they will regain their will power, confidence, and bodily energy. There is a detoxification process that occurs here, and we will explore more of that in the chapter **Mastering the Body | Health**.

The last perspective I want to share before we move on is relating back to the seeking of pleasure to avoid pain. Another way this can be looked at is the distinction between immediate gratification and delayed gratification. When we are seeking quick doses of pleasure, we are seeking immediate gratification or immediate results. This is the antithesis to success and growth in every area of life. We have to be very clear about what we are trying to achieve here. Do we want the quick, easy, and predictable route, or do we want success? We cannot have both because neither route leads towards the other. If one is going to heal themselves and recover from their addictions, they are going to have to earn it. If someone wants true freedom in their life, well, as my mentor Wade Lightheart told me, you are going to have to earn that freedom! This is so true and essential for success.

Delayed gratification is where we create a gap between our thoughts and our actions. We create a space between our urges and acting on our urges. The longer we practice this the gap between the two gets bigger, the urges lose their potency, and our mind becomes non-reactive. In order to shift the operating system from immediate to delayed gratification we must find our own sense of pleasure in all of the discomfort. I remember a friend saying something many years ago which was "if you fall in love with the work the results come naturally." If we fall in love with a greater purpose for our lives, then we seek a higher pleasure in life. This is the pleasure that only comes from living on purpose or another way of saying it is being moved by intrinsic motivation instead of extrinsic motivation.

Extrinsic motivation is the immediate hit of dopamine. It is being driven towards external stimulus, outward validation or approval, numbers in the bank account, etc. Intrinsic motivation is being driven from a deeper purpose within us and does not have a lot to do with what is happening outside of us.

In the case of addiction, it is a need to change the external in order to alter the internal. This will not produce long lasting pleasure and will only keep us on a hamster wheel of addiction. The real addiction here is being too plugged into the external world and all of its flickering lights to keep us distracted from what is occurring within us. If we do not get right within than we will never be right without. Someone who is truly sovereign and interdependent is someone who has accepted the responsibility of adulthood and is not dependent on circumstances or quick pleasure for their fulfillment. Dopamine also triggers the reward centers in the brain which is why it feels so good. Many people are seeking approval, inclusion, and recognition. When we are rewarded for something, we did we tend to repeat that pattern because it feels good. Our brain associates the 'something' with the chemical release of pleasure and thus we get into a reward-based operating system. This pattern does not allow for delayed gratification because it is too uncomfortable to wait for what we want, work for what we want, abstain from what is not serving us, and that is low and behold the major psychological collapse of our entire western civilization.

So, as we move forward here, understand that we are not simply talking about a simple physiological adaptation of the body. We are talking about using the knowledge of the body and brain chemistry to access greater depths of our mental capacity. It requires a tremendous amount of courage and will to reroute the operating system and it does not happen all at once. We will slip and fall, time and time again, but we will continue to make progress along the way. However, if we set ourselves up for success by implementing the health-based habits, we will discuss you will automatically experience greater discipline and intrinsic motivation. The pleasure reward center of the brain will begin to calibrate to a new normal based on long sustainable pleasure rather than the brain acting like a drug dealer or abused pharmacist. We will go from dependent adolescent to interdependent adult, and it all happens when we take command of the operating system of our body and the mind will adapt very quickly.

Let's explore the scientific basis for dopamine and how it operates within our bodies and lives.

A Scientific View on the Dopaminergic System

Dopamine is usually thought of as the pleasure and reward molecule of the body. This is only partially true and is a more emphasized factor in addiction. Dopamine is actually a very versatile and diverse neurotransmitter that plays a major role in the holistic functionality of our body and brain. Dopamine, like other neurotransmitters/hormones, is a chemical messenger and travels via neuronal connections assisting in executive thinking, voluntary movement patterns, cognitive function, and yes, reward and pleasure dynamics. This is an incredibly important molecule that helps run the entire system, especially motor function, speech patterns, and neuromuscular health.

The dopaminergic pathway system governs all of the dopamine production and transportation. There are 4 identified dopamine pathways that all have their own role to play. Dopamine is formed from the amino acid's tyrosine and phenylamine, which are building blocks to the pre-cursor molecule L-Dopa. When we do not have the necessary building blocks available to self-produce L-Dopa or dopamine our body will try to extract amino acids some other way. This is also why amino acid therapies have been so effective in all cases of cognitive decline or motor system dysregulation i.e., Parkinson's and MS. The number one reason for Parkinson's, for example, is a combination of a damaged myelin sheath and a dopamine depletion. When we overproduce dopamine multiple times a day in excess but have nothing to rebuild our reserves, the tank will end up going empty and this begins to negatively affect other aspects of our health.

Adrenal fatigue and dopamine depletion are tightly interlocked together, largely because they are both basically the same thing. The adrenal glands produce what are known as catecholamines which adrenaline, noradrenaline, and smaller amounts of dopamine are formed.

Adrenaline is the sympathetic hormone responsible for being able to stand and walk upright, or bipedalism. This makes us distinct from all other mammals because we are able to adrenalize and walk upright most of the time. When our adrenaline i.e., adrenals begin to go out our posture caves in, our enthusiasm lowers, and our ability to hold ourselves up against gravity weakens. In traditional Chinese medicine they would call this a qi deficiency which basically means an absence or leaking of vital life force. There are large amounts of dopamine receptors in the adrenal cortex, and dopamine is one of the main ways the body deals with stress. Once our dopamine goes, our upright ability goes, our adrenal glands start to go, and eventually our control over our motor function begins to go, too.

The number one pharmaceutical for Parkinson's disease is a highly concentrated L-Dopa (leva-dopa) prescription. This of course is not recommended since pharmaceuticals only isolate the active compound from the plant and synthesize it in a chemical form. It is completely void of the plants overall intelligence and co-factors built into it. The plant that is sought after for this though is an Ayurvedic herb called Mucuna Pruriens or Mucuna for short. This is called the dopamine bean because it is the highest naturally occurring source of L-dopa in the entire plant kingdom. It is commonly used for stress reduction, sleep, cognition, and sexual enhancement but truly what it is a miracle plant. The L-Dopa helps to create an endogenous production of bodily dopamine instead of relying on exogenous hormones such as hormone replacement therapies (HRT). Endogenous means to generate from within i.e., the body self-producing its own chemistry and not being reliant on exogenous chemicals to fill in a deficiency.

Now, let's address some of the misconceptions stemming from our "trusted" mainstream conventional wisdom. There are mainstream "scientists" who tell people that dopamine is the reason for their addiction and that they should be very careful about producing too much dopamine. This is absolutely preposterous, misleading, and dangerous to espouse when in reality it is the exact opposite. Dopamine depletion is the cause of addiction and compulsive urges leading to the immediate hit of dopamine producing activities. The addictions keep popping back up because there is a lack of healthy dopaminergic receptor activity and we are compensating for the deficit through our addictions. This is an issue that will not be solved by a pill or prescription. It must be worked out, over time, through the entirety of our lifestyle.

Everyone I have ever met that takes a prescription form of L-dopa (concentrated from Mucuna) is also struggling with some form of addiction. The most common I have seen are excessive smoking (tobacco or cannabis), alcohol use, attached to their phones, and pornography is a major one as well, but it is much more undercover than say smoking or being on the phone all day long. This all comes from having a reactive mind and the inability to find our still point internally. And, paradoxically to that, our mind is a response feedback to the overall state of our nervous system. Dopamine is a calming agent and helps to sooth the heightened electrical activity when the system gets overloaded, disorientated, or frazzled. Knowing this is important because excessive smoking or binge eating are attempts to sooth and calm down the systemic disarray. This is why fasting, and intermittent fasting are so powerful. This is also why cold showers and ice baths are so incredible. We can self sooth but should do it in ways that increase vitality instead of ways that diminish vital life force.

The endocrine system of the body is the chief hormonal production warehouse that is responsible for catalyzing all of our chemical messengers that feed into the bodies operating system. This includes all of our various hormones such as testosterone, progesterone, pregnenolone, adrenaline, noradrenaline, DHEA, thyroid stimulating hormone, human growth hormone, and all the rest. The endocrine system can be looked at as the bodies inner pharmacy that ensures a type of rhythmic harmony and equilibrium throughout the body. In short, this is our naturopathic inner physician that allows for homeopathic self-healing of both the body and the mind. The hypothalamic pituitary adrenal axis (HPA) plays a major role in the synthesis and regulation of our entire hormonal chemistry set. This has a lot to do with what is known as neuroendocrine adaptation to stress or in laymen's terms our ability to adapt to mental and physical stress. When the HPA axis is overworked or simply not functionally optimally it can create a significant stressor on the adrenals and thyroid, in particular. This is very important to understand.

When people have thyroid based metabolic challenges, they likely also have kidney/adrenal fatigue or exhaustion stemming from one thing

50

or another. Vice versa, if someone is struggling with adrenal challenges, they likely also have a thyroid challenge that is misdiagnosed or undiagnosed. The thyroid and adrenal glands work in synchrony with one another and act as direct feedback communication glands. The HPA axis should also include the thyroid as it is the master regulator of all metabolic processes and can play a significant role in how we navigate through our dopamine-based habits. If our endocrine system (which includes our liver/gallbladder) is out of balance then our ability to self-regulate our cravings/urges will be diminished and we will have to exert far more will power, which we know is finite and reliant on how much energy capacity is available in the operating system i.e., nervous system complex.

When our endocrine function is good to great and the chemical messengers are working correctly, then our reliance on temporary pleasure is minimized and our dopaminergic system is happy. Much of the same advice for recuperating a worn out HPA axis system is also similar if not identical to restoring adrenal health and neurotransmitter production. This is actually the case in most health situations for the simple fact that our entire body is one big holistic unified system and works in combination with everything else. When you positively effect one compartment you will create a positivity cascading effect which creates a healthy equanimity that spawns more of the same.

Remember, our bodies entire chemistry set are what should be viewed as 'sacred secretions' that all serve a unique purpose, work in synchrony with one another, and play a significant role in optimizing our human experience. When we abuse these secretions i.e., our chemistry production through self-indulgence, pleasure seeking, and filling in the void of boredom we end up diminishing the gift of life. These sacred secretions that form in our body are what provides the spark of life itself in order for us to animate our bodies and do all that we do, every moment of every day. When we are in an addiction spiral, we set up a feedback rollercoaster between dopamine, serotonin, norepinephrine, cortisol, and have to repeat the cycle in order to get through each day. When we understand the science of addiction and how our sacred life force is being affected it then becomes far more obvious that these impulsivity patterns can only lead us down one path: bodily depletion.

Towards the end of this chapter, we will go into a set of free energy producing exercises and practices you can begin implementing in order to rebuild the dopamine pathways, balance hormonal health, and increase self-respect through simple disciplines. These are titled free energy producing practices because your human body is a form of technology that operates on free energy magnetic pulse wave principles and these practices are entirely free and help renew our energy without costing us anything. The only thing they may end up costing us is our old habit of being tired, wiped out, frustrated, and unhealthy.

Before we dive into that, let's discuss the withdrawal process of addiction and how it relates to the dopaminergic perspective.

Transcending the Withdrawal Process

If I had to bet money on what was is the scariest part of addiction it may have to be the withdrawal process. No one that has a compulsive addiction that is clearly causing harm or stagnation really wants to keep the cycle going. But we do keep the cycle going, don't we? Why is that anyways? Well, I suspect the real reason is we are choosing immediate pleasure/gratification over temporary discomfort and recovery. It is the gap in-between that causes us to hesitate and procrastinate instead of just getting on with the process. We prolong the process simply because we are avoiding the process of healing and that process is found in the withdrawing from self-defeating patterns and thought loops.

The withdrawal can feel like no man's land. It is the great void inside of us that needs to be felt and experienced rather than constantly fed and filled. This is the great challenge every human being comes up against in one way or another. By withdrawing from behaviors that do not serve us we begin to remove the layers that were covering up our true Self. This is an opportunity to become better well aquatinted with ourselves, our feelings, our fears, our bodies, and our mental stories. The withdrawal process can be fast, or it can be slow. It can be easier, or it can be made harder. How we approach it determines the experience of it. If we keep resisting it, we will keep building up friction and static in our minds as well as pressure and tension in our bodies. If we keep fixating on dopaminergic response stimuli as a way to self-medicate our inhibitions, it will only become more difficult (and painful) once we make a break for it.

There is a very interesting phenomenon that seems to play out with core conditioning and addiction loops. Addictions seem to carry their own form of consciousness. It is as if the addiction itself knows everything about us and in some way is part of our mental processing unit. Addictions can form sub-personalities and make it very tricky to discern between who is running the ship at any given time. Once we begin to create space and separation from them, we feel a sense of relief and grounding. But this relief seems to be temporary because not long after we begin to experience it creeping back up on us, as if to whisper its seductive melody in our ears and influence the chemistry set of our body. Once we begin to back off from our addictions and make progress forward, they begin calling us back, and capture our attention through a form of a subtle hypnotic trance. This is the true battle we have with ourselves and the tug of war conflict playing out within our own mind.

Addiction withdrawal seems to function like a phantom limb. Even though the habit itself is not visible or detectable in our environment the urge still wants to be scratched. Similar or maybe identical to someone who has had a limb amputated and yet feels the presence of it still. They find themselves scratching or attempting to touch it because it is hardwired into their physiology. Although it is no longer physically there, the energetic imprints in the person's electromagnetic auric field still have that information codified (encoded) in it. The energetic imprints of our daily patterns and the physiological response it activates create informational signatures, not only in our body but also in our consciousness as a whole.

So, the withdrawal process is not just a physical rehabilitation of habits and patterns but also a rehabilitation of our consciousness as a whole. We have to be able to consciously track our habits and see when they arise, what thoughts creep up, what stimulation occurs in the body, and how easily we are likely to go into it. Our dopamine response patterns are being influenced and effected by our consciousness itself and vice versa. Another way to look at addiction loops is also considering an idea called consciousness traps. A consciousness trap is something in our outer environment, most pronounced on the internet, such as social media where our conscious awareness is being captured or arrested at any given moment. Aimlessly scrolling on Facebook or Instagram is a perfect example or forgetting what you were going to do once you opened up the social media app. Getting into arguments, debates, and all that is also another form of a consciousness trap.

This is when a portion of our conscious awareness or mental energy is being trapped, like in a digital box, and is then being harvested. That is actually a very accurate way of describing this phenomenon because it does trap our mental energy, compartmentalizes our awareness in the moment, and we can easily feel like our life force is being extracted i.e., having low energy, low will power. Avoiding the healing and recovery process is a byproduct of being in some form of consciousness trap. Having low energy every day, exhausted dopamine receptors, poor sleep, etc. are all indications that parts of our life force is being trapped. The good news is that we have total control of this. We allow ourselves to become trapped and used up due to the permission we give through the actions and habits we practice. This is a permission-based universe, and nothing happens without our conscious or unconscious consent. There are no victims here, in fact, playing a victim is directly tied to addiction and the victim never wants to take responsibility, because doing so is the only way to actually recover.

The way out of the consciousness trappings is fundamentally about becoming more aware of ourselves, our tendencies, and taking back the power of our operating system. When we notice ourselves going into an automated loop, we must pattern interrupt by shifting the energy. If we notice ourselves "checking out" of the moment, then we need to become even more present in the moment and this happens through our breath. Taking deep breaths create spaciousness in the system and eases the body into a state of relaxation. The inability to relax can also be traced to an addiction to stress and contraction. So, breathing into the tension and contraction will help relief the discomfort and allow for more energy to circulate in the body.

Instead of looking at the withdrawal phase as something unpleasant or even terrifying we can look upon it as an opportunity for self-initiation. We avoid those things that we feel will bring us pain or discomfort. In actuality, the discomfort is simply a growing pain, and it will subside as soon as we accept it for what it is. Accept the fact that you must initiate yourself in a developmental process of interdependency and self-sovereignty by detaching from the circuits that keep you imprisoned. The attitude we possess creates the framework for our experiences and can radically change the feeling tone of the entire process. Our attitude determines our altitude in life and interestingly enough our attitude also increases our aptitude. We are literally smarter, more cognitively capable, and mentally stronger when our attitude reflects that kind of optimism. So, see this as the opportunity for healing and transformation that it is by engaging fully in the process of withdrawing from what does not serve you.

The Epigenetic Factor in Addiction

> *"Epigenetics teaches that we, indeed, are not doomed by our genes and that a change in human consciousness can produce physical changes, both in structure and function, in the human body."*
>
> *Dr. Joe Dispenza*

Over the last two decades, the biggest innovations in the fields of both holistic health and natural medicine have been revealed through the dynamic influx of cross referenced and peer reviewed research. There was a time when it was almost unanimously agreed upon by experts that our genes were fixed and what we were born with was all we had to look forward to regarding the physiological health of our bodies. It was thought that disease conditions, along with psychological conditions, were largely due to heredity and if our parents or grandparents suffered from a particular affliction then the chances were strong, we would as well. It was commonplace to hear statements such as cancer or diabetes just "runs in my family" and without questioning this narrative people simply accepted this belief as a self-determining fact and a self-fulfilling prophecy.

This is a sad state of affairs to consider because if someone adopts the idea that the genetic dispositions, they inherit through their family lineage are set in place then it implants the seed of victimhood and helplessness in one's own consciousness. We now know through the advancement of scientific research on the inner workings of the human body that this is not only a simple misunderstanding but a gross error in judgement that has led to a laundry list of sicknesses and disease conditions that are all entirely preventable and avoidable. We now know there is incredible genetic adaptability and variability in all physiological conditions that are more dependent on the factors of lifestyle, nutrition, exercise, and recovery than they are on familial lineage. It is true that we inherit the genetic contents of both our mother and father which include the residual genetic information of their ancestry as well. This is an obvious fact yet the implications of this on our own potential for health and quality of life have been deterministically mapped out for us by this outdated and overturned theory which has produced an entire industry of sick care and disease management.

The discovery that our genetic blueprint has a tremendously untapped reservoir of healing potential is the single greatest breakthrough in the fields of health sciences and this science is known simply as epigenetics. Epigenetics teaches us that our genes are more influenced by our environment, both inner and outer, than they are by anything else. This discovery has brought forth numerous sub-categories such as nutrigenomics and social genomics. Nutrigenomics is the understanding that the nutrients in our foods, supplements, and liquids have a significant role in the activation of our genes and can determine whether we trigger the genes associated with longevity or trigger the genes associated with disease and morbidity. Social genomics shows us that our genetics are directly influenced by the people we spend the most amount of time with and are responding to the emotional content formed from the relationships in our lives. We've all heard the saying you are the reflection of the 5 people you spend the most time around. It appears this statement has far deeper meaning than simply influencing our attitude and mindset. It literally informs the biological template of our physical health and wellbeing.

Now, with this all said, there is a very deep exploration this can take us into the realms of addiction because our genes do play a significant role in how we adopt certain habits and how we navigate the addiction cycle. First off, if we believe that we are born into an unsurmountable circumstance due to factors outside of our control, such as being a victim to our genetic disposition than it postulates a victim identity and that is the psychological source code of all addiction struggles. We have to transcend the identity of being a victim to outside forces (or inside forces) beyond our control. It is true that we are born into the bodies we have, and these bodies come fully equipped with an inborn template which contains a variety of information that may or may not automatically work in our favor. If our parents and grandparents endured significant challenges and trauma in their lives it is possible that the residue of those unresolved energetics can be transferred over too us in the conception process leading to birth. It is also true that if our mother's bodies had any form of toxicity, nutrient deficiency, and any other obstructions, some of that may have been passed over into us through the umbilical cord during birth or even in the breast-feeding phase of infant development.

Each individual was born with a different set of circumstances, advantages and disadvantages, upsides and drawbacks, and some were more affected in challenging ways than others. This is very much true and should be acknowledged for what it is. With this understanding it is now far more important to know and acknowledge that regardless of the genetic drawbacks our bodies have the proven capability to override inherited genetic software programs and rewrite the genetic transcription all together. If someone did come into this world with very pronounced genetic challenges, whether it be physical, trauma based, etc., they may need to work harder to reroute the system than others. But knowing that we have the power to upgrade the genetic program, one way or another, is where the real power resides. Once we have the knowledge we then have to power to choose and all it takes is a convicted choice to turn around our entire destiny, both physically and spiritually. Once we vaporize the victim attitude and take total responsibility for our bodies, our habits, our mental states, and our consciousness to choose we then inform our genes that we are ready for a complete and total upgrade!

We are going to discuss the concept of epigenetic damage that is a byproduct from our familial inheritance, our genetic development from our upbringing, and its role in addiction but before we do that, I want to bring in a fresh perspective that comes from my colleague and friend Richard Rudd. Richard is the author of one of the most incredible spiritual growth books that is chalked full of metaphysical wisdom called the **Gene**

Keys. The Gene Keys is a road map for navigating the human experience unlike anything else ever created and, as the title suggests, deals with the genetic and epigenetic phenomenon geared towards transformation and evolution. I have had the good fortune to share many conversations with Richard over the years including conducting 4 interviews with him for my podcast show: The High-Performance Health Podcast. He also was gracious enough to write the forward for this book.

I want to share a few paramount teachings from the Gene Keys that come out of what is known as the 24th Gene Key and the chapter is called Silence- The Ultimate Addiction. In the Gene Keys there are 3 distinct phases that the human being or human consciousness goes through. The first is known as 'the shadow' which is where our addictions live. The second is called 'the gift" which is where our self-empowerment and motivational strength lives. The third is called "the siddhi' which is where our liberation and full authentic creative expression lives. You can study the Gene Keys more for your personal research and I highly encourage you do so.

> *"The 24th shadow, when correctly understood, explains much about the shadow state itself as well as why human beings find it so difficult to resolve the deeper repetitive problems in their lives. This is the shadow that keeps the psychology profession in business, and it is the shadow that big advertising companies take full advantage of. We humans come pre-programmed for addiction, and the main culprit responsible for this is our minds. A well-known urban myth states that we only use a very small percentage of our brains, but any neuroscientist will tell you that this is untrue. In an average day we use almost all of our brains. It is not how much of our brain we use; it is how efficiently we use it. As it stands today, the human brain is still such unexplored territory for consciousness."*

In this passage Richard is illustrating the understanding that we do, indeed, use the entirety of our brains at any given moment but at varying degrees of efficacy. This understanding helps us dissolve the notion that we are inhibited by the limitations of our genes or inborn brain cognition, and that those who are most gifted amongst us are the ones who have greater access to their cognitive potential. If our neurotransmitter receptors such as dopamine or serotonin have been exhausted by way of factors involving addictive habits, then we will not have as much cognitive accessibility as someone who's neurotransmitters are functioning optimally. This reminds us that the power is in our own hands and if we want something in our lives to change, we just need to adjust our mode of thinking.

The other golden nugget out of this is that we, as humans, came into these bodies with pre-programmed patterning that is primed for addiction. This does not mean we are born to be addicts but more so it means that we have genetic software programming that can make us susceptible to the formation and continuation of addiction. Since our brains are all synched up a bit different from one another the way in which this manifests itself will be distinctly different, but we all have a shared tendency to move into extremes, provided the necessary circumstances, and triggers are available. This is unique to each person but helpful to realize that our shadow nature is reflected in some kind of habitual repetitive pattern and if we want to move out the shadow frequency then all we need to do is shine a light of awareness onto the shadow pattern itself and choose our way out of it by raising our energy levels into the gift (empowered strength) frequency.

> "Nothing external can bring an end to your suffering, since it is rooted deep within your DNA. Only when you turn inward and look for the source of your suffering will you finally face the addictive quality of your own mind. The programming partner of the 24th shadow is the 44th shadow of interference, which is responsible for the dysfunctional relationships that occur across our planet and which are the current norm. This dysfunction is the by-product of a universal glitch in the genetic operating system of humanity and is reinforced by the 24th shadow. Addiction is the constant replaying of the same perceptive frame with no pause between frames and this is what happens at a synaptic level within the brain chemistry of

an average human. Like mice in spinning wheels, we
simply re-enact the same scenarios over and over without
realizing what we are doing."

This passage from the Gene Keys really hits the nail on the head right here. It details the fundamental understanding that our own personalized flavor of suffering is interlaced within our DNA pattern and is entirely unique to us. This helps to explain the struggle behind the addiction and why it can easily feel like we are the only one's going through this experience. In truth, everyone experiences their own version of it but that is where the wisdom clicks into place. We each experience our own distinct version of struggle and suffering because it is our own unique karmic triggering that is taking place in these instances. The deeper understanding of spiritual-psychology and trauma release therapies is that our addiction patterns are reflective of a karmic loop that is attempting to unwind itself from the DNA helix. The karmic information that is imprinted into us into this incarnation is stored in our DNA which is why Richard reminds us that nothing outside of us can bring an end to our suffering. The suffering (or sense of suffering) is simply feedback from the body that there is coiled up energy that wants to unwind itself and often times this happens through way of being triggered by something or someone.

If we do not have an awareness of this phenomenon than we tend to remain in the repressive shadow frequency, and this only reinforces the addiction. When we develop more awareness of what is happening and the underlining theme that continues to manifest itself, we can interrupt the cycle of karma. The Buddhists would call this cycle of addiction or repetitive suffering as the 'wheel of samsara' which is known as the karmic wheel of suffering through reincarnation cycles in order to finally learn the lessons we failed to learn in the past life or more practically speaking, in the past of this life. The epigenetic principle can be applied to any dimension of this conversation because it all traces back to the origin point which is the genetic information stored within the body. Throughout the book we go into great detail on how to navigate this process. In the chapter **Integration & Recovery** we will discuss and decipher the meanings of both our karma and our dharma as it pertains to getting ourselves off the wheel of addiction and set forth towards freedom.

A few years ago, I came across a great book by Bessel Van der Kolk, MD called **The Body Keeps the Score**, where he explains how the effects of trauma in our lives has a direct impact on our physical health. As the title suggests our bodies contain the store house of traumatic experiences and if we do not know how to exercise the traumatic imprints from our system, we can develop further health issues down the road. Taking this concept, a step further I also came across another book called **It Didn't Start with You** by Mark Wolynn. This took it to another level through the well-researched discoveries of transferable traits and attributes from one generation to the next via epigenetic factors. We already know that we inherit the physical genes of our parents and grandparents, but Mark explains how we also inherit the unresolved trauma of our familial genetic line as well. If our parents or their parents had a specific kind of deep seeded fear or persistent anxiety pattern, it can transfer into us via genetic redistribution during the conception process.

In his book and in public talks Mark describes many examples of individuals he's counseled who had a terrible anxiety or fear pattern that seemed to have no direct source or rational reasoning for. Mark simply ask's these individuals if anyone in their family had a similar or identical pattern. According to his testimony all these individuals discovered a parent or grandparent had a situation occur in their lives that created a fear or phobia that explained the anxiety pattern these individuals were experiencing and had no prior answers for. Once they had become consciously aware of this and utilized the tools available for releasing these stored genetic patterns of trauma-based information, they were able to move on with their lives. I have also witnessed this phenomenon occur more times than I can count and have even experienced it in my own life, regarding the unresolved aspects of both my mother and father. There is an aboriginal saying that states "the sins of the father are past down to the son". If our parents have carried unresolved trauma from their parents than it will likely be passed down to us in order to heal what they did not know how too in their time.

Now that we have unpacked the conceptual understanding of transferable traumatic patterns through our genetic lineage, it is time to discuss how to repair genetic damage that has accumulated as a byproduct of enduring the circumstances we have in this life. This will bring the concept into a grounded practical understanding and also discuss how our dopamine receptors are maladapted for addiction due to the epigenetic damage we may have experienced through our parents, their parents, and most specifically through the ways in which we were raised in our formative developmental years.

Repairing Epigenetic Damage

> *"Sometimes the most extraordinary biology lies hidden in the most apparent mundane of assumptions."*
>
> *Nessa Carey, Junk DNA: A Journey Through the Dark Matter of the Genome*

For almost the last decade or so I have been very intrigued by the conversation surrounding the epigenetic factors in all forms of healing, increased physical performance, mental cognition, and increased longevity of life. Once it became obvious and scientifically clear that the prior models of genetic determinism were only pointing towards a greater truth but not the whole truth, I became increasingly inspired about the potential for life we all have built within us. The idea of genetic determinism, also called biological determinism, is a belief that all human behavior is directly controlled by their gene's that are influenced at the expense of someone's environment such as developmental learning challenges or through the embryonic development process during conception and birth. Again, this is only a partial truth but does not point to the fact that our genes can be altered, in both positive or negative ways, through our environment, our diet, our exercise routines, our social circles, and through quality sleep.

Genetic alteration and adaptation are continual and ongoing biological processes that do not end at the moment of birth or even at the peak of puberty. We continue to grow and evolve every moment of every day in our lives, but the noticeable effects of this growth (or stunt in growth) are incremental and do not catch our attention, like it does in the first 12 years of our lives. We can be carrying a detrimental habit such as eating bad food, drinking contaminated tap water, watching pornography, smoking cigarettes, and consuming alcohol for many years, all while adapting to that lifestyle without noticing how bad we really feel. Depending on someone's genetic advantages or disadvantages the effects of a certain lifestyle will become much more noticeable much sooner. If someone had habituated to a set of patterns and lifestyle behaviors their biology will also adapt and thus produce the necessary amount of cellular energy required to maintain that lifestyle but nothing more. Once someone begins to make significant changes in their lifestyle then they will begin to notice the detrimental effects of the prior habits and the body will be forced to produce increased amounts of energy in order to compensate during the transition.

If someone does not make any of these changes and maintains the same detrimental habits over a long enough period of time their body will begin to send louder and louder feedback signals. The challenge is that all of these addictive habits are all forms of numbing and sedating, so the feedback signal is not always obvious in the moment. Most people end up noticing the long-term effects of wearing down their biological and genetic warehouse when they no longer have the cellular machinery to maintain the ill effects of these choices. A chronic injury will manifest itself, sore and worn-out tendons/ligaments can arise, respiratory problems become common, brain fog and lethargy creep in, and aches and pains become a daily occurrence. These issues will seem like they came out of nowhere and yet they had always been present in the system, but the overt symptoms were held off due to their genetic adaptation mechanism maintaining under the pressure of these ill-advised behaviors. The consequences of this kind of lifestyle is not evidence that our genes determine our state of health or our potential as human beings. They are evidence that our choices have a real and exacting effect on our genetic destiny and some people can stave off the consequences of their actions longer than others, but either way, the consequences come knocking eventually.

Genetic determinism is no way to live a powerfully inspired and empowered life. It is just another scapegoat the corporatized, reductionistic, scientific community has used to issue a blanket statement as to why we our bodies are flawed, why we get old and die, and how to sell us more pills for more ills in order to keep living with our vices of choice but never aspiring to live beyond our addictions. The information in this book and in this section is counterculture in this way. This is the access point to absolute inner freedom and physical vitality at the highest levels of human potential. Built inside of you is everything required to excel in every aspect of your life and to thrive as a whole human being; body-mind-soul. Your birthright is greatness, and your biological imperative is set to exceed all limitations. This is your user's manual for doing just that and healing the damaged DNA that has held you back from your potential and reinforced addictive cycles on the bio-genetic level.

What we need to address is that through our upbringing, as well as the inflictions placed upon us during the conception process, the birthing process, and tracing back through our familial lineage, we have developed genetic damage. In the case of addiction being our chief focus, we should discuss the direct damage that has been done to our dopamine receptors. The intolerance we develop to our vices is largely due to the inability for damaged dopamine receptors to receive the dopamine that is being produced in anticipation to the habit and from the habit itself. In the beginning we may receive a rush of stimulation and pleasure from any said behavior. Over time, we lose that immediate sensation and require much more stimuli in order to receive the same sensation. Eventually, we need a lot more of it and this creates the dopaminergic feedback cycle of addiction which also followed by lower energy lows when we do not have it or have prolonged spaces without it. Most of the focus on dopamine and its role in addiction is on the dopamine cycle itself but rarely addresses the DNA damage that is both caused by the addiction and was present prior to the addiction.

If our parents had an unhealthy lifestyle then it will influence the DNA and gene disposition we were born into. There are countless examples I can provide as to the disadvantages most of us experienced post-conception such as circumcision for boys, not enough mothers breast milk or artificial replacement milk, vaccinations, over sanitized as a baby, cutting off the umbilical cord too soon, malnutrition, and many others to list. The important thing here is to understand we were born into an aberrant situation where each individual has had disadvantages and any minor genetic defects can be overturned with knowledge and application. It is very common to see someone adopt similar or identical repetitive habits that their parents or grandparents have/had. This is not by accident. It was encoded into us by way of genetic transference and more significantly through the role modeling we received in our formative and pre-adult years. Our genes had adapted to this and so did our dopamine receptors. Once we begin repairing the dopaminergic damage, we then gain control over our behaviors and the rest of our DNA begins to heal itself automatically.

Remember, the brain is not a static piece of machinery. It is adaptive, flexible, and will adhere to the patterns we practice. There is tremendous neuro-scientific evidence to show that the dopamine receptors, over time, become tired and fatigued from too much stimulation without enough recuperation. We made mention earlier in this chapter that it is not that addicts have more dopamine which is problematic, but that they have far less dopamine and that is what is truly the problem. It has been shown time and time again that addicts of all kinds have far less dopamine in their receptors and also far less dopamine receptors left available to intake dopamine chemistry. The natural effect of dopamine (the reward system) becomes less and less excitable therefore more and more of it leads to a diminishment of receptors over time. The reaction is to "retaliate" by doing more and more of the behavior which leads to a new 'set point' being achieved in the brain and this becomes the new default setting or new default normal. The brain and all of its receptor activity is adapting to all of this, each step of the way, and this is what eventually causes the dopamine receptor fatigue leading to the receptor die off effect.

This helps to explain the intensified need for someone to take substances to feel normal. It used to be just to get high or alter their state by conscious choice. Now the brain has become maladapted, and it's become the new set point for feeling "normal". Once we have found ourselves in this state of affairs, we can be assured that there has been a significant amount of receptor atrophy and the only way to pull ourselves out is to aid in the neuro-regeneration of our brain as a whole. In the chapter **Healing the Brain | Rehabbing the Mind** we go into great detail on this whole subject and provide more tools for healing.

In the conversation about genetics and epigenetics we can look at all the patterns of gene expression and how that plays into the equation of addiction. There is no doubt that this is powerful and has tremendous value. However, if we overlook the factor of dopamine and receptor regeneration then it does not necessarily lead us to where we want to go. Which is the desired outcome of outstanding health, psychological empowerment, and activating the motivational triggers that make us better humans. Think of it this way. Increasing the dopamine receptors in the brain is like upgrading the hardware in a high-performance computer whereas increasing dopamine is like upgrading the software program. The hardware must be optimized in order to handle the capabilities in which the software program needs to perform. Increasing the numbers of receptors will create a long-term effect where someone is able to enjoy the smaller things in life much more and feel better with less external inputs. This also results in having more internal drive and motivation to pursue goals rather than needing a cup of coffee, caffeine pills, or whatever else in order to go after their day.

In the chapter **The Dopamine Detox Protocol** you will find a map broken down into three levels to reset the reward/pleasure system in the brain and begin the regeneration process back to whole health. In the next section in this chapter, you will find a synthesis of lifestyle tips to begin rebooting your body's natural inborn chemistry set which all play a significant role in repairing and producing additional dopamine receptors. What is really powerful about all of these practices is that they generally do not feel incredibly good while we are doing them but feel amazing after we have done them. This is the opposite of an addiction where we feel really good while we are doing it but feel really bad after we've done it. It is the inversion of an addiction cycle and exactly what is required to override the addictive impulses that hijack our pleasure/reward circuitry.

It takes discipline and persistence to rebuild our brain receptors naturally, yet this is also how we increase our confidence and self-esteem at the same time the body contains a self-organizing and self-healing design which is to say that whatever damage we have experienced, our bodies are pre-programmed to heal it and have all of the tools to do so. Our role in this process is to supply the body and brain with what it needs in the form of lifestyle modifications and high-quality nutrition. The epigenetic research has shown that the body can bounce back from extreme circumstances rather quickly depending on the commitment and conscious engagement of each individual. The more one commits to this process the more results they will experience and the quicker it will manifest for them. In the chapter **Healing the Brain | Rehabbing the Mind** we discuss specific protocols for repairing cognitive decline and neurotransmitter receptor damage.

"The more sophisticated an organism, the higher the percentage of junk DNA it contains."

Nessa Carey, Junk DNA: A Journey Through the Dark Matter of the Genome

Continuing with the revolutionary discoveries in epigenetic sciences I would be remised if I did not include a discussion on what is referred to as Junk DNA. In my original book, **The Holistic Health Mastery Program** I wrote an entire lengthy chapter on this subject and this section is a simple distillation of in-depth information I went into almost a decade ago. At one point in our recent scientific history there was a group of researchers who discovered that there was a vast amount of our DNA that did not seem to have any clear known function. This was termed 'non-protein coding DNA' because the DNA that was being observed did not seem to have 'coding instructions' for creating new proteins in a cell. Because of the conventional model of cellular biology and gene coding these DNA molecules did not adhere to the model and thus labeled 'junk' because they seemed to have no known function associated to them.

The Human Genome Project is an international research group whose goal was to conduct a complete mapping and understanding of all the genes in the human body and what their designed uses were. Perhaps the most surprising discovery this project made was to find that, accordingly to them, only 2% of our genome contains understandable genetic code. There has been a tremendous amount of research in this field conducted since but just to illustrate the point we'll leave it at that. Beyond this it had been a long-held assumption that at least 80% of our genes were inactive, non-functional, or as has been described "junk". This seems like a pretty monumental assumption to make in light of the fact that we are still only scratching the surface of what we know about human psychology (and everything else!).

Now, what is extremely interesting in following this research it was discovered that there was a discovery that our genome had 20% of what is known as regulatory genes. These genes are very unique but were not immediately understood because they do not make up the protein molecules in our bodies that basic genes do. These genes act similar to enzyme molecules in the body where they turn on, turn off, activate and deactivate the other genetic switches that are responsible for building out the structure of the body. These regulatory genes are something of a genomic control panel that contain up to 4 million control switches that determine which genes are put to work and which genes are put through a process known as apoptosis which is the pre-programmed death of a cell. This is a truly remarkable discovery and leads us into the realization that our epigenetic triggers are far more impactful on our gene expression than the set genes we inherited to begin with. If you want to dive deeper into the overall health implication and study this further, I suggest looking up the topic on telomeres and the telomerase enzyme associated with repairing and activating dormant strands of DNA. You can also look into methylation as part of this topic, and we'll elaborate on these ideas in the chapter **Mastering the Body | Health**.

It turns out that the so-called junk DNA or non-protein coding DNA are carrying out far more miraculous and sophisticated functions than the simple genes of our prior scientific paradigms. These are the master switches that control the regulatory mechanism that help our body maintain all of its intricate and complex functions, second by second. This is truly where the emergence of epigenetics comes to the forefront of our understanding of human health, addiction cycles, and unlocking the possibilities of the future. It turns out that the vast majority of our DNA is lying dormant inside of us. It is inactive because it has not been forced to turn on through necessity. You see, when we become addicted to a specific stimulation feedback cycle, we are priming our bio-genetic needs to support and reinforce that particular behavior. All of our internal processes begin to conform in service of repetition and prime the chemistry set of the body for repeatability of behaviors that induce a preferable (pleasurable) experience. It is only when we force our biology (and physiology) to break out of its dormant comfort zone that we begin to turn on other mechanism that are needed in order to carry out the new behavior.

There is no junk anything in the human body outside of the junk we put into it. The epigenetic phenomenon states that our physical environment, our dominant emotional states, and the substances we put into our bodies plays the biggest role in activating or deactivating regulatory genes. Epi means above or outside and combined with the word 'gene' means what is outside of our genes plays the biggest role in what happens within the cell that the gene is controlling. In my **Holistic Health Mastery** book, I did an extensive breakdown of how minerals are the primary nutrients that have the biggest activation catalysts for genetic signaling. If you want to dive deeper into that topic you can read my book or look into the work of Charles Walters Jr, in his book **Minerals for the Genetic Code** where he provides Dr. Olree's genetic mineral chart which overlaps the 64 codons that our current scientific understanding supports. You can also go through the work of Richard Rudd in his **Gene Keys**, who I referenced above whose work is likely the most useful and paramount in terms of the holistic human transformational experience and transcending our addictive shadow patterns.

So, in conclusion of this entire exploration let it be known that the process towards self-healing, addiction recovery, dopamine recuperation, and genetic revival is truly, truly simple. It is very sophisticated and full of incredibly fascinating research to entertain ourselves till no end. For all practical purposes though, let's rest assured that the fundamentals are easy to implement, basic in scope, and with consistent execution of the basics profound life lasting results can only follow. The knowledge that you have now gained in this short part of our journey in this book is already light years ahead of where most addiction recovery books or teachings will ever take anyone. We, after all, are not interested in making simple progress, although simple progress is key, it is not at all where the finish lines reside. In fact, there is no finish line in sight because the miracle of the human technology we call a biological body has no limits and neither do you, my friend. You are truly an unlimited being and the sooner you get on board with that understanding the sooner you will be experiencing the palpable effect of dormant genetic switches being turned on and bursts of motivational energy flooding your sensory system.

The drive for immediate stimulation that dopamine provides us is only a mild sensation that is available to us to experience. It is like the tip of the iceberg, but we get caught up in chasing the peak experience because we are not visibly aware of the entire glacier of human experience (or human DNA) that is available beneath the surface of the conscious mind. This is why we are tapping into what is available by delaying immediate gratification and delaying immediate pleasure as a way to invert the addiction cycle. Our internal biology has to be reprogrammed and our behaviors need to be re-patterned in order to begin experiencing what it is like to turn on our full gene expression which comes as a result of repairing and rebuilding our dopamine receptors.

Following this theme, we are going to close out this chapter by talking about self-producing dopamine strategies. Every one of these activities has a powerful effect on this process and if carried out every single day can have immense benefits in your life (and your health). Just like addictive patterns form their own lifestyle adaptations inverting the addiction cycle through empowering and healthy patterns also form a lifestyle which is based on self-reliance, self-empowerment, and increasing our bodily resilience to all forms of stress and discomfort which in turn allows us to become a greater (and healthier) version of ourselves.

Self-Producing Dopamine Strategies

The key to taking back our power from addiction to dopamine impulses is to disassociate ourselves from the habits that create the chemical stimulation and exchange out poor habits for better habits. This really means that we get to upgrade our entire lifestyle and all of the habits that make up our daily mode of operation. This is extremely simple but not always easy and at this point it should be clear why that is. Remember, this is not about perfection. It is about progress and daily progress leads to better and better results. As we stack on the upgraded habits, one after another, we begin to develop a greater sense of self confidence which can lead us towards self-mastery. Mastering our addictive impulses and urges leads us to mastering ourselves which is the ultimate point of all spiritual teachings and personal development philosophy.

Below are some of the best tools each of us has at our disposal to create a life of mastery and a lifestyle of optimal health and inner freedom. These are the foundational pillars of optimizing our physical health, our mental - emotional wellbeing, and creating more discipline in everything else that we do in life. Before marching off to accomplish some big, hefty goal, I suggest starting small and implementing the action steps below to build incremental solidarity with your routines. It is not required to do all of this at once, but it is advised to take on a few things together as all of these practices work in total harmony and synergy with one another. Once enough positive energy is moving forward in your upgraded practice the discomfort of letting go of the old dissipates and the momentum of the new takes over. Consistency is always the main thing to focus on and the beneficial results quickly follow.

Last thing here is to understand is that these practices (among many others not listed) serve mainly as pillars or anchor points for a deeper interpersonal growth process. None of these are magic bullets or cure all practices for overcoming addiction. They serve to help you grow into someone who exerts discipline, commitment, focus, and follow through towards your purpose. Without healthy replacement habits overcoming prior habits that have a downward momentum effect is virtually impossible. The body will still seek that immediate impulse of dopamine from the quick fixes that it was accustomed too in the past. Just sitting alone by ourselves, trying to talk ourselves out of the tension and discomfort of not giving into those urges tends to rarely, if ever work. This way we are redirecting the energy, changing the mental focus, and exerting enough will power to exhaust out the old tendencies until they no longer have a hold on us in any way.

Remember, finding pleasure in the discomfort of a positive habit adaptation is a corner stone to success. Smile into the discomfort, laugh into the temporary pain, breath into the wrestling tension, and, if needed, pray from deep in your heart when you feel the body go into a fleeting moment of shock because that is when you are right on the edge of where freedom resides.

Push Up Challenge

Push-ups are a great quick way to get your body (and mind) into action. Sometimes we may find ourselves reaching out for tobacco, coffee, or some other substance for a quick stimulation in order to get ourselves "going". Before you do that try challenging yourself to drop down and do as many push-ups as you possibly can. This will create an immediate hypertrophic effect where your muscles fill up with blood and oxygen causes an increase in bodily energy. Push yourself to do more than you think you can and keep going until your arms simply cannot do anymore. Once you stop, catch your breath, ask yourself do I really want a smoke or cup of coffee?

Morning Journaling

Morning journaling can be very helpful to trigger new ideas, insights, and solutions to any challenges we may wake up too. One of the reasons we can experience brain fog and mental overwhelm is because we simply have too many unprocessed thoughts contained in our head and they need to be unpacked. Journaling can help you take what is in your head and put it out on paper. Sometimes the things we are concerned about are simply condensed forms of energy bound up within our mind and once it's out on paper we realize how trivial these thoughts really are.

Meditation

Having a daily meditation practice is one of the most important rituals anyone can implement into their lives. Preferably first thing upon waking up, in-between the day, and prior to going to bed for absolute best results. Meditation is simply closing your eyes, stilling the mind, and breathing in and out. This is as simple as simple gets. This allows you to become an active observer to your thought patterns and detect the emotional energy that arises in the body. All you are required to do is breath and sit still. It is recommended to maintain a 15-30-minute practice but 10 minutes minimum if that is all you have in any given moment. Starting the day this way can change the entire dynamic of your day and ending your day this way helps to transition the mind from being active and awake to slowing down the brain waves, preparing for a deep night's sleep.

Fasting

Fasting is a principle of abstaining from a certain activity or set of activities for a certain duration of time. There are all kinds of forms of fasting one can practice in order to help reset the body, the mind, and the bio-chemical relationship our bodies have developed to specific activities and/or substances. The most common form of fasting is to abstain from certain types of foods or all food together. Fasting is one of the most powerful ways to rebalance the body by initiating the body's innate healing metabolic functions. The easiest way to begin with fasting is to start with intermittent fasting which is basically abstaining from solid food through the morning (until 11-12 noon at least) and only consuming liquids. This will be explored more in detail in the chapter **Mastering the Body**.

Breath Work

Perhaps the single most powerful tool for shifting one's mental and emotional state is having a consistent breath work practice to rely upon. Breath work is not complicated nor is it hard to start. We are always breathing, every moment of every day, but we tend to take autonomic shallow breaths instead of conscious deep diaphragmatic breaths which can help us reset our inner state and regulate our nervous system. There are a lot of breath work techniques to experiment with. You can easily go online and search "breath work" to learn more about different ways to begin. What I recommend is simply to take ten deep breaths each morning, upon waking up in bed before getting up for the day. Place one hand on your heart and the other over your stomach. Breath from your belly and into your heart. Slowly exhale the breath out of the mouth as if breathing out through a straw. You can take this into your meditation and at any moment in the day where you feel stress or cravings emerge to medicate the sensations that emerge in the body.

Cold Showers / Ice Plunges

Out of all of these tools presented, the act of getting into a cold shower is easily the most powerful method for quickly shifting one's internal state, regardless of whatever emotional or energetic discord may be going on. This is also one of those things that many people feel very resistant too because it can feel very uncomfortable at first, especially if they are sensitive to cold temperatures. We are so used to taking hot showers because of the comfort and ease it provides but this can also create a lethargic energetic in the body and in the mind. The cold water helps to stimulate the central nervous system, thus energizing the body and providing a pattern interrupt for the mind. When you get into a cold shower or into an ice bath there is literally nothing else someone can think about other than the present moment, they are in. Go ahead, try it. Try to obsessively think about anything that is bothering you. No go into a cold shower and try to keep thinking about it. If you stay in the water, you will be unable to focus on anything except the immediate sensations of the body and the breathing cycles your respiratory system involuntarily goes into.

Cold exposure therapy was popularized by Wim Hof who is also known as the ice man who has broken all kinds of world records for staying in the coldest conditions of any human, longer than any known human. His work and message has spawned a huge movement of health enthusiasts who love to do 'ice baths' or 'ice plunges' which is submerging the body in a container of water filled with ice. It's best to begin this practice with cycling hot and cold in the shower, until you get do entirely cold. It took me months to adjust to it, while finding myself slipping back to the comfort of the hot warmth in the morning, but I just pushed myself to keep going, and now cold showers are a daily routine for me.

The Addiction to Struggle

"Every time we give away our attention to these
distractions - smartphones, alcohol, drugs- we are actually
giving our power and energy to them because where our
attention goes, our energy flows".

Charles Clay

We have made our way through some of the most important discussion points in the entire realm of addiction, both the subtle nature of how addiction begins and also the bio-chemical aspect of how our dopamine neurotransmitter system is affected. Now we get to unpack the not so obvious psychological aspects that exist beneath all forms of physical and emotional addiction cycles. Below the surface of our overt habits that form over time through repetition is the psycho-emotional drivers behind what I will later describe as the addiction frequency is the root causation for why we do what we do and also why it is so challenging to pull ourselves away from habits we know are not serving us.

There is a more nuanced addiction that rests below the surface of all other addictions and it is one I have identified to be at the core of all others. This addiction I am referring to is the addiction to struggle or another way of saying this is the addiction to hardship. This may not seem entirely obvious or even make a lot of sense at first glance. In order to identify this tendency within ourselves we need to go beyond the habit itself and begin to observe the motivational force that enacts itself through us as we find ourselves reaching out for "the thing" that lowers our energy, weakens our resolve, chips away at our discipline, and imbalances our health. In everyone I have ever worked with and observed that struggles with addiction has this pattern. This pattern is more of a mental program that tricks the user into believing life is a struggle, life is meant to be hard, and in order to succeed we have to punish ourselves as a way to reach the finish line.

The problem with this program is that the proverbial finish line is ultimately unachievable, largely because it is fundamentally designed for failure. You see, within our high paced culture we have been taught to struggle towards success, but we have not defined what success really is and our strategy for getting there is based on bad information. There is a brilliant saying from Alice in Wonderland which is if you do not know where you are going than any road will get you there. If we are operating from a program of struggle and hardship than we will continually create situations and circumstances in order to reinforce that program, despite how illogical and counter-productive it is. It's like digging a hole for ourselves, putting ourselves in the hole, only to exert the effort needed to pull ourselves out and repeatedly doing this, over and over in order to feel like we are making progress towards our goals but ultimately going nowhere. Does this pattern sound familiar at all?

This is an example of what we could call the self-sabotaging cycle of addiction. We set our aim for a certain goal/destination, begin to set good intentions to get there, get motivated to do the work necessary, and once we begin to feel like we are making progress we find a way to fumble it all up. This can show up in all kinds of ways. It can show up in our relationships (and often does!), it definitely can show up in our recovery from substances, as well as our health and fitness goals, for sure. It is the same thing that happens when people make new year's resolutions to change their lifestyle habits, take on a new diet, or begin working out at the gym. We have all the best intentions in the world and feel super motivated, for a while. This of course wears off within a few weeks or for most within a few days. For some people who have dug themselves into an especially deep hole of their own making it can last for only a few hours.

We all find ourselves wondering why we experience the extreme highs of motivation and consequently go through the deep lows of demotivation. We ride the momentum of inspiration only to find ourselves soon after losing that charged up energy and reverting back into the same old habits, we told ourselves we were ready to leave behind. There are multiple reasons for this, and we will unpack them all within this chapter. The important concept to ponder though is this addiction to struggle and hardship as a force that repeatedly shows up in our lives every time, we make headway towards recovery and success. If life feels rather hard and it seems as if you are constantly struggling in one way or another, than you need to consider that you may have a belief program operating unconsciously that tells you in order to achieve anything in life that you must struggle in order to get there.

Sit with this for a moment. Take a deep breath.

Now, let's look at this a bit closer.

The reason why an addictive relationship to anything forms in our lives is not entirely due to the addictive nature of "the thing" itself but more so the relationship we have with ourselves. There are countless examples of people who experiment with all sorts of "addictive substances" and do not seem to have a compulsive repetitive relationship to those things. And then there are individuals who absolutely cannot go near certain substances, otherwise the "uncontrollable" urge to repeat the behavior manifests itself and becomes a serious problem. Think of alcoholism for example. Some people can have a drink once in a while and others have one, which becomes ten and then becomes an out-of-control spiral. You can chalk this up to some kind of genetic defect in certain people's genomic makeup or inherited patterns from their familial line. This is a basic fact and one that makes more sense from discussing the epigenetic aspect in the prior dopamine dilemma chapter. But the point I am driving at is that what influences our genetic and epigenetic factors is the belief program operating behind the genetic switching station in the first place.

The simple point I want to make here is that all functions of our physical patterns are a byproduct of our psychological patterns. Every addiction that plays itself out in our lives is derived from a pattern that has been playing out in our mental lives. Essentially stress is the cause of all of our addiction patterns and our "self-destructive" habits are actually ways in which we attempt to sooth the tension we feel in our minds. This is all unconscious until it is made conscious and once, we become aware that this pattern exists we become empowered enough to do something about it. This is also why simply trying to change the habit itself usually does not work because there is a stronger driving force that keeps the habit alive and causes us to seemingly forget about the original commitment, we had made about quitting it. This is why the withdrawal process is so difficult

We are now going to explore the deeper causal roots of this nuanced 'addiction' to struggle and hardship. Remember, this is not your fault or some kind of blemish against you as a competent human being. This is largely indoctrinated into us through the conditioning of organized society and consumer-based culture. Phrases such as 'life is hard', 'suck it up', 'don't be a wuss', or 'money does not grow on trees', or whatever other absurd memes we were told by our trusted parental figures or authorities had an effect on our impressionable minds as children. So be easy on yourself and those around you who also are in a recovery process from the hardship program and transitioning into a much more effective and graceful process towards life.

The Upper Limit Problem

Moving onto the next phase of this conversation we are going to explore an important principle simply described as the upper limit problem. This is something that we all encounter at different stages in our life and most certainly in the recovery process from addiction. The upper limit is likened to our general comfort zone where we adhere to the behaviors and psycho-emotional states that we find comfortable and easy to maintain. As human beings, we tend to become creators of comfort and what is familiar to us. If we have rehearsed certain patterns over enough time, we will find ourselves reverting back into those patterns when we experience states of discomfort or pain. This understanding is the key principle to overriding rehearsed behaviors and adapting our minds to a whole new set of behaviors and skill sets.

The upper limit problem was coined by an author named Gay Hendricks. He has a lot of great perspectives on this and does a great job at explaining how we can easily self-sabotage our goals through hitting the 'upper limit'. The upper limit is basically our personal threshold of what feels comfortable in any given area of our lives. You know you are reaching your upper limit because sensations of tension, anxiousness, and contraction can manifest in the body. Feelings of fear, doubt, worry, or even panic can arise in us when we are pushing against our edges. This is usually the point where most people will either freeze, turn away, or fight their way through it. Each of these responses produces a different result and each is a reaction from the nervous system that is signaling the fear response in the body.

When it comes to the topic of addiction this concept should feel very relevant right now. The underlining tension that can creep up when you begin to make a clean break from the habits that have formed in your life. Becomes something has been normal and familiar to us it also begins to become a part of us. What we continually spend our time and energy with fuses itself with us, including all of the habits we know are slowing us down. The fact that addictive habits do slow us down is likely one of the reasons we find some kind of value in them. If we did not have these things to slow us down than we would have to face our upper limit thresholds, because we would not have anything blocking up the flow of energy. So, our habits keep us safe in our comfort zone, even if our comfort zone is secretly keeping us uncomfortably comfortable and holding us back from experiencing true liberation.

Another way of thinking about this idea is to consider that each of us has an internal thermostat that ranges from extreme hot to extreme cold. Most people tend to live their lives in the lukewarm place in-between the extremes. Some rare people live their lives with a passionate fire and stay in the hotter side of the thermostat. Some others seem to have no passion or energy whatsoever and live their lives in the cold end of the spectrum. Every person has a different temperament which causes them to run a bit hot or maybe a bit cold. Hot represents high energy and cold represents low energy. Somewhere between the two extremes is where most people spend their time. This in-between place is a form of a comfort zone where it's not too cold and it's not too hot. It's lukewarm and does not require a whole lot from the person in order to maintain consistency and normalcy.

There is a temperature that most people feel when they reach outside of their comfort zone and it tends to feel hot, like a heating up in the body when you are in an intense workout, a breath work practice, or in a sauna for a while. This is what we call putting our feet to the fire. When we begin to reach that upper limit, our internal thermostat begins to heat up. This is actually the place we want to be, always with a healthy amount of pressure or discomfort but never enough to completely flat line our efforts. This heating sensation is the energy we get to sit with, fully embrace, and master inside of us in order to reach a new normal. The new normal is the upper limit we are uncomfortable with but now has become our new comfort zone. This means we can just keep upping our upper limits instead of being held back by them.

The best way to engage with this upper limit upgrade process is to gamify it a bit and make it fun for yourself. Of course, it's going to be uncomfortable, and you will feel awkward at times, but that discomfort does not last forever. It's temporary and if you focus on where you want to be opposed to obsessing about how uncomfortable it is where you are at then the sensations can move pretty quickly. As long as you know where your upper limits are than you will not be surprised when you experience them. This is why organizing your lifestyle in a way that supports your overall health, mental focus, emotional balance, and keeps you productive is the formula for cruising past these upper limits and maintaining a comfortably hot inner thermostat.

There are a few key concepts we need to discuss in order to observe the belief programs and 'memes' operating within our own consciousness, that are not easily detectable using our normal adapted methods of perspective i.e., our lifelong viewpoints. We have to adjust our lenses a bit and turn our belief systems upside down in order to see things right side up. This comes from adjusting what we are seeing playing out in our lives which leads to a greater degree of clarity and potency of truth. I am going to call this process the eagle eye perspective shift. This 'process' basically allows for us to take a broader view of the landscape of our lives and to witness all of the moving parts, not as we think they are but exactly as they are, for exactly what they are. This can be the hardest part of any transformational initiation because we can become so attached and identified with the stories playing out in our lives that we lose sight of the truth and simply settle for a version of the truth, which usually has an addiction frequency associated with it.

This eagle eye perspective attitude requires us to identify our own blind spots, to sit in the discomfort of whatever new information emerges, and then to let go of outdated information or beliefs that do not align with the new information that has proven to be closer to the truth. Essentially what I am getting at is that in order to rise to a higher perspective of our lives we have to go through a bit of an ego reset process thus allowing ideas that do not serve our future to fall away. This requires developing neutrality and balance towards our long-held ideas, beliefs, and even the addictions themselves. Neutrality is a state of balance, equanimity, and poise. Addiction is a state of imbalance, one sided perspective, and impatience. It's hard to gamify our recovery process or to sustainably raise our internal thermostat (comfort zone) if we are still caught in the sea saw of emotional charge (right to left - extremes). This process requires a tempered discipline of striking that internal balance point and that is what neutrality represents.

The upper limit problem is really pointing to a fundamental imbalance within an individual's perspective. Our perspectives shape our internal experience and if we are experiencing internal states of anxiety, worry, restlessness, or chronic stress then we can be assured that we are operating from an imbalanced perspective in our lives. This phenomenon creates another issue which I call the addiction to the energetic roller coaster. This is very much like the addiction to struggle or hardship but it's a uniquely chaotic version of the same thing. We can get addicted to the adrenaline and cortisol stimulation that comes from chaotic experiences and misinterpret them as an energy source. In reality it is just one extreme swinging back to another in rapid fashion and the result is lack of composure, stability, long term clarity, and certainly ill health.

The road back to holistic health recovery requires us to step off the energetic roller coaster and renounce our unconscious addiction to extremes. We, as human beings in times of great uncertainty, are being called to balance out our inner state and create certainty from within. Trading out the higher highs and lower low's template for the sustainable and calm energy levels is the map for a life of success and balance. It really does all come down to balance at the end of the day. Life itself is never really perfectly balanced but our attitude and perspective about our life can be truly balanced which creates the inner balance we are seeking. For most people, their biggest upper limit challenge is not some audacious goal to achieve or a mountain to go climb. It's actually just sitting alone with themselves long enough to feel everything their body has been trying to tell them and to organize their mind in a way that creates clarity and composure for the future.

The Normalcy Bias, Certainty Bias, & Compensatory Strategies

In different conceptual frameworks surrounding developmental psychology & cognitive development principles there are some terms you likely have heard before. Terms such as cognitive dissonance, certainty bias, cognitive bias, etc. The term cognitive dissonance is defined as *"the state of having inconsistent thoughts, beliefs, or attitudes, especially as relating to behavioral decisions and attitude change."* This essentially means thinking one thing, having an unconscious or conscious belief paradigm that is different, and consistently behaving/acting in a way that contradicts the belief. Cognitive dissonance is very common in the psychology of addiction and is almost always rooted in some form of trauma, whether it be mental, emotional, or psycho-emotional in origin. This speaks to a form of compartmentalization between the individuals adopted identity (the social self) and the underlining identity (the private self) which is lacking an integration between the two (integrity of identity).

This is an origin point of where many people, especially those struggling with addiction recovery, experience their strongest bouts of stress. The internal conflict of contradictory beliefs, ideas, or values that are not being exercised and entirely embodied in their actual lives. This also explains why there is a sudden sensation of stress or distress when someone in this situation begins to go against their subconscious "programming" and hits what we have described as the upper limit effect. If one is experiencing this issue in their lives and wondering why it keeps on looping back and forth, well this is a pretty solid explanation to consider. This is the same phenomena that occurs when someone is told by their doctor that smoking or drinking is detrimental to their health, yet they are bombarded by corporate advertisements and billboards that are glamorizing alcoholism and cigarette smoking, as a common example amongst many. This can create a contradictory framework inside someone's psyche that begins from a very early age. Especially if they witnessed their parents drinking and smoking. Or worse yet, one of their parents modeled that behavior and the other parent was strongly against it. Talk about a cognitive developmental glitch or schism that could occur in someone during their formative years of development.

The solution for this disconnects is multi-layered and presented within each and every chapter of this book in various ways. Ultimately, the simple answer is to bridge the unconscious desires/impulses with the conscious operating system and integrate the two together. This sounds profoundly simple and in theory it is, yet the human condition (through social conditioning) presents us with a bit more complexities than meets the eye. That is why this book is far bigger than a few pages or even a few basic chapters. Over the course of our developmental years from childhood to adolescence into adulthood each of us has adopted compensatory strategies in order to manage stress and move on with our lives. Due to the lack of psycho-emotional integration or conscious-subconscious integration we develop habits and behaviors to compensate for the inner conflict i.e., emotional disconnection within. This is what the entire industry of pharmaceutical and psychiatric drugs is attempting to address (without admitting it).

Compensatory strategies can often manifest as ways to numb, medicate, or negate the internal tension that we call stress. The longer we carry this "stress' around with us the stronger the need and desire for compensatory tactics becomes. Virtually anything that helps to mitigate, buffer, or reduce stress (in all of its forms) can be considered a compensation strategy. And these compensatory strategies/tactics increase their stronghold in our lives because of something called a 'normalcy bias'. Normalcy bias is similar to what is known as a cognitive bias or a certainty bias. A cognitive bias is explained by Wikipedia as *"Individuals create their own "subjective reality" from their perception of the input. An individual's construction of reality, not the objective input, may dictate their behavior in the world."* This basically means that someone can create their own personal reality out of the information that resonates or aligns with a subjective bias they have about themselves, their surroundings, or the world (or any topic) and tend to filter out/exclude any information that competes or contradicts their pre-conceived bias's.

It should be pretty straight forward to see how that kind of mentality plays itself into the addiction cycle. This also explains the challenge (and sometimes turmoil) of reaching the upper limit of one's own psychological comfort zone. When we have a cognitive bias, we essentially have chosen ahead of time what is true, what is real, and in effect who we believe we are in every definable manner of what that means. We are not open to outside perspective or conflicting information which therein lies the fundamental challenge with an addiction that someone says they want to let go of but internally are getting compensatory value from it each time they do it. This ties together the cognitive dissonance and cognitive bias concepts along with the utility of compensatory tactics being the glue that holds it all together. Moving on into the normalcy bias concept we also want to become aware of this other idea called a certainty bias. This basically means that we can assume something is a concrete fact or a certainty when it may only be a probability or even merely a hunch.

This can express itself in erratic behaviors of extreme highs followed by disappointing lows. This issue can cause people to get really excited about something they have not properly thought through or thoroughly researched to determine if it is legit or not. This is extremely common in the nature of gambling addictions where someone impulsively gambles large sums of money on a rigged game and convinces themselves that winning is a certainty or at least high probability. This is another example of the imbalanced psyche where we defer to extremes instead of objectively looking at reality from a balanced and integrated perspective. If these individuals look at this situation from a balanced and neutral perspective, they would be able to calculate the probabilities of loss and access the risk vs reward ratio before thrusting their life savings in a moment of chance. The entire industry of gambling, whether it be casinos, slot machines, online apps, video games, or lottery tickets all rely upon people who have a strong certainty bias and are willing to gamble their long-earned resources (or someone else's) in a moment of bolstered confidence.

So, now that we have thoroughly explained these concepts and ideas, let's move onto the normalcy bias as it represents the wholism of each of these aspects relating to addiction. Normalcy bias is defined by Wikipedia as *"Normalcy bias, or normality bias, is a cognitive bias which leads people to disbelieve or minimize threat warnings. Consequently, individuals underestimate the likelihood of a disaster, when it might affect them, and its potential adverse effects."* This means that due to a biased attachment (i.e., addiction) to life as it is and has been, someone will ignore probable upcoming threats or simple warnings as a way to avoid disrupting their common place reality. This is the most dangerous psychological space to be in because it involves every other bias condition mentioned and takes it to the level of someone becoming a complete sleepwalker. The term sleepwalker is not meant to be an insult but more of a description of those who have fallen so deeply into the addiction of their own normalcy confirmation bias that they are essentially living in a dream (i.e., their minds) and disassociated from reality outside of them, including the consequences of this disassociation itself.

The only way to root out these subtle nuanced psychological confirmation biases' that underlie all forms of addiction is to address the compensatory strategies themselves. Like so much of what we have discussed and will continue to unpack throughout the book, these compensatory strategies are a form of medication to numb or subdue the psycho-emotional tension within the individual's experience. With every form of addiction there is an emotional root cause, just as there is with every physical health issue we may experience. Everything is interconnected between the mind(thoughts), the body(feelings), and the heart(emotions). In the book **Power Vs Force** by Dr. David Hawkins brilliantly explains what he calls the levels of human consciousness which are described on a numerical scale from 0 to 1,000. 1,000 represents total enlightenment such as what we associate with Christ Jesus i.e., Christ consciousness (enlightenment) and closer towards 0 is a complete absence of consciousness. He was able to 'calibrate' human emotions at their resonant frequency signature based on this consciousness model and at the lowest of all human emotions he found that shame, which resonates at 20 out of 1,000, was the bottom of the emotional spectrum.

I am bringing this to our awareness because what I have found is that built into the metaphysical fabric of all addiction energetics is the emotion of shame and guilt. There are more but these two represent the bedrock of which all addiction challenges stand on. Guilt just so happens to be the next up in the emotional octave resonating at an energy level of 30. This is the lowest of a human being can drop down into before completely checking out of the human experience all together. And just for a disclaimer, if you want a detailed perspective on the dynamics of guilt go to the later chapter in the book called **Integration & Recovery** where we dive deeper into the guilt complex. We are going to focus on the dynamics of shame energy right now because underneath the cognitive dissonance, normalcy bias, and compensatory tactics that hold that all together is an unresolved aspect of trauma-based shame.

We are going to unpack the emotional roots of multiple aspects of physical health and associations to addiction in following chapters in the book including the chapter **Healing the Heart**. In his book, *Power vs Force*, David Hawkins has some very interesting insights about shame and its influence on people's lives.

> *"The level of shame is perilously proximate to death,*
> *which may be chosen out of shame as conscious suicide or*
> *more subtly elected by failure to take steps to prolong life;*
> *as in "passive suicide." Death by avoidable accident is*
> *common. We all have some awareness of the pain of*
> *"losing face," becoming discredited, or feeling like a*
> *"nonperson". In shame, people hang their heads and slink*
> *away, wishing they were invisible. Banishment is a*
> *traditional accompaniment of shame and, in the primitive*
> *societies from which we all originate, banishment is*
> *equivalent to death."*

What Dr. Hawkins is explaining is an idea that I have been researching for many years called the subtle death habit syndrome which was coined by Dr. Leonard Orr. This is where someone has unconscious suicidal tendencies that would never be considered suicidal such as socially acceptable choices i.e., drugs, junk food, cigarettes, alcohol, pornography, gambling, etc. that only have a net negative effect and create detriment in people's lives. When the emotional frequency of shame is living underneath the surface of one's psycho-emotional wellbeing the behavioral tendencies that matches that emotional state will not be far beyond it. When one carries unresolved shame and/or guilt they will likely turn to compensatory strategies that medicate the emotion but further the shame and guilt which most, if not all addiction patterns tend to do. If one has become too comfortable and normalized to this state of affairs (state of being) the confirmation bias and normalcy bias will likely reinforce itself in that person's unconscious framework. Therefore, unless the emotional signature of shame/guilt is not addressed, discharged through somatic processing, and healed/integrated there will continue to be an inner divide/disconnect that remains the access point for further compensation/numbing mechanisms to fall addicted too.

"We change the world not by what we say or do, but as a consequence of what we have become"

David R. Hawkins

Psycho-Emotional Masturbation

"Worry is a habit that shatters our peace of mind and needlessly drains our energy, a form of mental masturbation without any benefit."

Sue Patton Thoele

As I was contemplating this concept I am about to share, I was not exactly sure where to place it within these chapters. The obvious inclination was to include it in the chapter **Pornography | Sexuality** but after reviewing all that has been written in that chapter, I realized nothing more needed to be said in terms of overt sexuality itself. The term masturbation tends to make us think of one thing and one thing only but the roots of sexual addiction or simply sexual urges itself are not entirely basal desires of the carnal body. As I began to unpack this idea of psycho-emotional masturbation in my mind it became quickly apparent that the root of "masturbation" comes from the imbalance between our mental state and the sensory stimulation we experience as emotions. I am going to really delayer this concept for you because at the root of this problem it is most certainly originated from the addiction to struggle and that is why it is perfectly placed in this chapter.

Psycho-emotional masturbation as I am terming it is a form of mental masturbation that can take different forms internally. Essentially it is an energetic that takes on the flavor of consumerism, immediate gratification, and impulsivity. That is the overt form it takes when it comes to the more obvious sexual connotations and especially in terms of masturbation of the genitals, which we are all very well familiar with. What is not as obvious is the awareness of how we perform the same behavior mentally and also emotionally. We do this because we do not have solid boundaries around our mental-emotional entertainment tendencies. This shows up most commonly in the form of fantasy projections, usually of some enticing event in the future, or in some grasping of a past event. Mental masturbation is playing 'with ourselves' while living in our heads and not being anchored fully into our bodies. The sexual stimulatory response most men in particular experience that leads to excessive masturbation is a built-up energy in the body seeking an easy pressure release valve.

The more energetic pressure that is built up in the body (and the mental body) is always going to seek out outlet point. We can find many outlets for our internal energy but if we are not consciously aware of the mechanics at play then we will likely find the easiest and less optimal way to release accumulated pressure. What makes this more challenging is when we are constantly reinforcing the source of our pressure without putting a stop to it. This is the same for people who get onto a juice cleanse or detox program but never make the overall dietary changes needed to live a healthier life. They keep re-toxifying themselves with poor food choices and lifestyle habits that require them to constantly go on fasting protocols. Just like physical toxins bio-accumulate in our bodies tissues this also happens within our mental and emotional bodies as well. In order to stop reaching out for the pressure release valve, i.e., masturbation, we have to stop creating pressure in the first place.

This pattern is deeply rooted in the hardship or struggle program that is encouraged and reinforced through societal confusion. We are taught on one hand to restrain our urges and yet we are bombarded with contradictory messages about indulging in our shadow temptations. We are taught through societal moral frameworks to adhere one way and also programmed through organized religion that sexual expression or even masturbation is a hardcore sin. Is it any wonder that people feel so pent up inside? That the tension meter for most of us, especially men growing up in organized society and potentially in a single parent household feel so confused? Eventually this kind of confusion between social ethics, religious morals, and the overt indiscretions of our extravert and wildly undisciplined entertainment icons wears down on one's will power. This leads to a lot of experimentation through our adolescent or even young adult years. This is not inherently a bad thing but, in most cases, from what I have experienced and seen, it tends to lead to a lot of wasted time and energy.

One of the big ways mental masturbation has played out in my own life is the hyper intellectual pursuits I have dove into in search of information and knowledge. I have spent countless months, which have built up to years of intensified research, endless internet rabbit holes, uncountable conversations that may or may not have been of much use, oh and of course, spending way too much time on social media and YouTube. We, as a culture, have been put into a very perplexing situation for the simple reason that our developmental skills to handle the amount of digital exposure, increased pace of economic life, and the voluminous amounts of information that we can sift through daily has not been well worked out. It can become very easy to detach from the lived experience of our lives and defer to consuming information about information, researching ideas about ideas, and pontificating about life yet very rarely fully experiencing it as it is happening. This is one of many challenges we find ourselves in today. And you can go deeper into the digital addiction aspect of this in the chapter **Virtual Simulated Reality**.

The pursuit for knowledge and information for its own sake eventually leads to the realization that no amount of information can make up for a life unattended too. We can escape our situations as much as we want through acquiring more information but at some point, we have to apply the information or else it just congests the mind. We can layer idea on top of idea in order to help make sense of our lives and the world around us, but this does not inherently make our lives better. The way to reroute this pattern is to only focus on information that furthers our personal goals. This shows us the true measurement and qualitative value of the information we are acquiring. It is a tragedy of time to spend years on top of years studying and building idea structures in our mind only to discover it was based on a false premise and we now have to tear it all down. Inserting consistent meditation practices, work out routines, and mapping out a daily routine for where our energy goes can help us step out of the cycle of intellectual masturbation and really begin living our lives fully.

Emotional masturbation can play itself out in the form of indulging in our emotional responses and creating a story line around them. As strange as it may seem, we all have some sort of personal mythology about ourselves build up in our own minds and this can lead us to making unconscious decisions based on emotional urges. We can become extremely excited about a new sexual/love connection that shows up (or is just imagined) and dive headfirst into it because it feels 'good'. This is really just another dopamine response that our brain gives us because it feels better to do that than it does something else. The something else sometimes being objectively looking at a new possibility from both sides, pros and cons, before blindly jumping into something out of pure emotion. This also works when we get emotionally bound in negative feelings and create subconscious stories that fit perfectly with that. We can spend so much time and energy marinating on either past experiences or future projections and fail to realize none of it is even real. But we make it real through indulging in our imagination and living from our emotional response patterns instead of being objectively present, moment by moment.

A concrete example I can give from my own life experience of this is getting deeply invested in new and seemingly profound romantic connections. This had become a bit of a pattern for me in my late twenties as I was navigating the spiritual and health orientated communities which compromises of people who are on all spectrums of their own healing journey. This tends to be a much more heart centered, open minded, and 'open energy' community than what we typically find in the rest of society. When new and exciting romantic connections would form, I found myself, at times, getting really excited about the connection and indulging in all kinds of deep emotions that would draw me into the idea that this person was my soul mate or my twin flame (twin soul). I was still in my own awakening process and becoming more familiar with the concept of what a soul mate connection or what is called a twin flame connection was. When I would encounter such potent and unavoidable emotional bonds/resonance points I could find myself jumping into an entire relationship without ever going on a first official date.

I suppose in those dynamics the idea of conventional dating does not necessarily apply anyways. It's very much a spiritual connection but easily construed into a romantic longing, depending on the amount of healing work both individuals (her and I) had done at that point. And sometimes we can magnify people, especially romantic reflections at the level of our unresolved/unhealed wounds/shadows. This can also be where the highly polarized electric charge between two people who stumble upon each other resides. On the surface it is a very powerful connection with chemistry, attraction, and possibility. Underneath the surface, the deeper electrical charge can sometimes be two half pieces finding a whole, in one another but those half pieces are parts of the each that have not been fully healed and made whole in of themselves. I discovered this happening in many of my potent encounters with the opposite sex and realized it was a form of wound bonding that was merging us together. If I did not so easily indulge in my emotions and allow my mind to wrap around fantastical stories about what this connection was or could be, I would have been able to be much more present and objective. I would have also been able to simply take my time, step by step, without hurling myself into a deep love affair, only to go so deep so fast that it took years to work myself out of (literally!).

The addiction to an underlining struggle pattern can be found in some of these dynamics I am sharing. I have witnessed it in my own life and see the same pattern recognition in everyone that struggles with any manner of addiction. As I mention throughout this book, an addiction to one thing is never really the addiction itself. It is always an underlining energetic pattern that holds its own resonate frequency signature and expresses itself in a variety of ways. In our relationships is where we tend to discover the immediate reflections tied to our psycho-emotional (energetic) tendencies. This also can put stress and pressure on people who are experiencing the merry go round of reoccurring relationship challenges and cannot identify what is causing it. There is usually some unmet need, desire, or hidden thought form that is rooted in the masturbation patterns of the mind. Engaging with conscious or subconscious ideas or desires that are not appropriate or agreed upon by both people within the relationship container. I have certainly experienced this reoccurring pattern and that is why I can speak to it so easily.

The energetic pattern tied to 'masturbation' (in whatever form) is an avoidance strategy from what is happening in one's experience/body. In order to reroute from this habit pattern, we have to identify what we are doing (or what in our life) that is causing this buildup of pressure. Is it due to working too hard and not resting enough? Is it due to fantasizing about a life other than the one you are living now? Is it due to repressed desires or unfulfilled experiences you are itching to get too? Whatever it is, just know that there are many alternative ways for you to redirect the energy into things that are productive and build a consistent momentum for your life. The trick is to simply keep directing your energy into the things that "are working" and starve out the temptations that lead to sabotage. You just need to catch your rhythm in what you are doing and keep riding that energy, regardless of how awkward it might feel along the way.

I have found in my own experience that I have been most prone to "compromising" situations due to poor judgement when I was already in a state of psycho-emotional imbalance. When I was not focused on my goals and steadfast in my life direction. When I was being dodgy about my own integrity and following through on my personal commitments. The times where I felt a wobble in my life and had allowed myself to indulge in emotional masturbation too long. These had always been the times where I was most susceptible to addictions resurfacing and regaining a foot hold in my life. Because it takes real discipline and commitment to overcome addiction. It requires us to completely overcome ourselves and the version of ourselves that likes to create patterns of hardship just so we can climb our way back up the mountain top in order to feel triumphant. Falling from grace only to pick ourselves back up again. This is the addiction to a struggle cycle and where it originates is in our psycho-emotional masturbatory indulgences.

> *"It's what I call "mental masturbation", when you engage in some pointless intellectual exercise that has no possible meaning."*
>
> *Linus Torvalds*

The Eagle Eye Perspective - Neutrality

> *"The moment you realize you already have everything you're looking for the universe gives it to you."*
>
> *Dr. John Demartini*

We are now getting into a mental framework that is very near and dear to my own transformational process I have undergone within myself and continue to find new layers being revealed all the time. First of all, what is the eagle eye perspective and why am I calling this process, if you will the eagle eye perspective. Again, everything in our life experience seems to come down to perspective and the physiological sensations we call feelings/emotions tend to come alive within our bodies in response to the perspective/viewpoints we are holding in our minds. When we feel states of empowerment, we tend to have a particular attitude or consistent perspective we are holding that triggers the sensations we experience. This is also true if we are holding a disempowering perspective that causes us to feel as if we are a victim to circumstances and the resonant sensations cascade from there. Ultimately, whether we are holding a very high perspective or very low perspective, we are operating from an imbalanced perspective in relation to what is accurately true.

Let me unpack this idea a little more for you.

The human potential and behavior development specialist Dr. John Demartini has some really incredible insights into this idea which have bestowed many benefits in my own health/addiction recovery process. His entire body of work over the last 4 decades has been about helping people discover their core values in life and also to integrate the imbalances we all hold in our mind from time to time. He states that each human being is intrinsically motivated from within to fulfill their core values and to the degree that someone is living authentically vs inauthentically in their value system determines the happiness/unhappiness, success/lack of success they experience. You can explore his value determination process to learn more about determining what your core values are by visiting his website www.drdemartini.com. The insight about living from our true values instead of living from false values (social pressures) is also explained in another way in the chapter **Integration & Reconciliation** when we discuss karma and dharma.

The most important idea for us right now is finding the balance point or equilibrium between our misperceptions (imbalanced perceptions) and seeing the truth that exists in the neutrality point. Neutrality is a state of equanimity and balance whereas anger, sadness, despair, frustration, hopefulness or even hopelessness are emotionally charged states that have their highs and lows. As human beings we tend to experience a spectrum of emotions in any given day, week, month, and years which can inform our operating system (nervous system) how we should respond in relation to the emotions we experience. Especially if these emotions arise in stressfully charged situations that have a real effect on our equilibrium and confidence/certainty about the safety of life or that of our ourselves. The addiction cycle exists on an emotional roller coaster full of highs and lows but cannot take effect when someone is in a regulated state of neutrality that does not contain an emotional charge in either positive or negative direction. Another word for neutrality could be integration which is also another way of saying integrity.

Integrity is not simply a moral concept to intellectually access whether we are in integrity with ourselves or out of integrity with ourselves. Such an example would be whether we are in integrity with our decision to let go of an addiction or are we out of integrity with that decision by going back to it. This is usually where most people get stuck or simply stop because it's an intellectual pursuit but not a bodily integration process. Shame and guilt can emerge within one's mind if they feel they are out of integrity with their commitments, yet most people do not tend to go much further than this repetitive cycle. This is what we all must understand about the nature of integrity and its role in whether we grow out of our patterning or if we remain hostage to our conditioning i.e., addictions. Integrity is not simply a mental framework or concept but more so it's an internal guidance system that is synched up to our physiological nervous system. Remember, the word integrity means to be integrated and to the degree our core values are integrated within our behavioral patterns (consistent actions) determines the degree we are in integrity with ourselves (our true self!).

Dr. John Demartini has a unique methodology for helping people integrate the fragmentations of prior life experiences, subconscious traumas, and imbalanced perceptions which he calls The Demartini Method. Without going deep into the ins and outs of what that entails, the end result of doing this process correctly is that an individual reaches a state of internal equanimity and neutrality around whatever was previously bothering them, whether it be small or large. Demartini says that you know you have healed yourself when you reach a point where all you have is gratitude and thankfulness for every single thing that has ever happened to you because you can see the divine implicate perfection in it all. Gratitude is the emotional state that results from becoming truly integrated within ourselves and all of our past experiences. Our integral navigation compass is seeking out spaces within ourselves that we do not feel whole or healed and will bring those to our attention in order to rise into a higher state of integration i.e., wholeness and healing.

I call this state of being **the eagle eye perspective** because what happens is that we no longer are pigeonholing ourselves in the myopic details of our pains, wounds, and stresses but instead we are seeing the entire situation for what it really is, from an eagle eye vantage point. There is a saying in business which is you can either work in your business or you can work on your business, but you cannot do both at the same time. Most of us get stuck working in our lives but rarely zoom out of the details to work on our lives and see what is not working for us from a much broader perspective. The only time we tend to get emotionally charged or stressed out about what is occurring in our lives is when we are stuck working in the circumstances. We bump up against situations that cause us stress and can easily get stuck. It's only when we learn to step away from the situations that challenge us and zoom out enough to see the entire picture that we discover how easy and obvious the solutions really are. This is the difference between having a subjective perspective of life vs having an objective perspective. Subjective usually has a lot of personal attachment and emotion tied to it. Objective simply sees a situation or set of situations for what it is without the emotional charge and personal attachment to right or wrong. What simply just is and the solution is easy to spot out.

The Quantum Collapse Process

I developed a self-integration process of my own to assist my clients (and myself) in rapid integration between the happenings of the mind and the processes of the body. This essentially helps with mind-body integration and the method is called the Quantum Collapse Process. This is a simple yet incredibly powerful practice that is designed to support the body in emotional processing while teaching the nervous system how you want it to feel instead of being at the effect of circumstances. The way this works is that you can either sit up straight or lay on your back. Place your right hand on your stomach (around the solar plexus) and the left hand on your heart. Begin to inhale from through your nose and from your right hand (the belly). Raise the breath into the left hand (the heart) while slowly expanding the chest cavity and slowly exhaling from the mouth in a controlled and steady manner. You are going to continue this cycle like a bio-feedback pattern, back and forth, back and forth.

You will notice a lot of energy begin to move. The key is to focus entirely on your breathing cycle and allow the body to circulate the stagnated energetic knots that have built up in different regions of the body. You may notice tension or resistance in the solar plexus region. This is where the sensation of fear animates itself in the form of contraction or resistance to moving forward. Ironically, this is also the region where courage and excitement reside but buried underneath the density of fear we have not dealt with. So, keep breathing from the belly into the heart and allow the chest to open up, as if you are handing off the resistance in the body to the heart so it can dissolve it for you. Throughout this process you are increasing blood oxygen supplies to all of your muscles and to the brain. This will only increase the healing potential of the body and assist in increasing your overall bodily energy.

The next aspect of this practice is to begin reprogramming the cellular information database of the body through instructing your body on how you want it to feel. Yes, how YOU want your body to feel! All states of emotional consistency are really just programmed rehearsed states we adapt too over time. Stress is one of those rehearsed and repeated states. You have the power to exit out of that repetitive loop but it's going to take some work. So, as you are breathing begin to tell your body how you want it to feel.

For example, in your mind, ask yourself:

How does it feel in my body to feel confident?
How does it feel in my body to feel healthy?
How does it feel in my body to feel powerful?
How does it feel in my body to feel pain free?
How does it feel in my body to feel supported?
How does it feel in my body to feel inspired?
How does it feel in my body to feel successful?

And on and on you can go with this practice. There is literally no limit and no end to how far you can take this. The only thing you need to be aware of is the tendency for the mind to raise a skeptical brow to this process and try to talk you out of FEELING. The solution to this is to observe the thought but give it no energy. Simply keep breathing hand to hand, belly to heart and back and forth until the resistance subsides. And it will subside, it always does.

You can also perform this practice with a guided meditation you enjoy in the background. Dr. Joe Dispenza has some excellent guided meditations. I have also created a series of guided meditations that are specifically oriented towards the Quantum Collapse Process you can access and have fun with.

Purpose | Goals | Vision

"Where there is no vision, there is no hope"

George Washington Carver

It has been said that the quickest path from one point to another is a straight line. This is actually a strongly held scientific belief based on the theory of relativity and the idea that information travels at the speed of light. Without going deep down that rabbit hole what I can say about the basic assertion is that it is only partial true. Yes, when we are thinking about an incremental progression towards an outcome, logically it makes sense to say it is a straight line from here to there. However, that framework of thinking only allows for straight lines and a bit of a reductionistic model of reality which in my experience, is not a lot of fun, and does not allude to what our true potential as human beings really is.

The quickest way from here to there is actually not just to move in that direction. It is actually to assume the future outcome in this moment, exactly where you are and not postpone it for a later date. This is where the fancy mess of goal setting comes to mind. Set a goal, get a goal. Don't set a goal, don't get a goal. Sounds nice but really has no depth or meaning to it. This will be unpacked to its core in the section below. It is not necessary to wait for a time in the future to be anything, do anything, or experience anything. Let me go deeper on this one.

We could take the example of electricity and magnetism. We live in a world where people have been entrained into the science and understanding of electricity. In fact, a huge part of our world view is influenced by the idea of electrical phenomenon that is completely excluded or simply does not understand the most powerful force which is magnetism. Health is based on magnetism. Aging is based on electricity. We live in a very masculine dominated world view. We are missing out on the embodied harmonious whole of feminine wisdom. Electricity is masculine. Magnetism is feminine. As two complimentary opposites they seek attraction and want to parabond to birth a more powerful amplifier field called electromagnetism. This is where all of the energy or information in the quantum field (emotions, thoughts) self-organize, feed off each other, and amplify into any physical territory the energy generators are in.

When I say energy generators, I mean to say the people themselves. We are designed as a free energy generating technology i.e., the human body. The energy we experience, cultivate, direct, and pulsate emanates from us and reverberates far beyond our measurable devices can detect. So, when I say we have been made to think in only electrical terms, I mean to say we have been conditioned to become left brain dominant and to live mostly in our analytical minds. The right hemisphere of the brain is magnetic in nature and contains the vast amount of stored information that the left brain is constantly trying to filter or decode. The left brain requires far more rest, sleep, and time off than the right brain does. Electricity is not a self-renewable energy source. The right brain is completely self-renewable and seems to have no limits to how much energy it can produce.

So, what exactly am I saying with all of this? What I am saying is that due to our upbringing in education, scientific half-truths, and world view of things we have been seriously disadvantaged in our understanding, well basically about everything. In order to fulfill what you are truly capable of, increase bodily vitality, increase clarity in your life, and accomplish the goals you have set for yourself you are going to need to operate on a brand-new level. Magnetism and electromagnetism are the fields of study we must engage ourselves in. After all that was the entirety of Nikola Tesla's work and he was likely, if not definitely, the single greatest scientist we have ever seen, and his technologies are incomparable to anything we have seen using other methods.

So let me complete this train of thought for you...

One way to go about this is the typical AA (Alcoholics Anonymous) route, which is to admit you have a drinking problem, come to aa meetings every week, get on support calls, oh! - and also repeat that you are an alcoholic, will always be an alcoholic, and the best you will ever do is to be a recovering alcoholic. It should be halfway obvious to see all the encoded messages of mediocrity, codependency, and victimhood symbolically placed into the subconscious of the recovering individual.

For the immense value this organization and others similar it has been to countless people what I would like to illuminate for everyone is that these methods are outdated, antiquated, and only serve the left-brain electrical reactivity of the ego identity complex. If our identity is that we are "a recovering anything" than that is all we can hope to be.

We need to engage the full utility of our brains here and this will include later on a discussion on brain wave states, head-heart coherence, and plant medicines as well. For this discussion's sake let's begin to shuffle up the deck of cards in our overactive minds and explore a new way of thinking. We need an entirely new deck of cards, with new messages, new symbolic illustrations, new intentions, and a renewed sense of possibility. This only happens for us when we begin to exercise the right regions of the brain and go from electrical impulses to magnetic fields. A magnetic field encompasses everything within it. Our earth plane is held together by way of an 8 shaped toroidal magnetic field and it is fully sourced by the complimentary elements that also fully source our own magnetic field (earth, air, sun, water, minerals, photons).

In order to move much quicker from point a to point b than traveling incrementally on a straight line we move begin to move instantaneously. This happens from holding your electric charge at point i.e., where you are/who you are and generating a magnetic field that crosses the distance of space and time all the way over to point b. This is called exponential growth and expansion. The prior approach is called incremental growth or slow expansion. Another phenomenon you are likely familiar with is contraction and expansion. Cold contracts, heat expands. Lifting weights creates contraction, letting go of the weights allows for expansion. Sitting with the urge to perform a taboo habit is contractive, releasing the urge all together is expansive. We must learn to expand by also learning to be with the tension of contraction.

If you want to achieve something in life you can work incrementally and contract yourself towards it and this may or may not end up panning out for you long term. It takes such a long and arduous road to get there that you may not have the energy to hold the electrical charge (tension/will power) once you get there and as we see with so many people, once they get what they want, they end up losing it, abandoning it, or completely sabotaging it because they are now running on empty. Again, Magnetism never runs out of charge because it creates the 'field effect' and pairs up with other elements within its proximity that continue to source its expansive nature. We need to begin adhering more into our magnetic and electromagnetic capabilities because inertia/stagnation blocks the flow of life force and momentum carries the flow of life-force forward.

"The essential element in personal magnetism is a consuming sincerity - an overwhelming faith in the importance of the work one has to do."

Bruce Barton

When we begin to instill a more heart felt purpose in our lives, we begin to broaden the electromagnetic field (aura/bio-field) and all of a sudden, the things that come into our lives are based on another principle called resonance and dissonance. Resonance is the feeling when the body perks up, something lights up inside, the aha moment arrives, or we simply feel the truth in our gut i.e., a gut instinct/guttural intelligence. Dissonance is the counter opposite which is when someone, something, somewhere does not feel right or feel correct or does not sit right with you. The ego identity tends to overlook this principle and simply proceed based on facts, probabilities, statistics, and security. How many times have you made a decision to move forward with something even though you felt in your gut it was the wrong move, but your mind convinced you otherwise? How about any times where you felt excited and naturally motivated towards something but either your mind or someone else (which is still in your mind) warned you not to go that route, said how unsafe or unreliable it was, and you chose to heed that cautionary advice only to discover it was the right move or the opportunity become a big success with you?

The master key to this philosophical lock is to simply become the person that exists all the way over there on point b. If you were gifted with vision and foresight to see who you can become, that means it exists, **you are right now.** At this exact moment! This is where faith comes into play. Faith is the unseen but seen from within; it's the acorn seed that wants to grow into a massive acorn tree, figuratively speaking (and literally). We do not get to electromagnetic proportions by playing on the sidelines, worrying about the future, indulging in the past, and not even by taking all out massive action. We get there by stabilizing our own energy, in this exact present moment, and exercising our ability to stretch ourselves, in whatever way is required, in order to catalyze an internal shift that allows for the future to become a present state experience. We need to bridge the future into the present moment and relax our nervous system, layer by layer, to begin accepting the updated informational instructions based on who we are becoming, no longer only being informed by who we have been.

In practical terms, we have to have a vision of our future, who we must become in order to live into that vision and develop ourselves in service of that future. We have to develop new skill sets and we may associate that as setting new goals. We have to be powerfully moved by a motivational force and we may associate that as purpose. We also must develop an inner clarity of productive imagination and we may associate that as having vision. These three components working together in unison create the electromagnetic charge in this equation and our ability to hold this charge via a fully optimized vital body creates the inevitable future. In simple terms, you must exercise purpose, direction/goals, and vision along with investing in quality nutrition, organic chemical-free supplements, living spring water, movement, time in nature, and restorative sleep.

Now, with all of that out of the way let's move onto the next part of this journey.

"If you want to understand the universe think in terms of energy, frequency, and vibration."

Nikola Tesla

102

Purpose

"People take different roads seeking fulfillment and happiness. Just because they're not on your road doesn't mean they've gotten lost."

Dalai Lama

In all of my years doing the work I do, the biggest concern I hear from people, whether they say it or not, is they feel a total lack of purpose in life. The conversations take all different forms, and the nature of these conversations is very diverse and unique. For ten years my primary focus professionally was on the fields of living foods nutrition, detoxification and cleansing, and whole-body optimization. I've talked to thousands of people during my country wide speaking tours, international health retreats, hundreds of client work, hundreds of students through my online courses, and countless others from listening to my worldwide podcast show.

Using health as the best example, people experience a wide range of issues and some much more severe and specific cases of health abnormalities. In all of these years I have observed a very interesting pattern that has arisen from seeing a bifurcation between the people who tend to heal and get better and the people who tend to get a little better or much worse. This was an enigma within the logic of my nutritional understanding because it seemed obvious that if people just did the protocols that work for others in similar situation then they should heal just the same. I was operating from a type of perspective I had picked up in my entrepreneurial development, which was if you want success, find someone who had done it before, do exactly what they did, and you will get the same results.

Well, my friend, I am here to share with you my report of findings from thinking that way. It not only proved to not be true or totally accurate, it proved to be dangerous in some respect due to the fact that each human being is totally unique. We say this or we hear this kind of thing, but it had taken me many years to fully comprehend its complete meaning. The reason some people succeed, whether health, business, athletics, or any other pursuits, and a vast majority of others simply do not succeed, or the road to success seems to be much harder and filled with frequent obstacles, is actually simple. Simple but sophisticated in depth. By simplifying what is truly sophisticated and multi-factorial we have boxed ourselves into belief systems, binary black and white thinking, and have lost the very thing that is responsible for all healing; expanded perspective.

You see, it's never the problem itself that is the problem. It's our attitude about the problem that is really a problem. The people who I observed getting the results of the work had a great attitude about the work itself. They were positive, forward thinking, humble, and even some grateful for the challenges they were overcoming. The one's that do not do well tend to be pessimistic, backwards thinking, unwilling to let go of resentment and bitterness, and in some cases were using their dysfunction as a way to garner more attention from care takers, therefore what they really needed was love but enabled their situation as a way to stay stuck. In other words, they did not have a true conviction to heal, let alone any real intention to heal or advance themselves in their lives.

So then, what exactly heals us after all? What about prescription medications? Psychiatric medications? Do pharmaceutical drugs really help me or just harm me? Does my dental history or mercury amalgams have anything to do with this? Am I supposed to be vegan, vegetarian, pescatarian, omnivore, or even a carnivore? Do I need a hair mineral analysis to see if my copper levels are too high? Am I missing that one tiny nutrient at the bottom of Mendeleev's periodic table of the elements? Sigh…. I think you are starting to catch my point. Let's continue...

Without going any deeper into the nature of these questions (and they are valid ones!) I want to really drive this section of the book home for you. Remember, towards the end of this book is a fully detailed blueprint for dialing in the chemistry set of the human body, supplementation, dietary information, and effortlessly releasing the chemical assault of the damaged cells in order to restore optimal physiology and vitality. Moving forward, the big distinction between all of these people is one fundamental game changer and that attribute is calling having a purpose.

Purpose is everything. Faith in action is what creates miracles. Faith is a by-product from the spirit that comes online when we have another ingredient in the mix and that is called courage. Courage is the ability to see something for what it is, arrest all doubt in the moment, and powerfully (or even wearily) move forward. In fact, without fear there is no need or possibility for courage to arise. In the next chapter we will be diving very deep and in-depth into the nature of fear and how it plays a crucial role in the retainment of addicts worldwide. That is no longer an issue for you though, you've already demonstrated heroic qualities by receiving this book, opening its pages, and following along on this journey together. You are already healed! Your body and mind are just catching up because the body exists within time and space which means there is a bit of a lag time. More on that also, later.

What is purpose anyways? There is so much talk about living a purposeful life. Being on purpose! Or how about this one; FIND YOUR PURPOSE! Tell me if I am wrong, but is that not the most commonly used phrase in all of self-help, personal development, spiritual growth books, seminar talks, new age publications and snow-flakey millennial influencers on the internet? I do not know about you but for me personally I have never, ever, found this notion of needing to go find my purpose helpful, not in the least. In fact, as you may have found for yourself this only pushes more distance between myself and my purpose than brings me closer in alignment with it.

Now, grant you, there is much benefit in internalizing this question, meditating on it, feeling our way through ourselves with this in mind. But there is one important nuance I think we should consider and that is what is my energetic association to that inquiry. Do I feel lack of purpose, lack of vitality, the absence of support or prosperity, or the absence of good health while I am asking the question? For some, and I have been there, this is the only starting point we have. This question may be the life raft your hanging onto and using it as a way to keep afloat until more help arrives. That too, is so powerful, so important, and so faithful. Even within that situation, you'll see upon closer investigation, carries the energetic of faith. Sometimes it's faith under fire but faith is holding it all together none the less.

Consider this though, if we are living our lives in a codependent manner meaning we voluntary depend on hand outs, more help than we need, emotional support, psychological stability, or financial survival than our faith is put to rest because we have become irreparably lazy, energetically stagnant, and in extreme cases physically immobilized due to this way of living. I'll let you in on another secret to optimal physical health and unlimited vitality which also translates into accelerated longevity, without drugs or interventions. Are you ready for this one? Because this is the truth and nothing but the truth... Read this very carefully.

The human avatar technology that we call a body is fully capable, self-reliable, and perfectly designed to heal itself, regenerate damaged skin cells, muscle cells, organ and glandular cells, immune cells, nerve cells, brain cells, heart cells, and red blood cells with little to no external interventions necessary. This is a very deep truth and one that does not monetarily support institutionalized medicine or the big agricultural cartels because they depend on you to be sick, addicted, dependent on them, and in a moderate to low level of energy. Again, more on this in detail towards the end of the book but the point must be made and sometimes repeated here. Your body is not solely dependent on nutrients for its optimal function, first and foremost the human technology is powered on by an electromagnetic force which is the human soul.

The soul interwoven into the physical body is what powers it on each morning, carries it through our every day, and also down regulating the mind softens the energy output, and while the soul attends to the dream realm, the physical body is able to go offline and begin all of its incalculable processes for healing and restoration. This is the fundamental truth of our body's innate intelligence and also the distillation of all the greatest work on the subject.

So, why am I telling you this in a conversation about purpose? Perhaps it may feel like I am going on a tangent or two, but I assure you this is a coherent stream of consciousness leading to the deeper meaning of this topic. So, when you begin to sense the energetics of your body after you take a good few deep breath, what do you feel? When you place your hand on your heart and breath into it, what happens for you? If I am to guess you begin to become intimately aware of your body and the present moment it is resting into.

The quest to discover our life's greatest purpose is a fool's errand. It is an impossible venture into a windy road of the mind that eventually leads us right back to where we started. In the here and now. Wherever we go, there we are. So then, our truest of purposes is always in this exact moment. It is never far off into the future and it certainly cannot be found and excavated from the artifacts of the past. Sometimes our only purpose is to breath. To take a deep breath and place our hands onto our heart. Sometimes the greatest purpose is simply to pray.

In order to make our way towards addiction recovery and aligned with the process of healing we have to allow the mind-body complex to settle into the felt experience of life. When we avoid feeling our own experience, we blunt out sensations that would otherwise guide us to our next destined moment. We can easily lose touch with the purpose that is for us right here. By not being present and anchored into the flow of life, we can easily miss out on incredible opportunities that other people seem to "attract" easily and effortlessly. Did they attract those things because they were special or perhaps it was simply, they were ready for it when it came?

If you're reading this book and on such a quest seeking more meaning and purpose, I want to let you know exactly what that is. Your only purpose right now is to heal yourself. To be good and kind to yourself. To take an honest inventory of your life, your relationships, your finances, your occupation, and then begin listing out the habits or patterns that are unnecessarily getting in the way from your ideal vision. And soon we will dive deeper into vision because purpose is like the inextinguishable fire that holds steady, burns bright, and powers on the body at peak capacity. The next step is to direct that energy like a laser beam that is insulated and properly directed by achievable goals. All of the benefits and results we are able to manifest for ourselves and the energy it will require to make dreams come true is led by the boldness of our vision.

Goals

"The major reason for setting a goal is for what it makes
of you to accomplish it. What it makes of you will always
be the far greater value than what you get."

Jim Rohn

In the wide world of goal setting there are a lot of ideas and approaches on what is best practices are for achieving our objectives. I do not dismiss anything in this regard because they all have merit and have worked for many people over the broader landscape of human experience. As described above, however is a simple perspective shift that I believe is a bit more important than the tactics and strategies themselves. We have also heard a lot in recent decades about attracting our goals, attuning our personal vibration as a tuning fork and allowing our goals to come to us. This is a very useful idea but can only take real effect when we have the complete formula understood and that brings us back to electromagnetism.

Let's revisit this concept for a moment. Electricity acts as an outward force when it is directed or executed. It is a non-renewable force of energy that requires a conductive circuit via a fuse board, for example, to run the engine (produce energy) and this requires a battery in order to power the circuit board, otherwise there is no sourcing of power for it to operate. So, think about this for a moment. Electricity requires a battery in order to power it on. Well, let's take our bodies for example. We have battery packs within us that allow for this process to happen. We can think of our adrenal glands as battery packs, and we may even think of our cells as water filled conducers of energy via the mitochondrial energy production transport chain. As long as the holistic system is operating in relative functionality than the electrical energy is sourced and sustained but here is where the problem begins.

In the cases of when a human being has abused their body through way of recreational drugs, processed foods, contaminated water, lack of mobility, lack of sun exposure, pharmaceutical drugs, alcohol, and all the rest, the voltage meter on the battery pack is likely at a very low point and does not have the full capacity to hold a strong enough electrical charge to allow for the actions, strategies, and tactics of goal setting to be executed. If our physical body is out of order than our mind will be out of order, and thus our ability to focus on setting goals, think through our goals, and execute upon our goals will only lead to further exhaustion and burn out. This is my main concern when it comes to the general conversation of goal setting and relying on a certain strategy or plan to get us from point a to b.

If someone is recovering from addiction than their main goal should be to fully recover which really means to uncover the source of trauma within themselves in order to recover the soulful pulse that exists below the surface. I have seen all too many times in the self-help world seas and seas of people flocking to seminars, workshops, and conferences in pursuit of getting another step closer to their proposed goals. There is a less than 3% success statistic in even the highest attended personal development seminars of people who actually change their lives and what happens to the other 97%? They fall back into the default program response patterning of their core wounds and unhealed traumas, to put it bluntly. The event made them feel good, because it does feel good to be around possibility minded people and to envelop ourselves in a highly charged co-created atmosphere for a weekend. There is an electromagnetic field effect that takes place at events but when we come back home that field effect begins to lose its charge and why is that?

Again, because our personal battery pack did not have the juice to hold that energy on our own. When we were in that shared experience it was much easier to feel carried by the magnetic pulse of highly organized energy. In fact, which is the role of any good event producer is to create organization of highly charged energy, such as a magnetic field and when the electricity of the audience pulses, we then have a full-blown electromagnetic phenomenon take place among hundreds or thousands of human beings. Everyone is providing their own battery packs to the party and it's being amplified by the event itself. But notice this, how many times have you felt the highest of the highs at events but began to feel a bit drained, wired, and exhausted at the end of it or shortly after the event had concluded. Sit with this for a moment if you will.

What I am attempting to explain to you is that in order for us to even get to a place where we can effectively set goals for ourselves, we have to evaluate how much juice is running in the system at any given moment. Just like we check our oil, our fuse box in the car, or monitor our gas tank. We have to do this same thing with our own bodies. Think about those times at those seminars and all of the amazing ideas you had, all of the inspirational beliefs, the new possibilities you felt and saw for yourself. Those were all very real and within grasp and still are by the way. But why is it after these events or even after a really vivid dream we have a hard time recapturing the clarity of that moment and where did all the motivation dissipate too? It is also based on energetics within the moment, and you can still recapture all of those novel ideas and possibilities but it's going to require changing your external environment in order to do so.

When you think about setting goals it's important to consider multiple types of goals. Think of it this way. You have outcome goals which are specific outcomes you want to achieve, and they have a certain timeline defined. Ok great! For example, writing this book there is a clear outcome which is to have it completed, edited, proofread, and in the publishing process at X date. We always allow space for life to happen though because as the famous saying goes life is what happens when your busy making plans. But that is a clear outcome goal. The outcome goals are very specific, direct, and should not require very much of your time once established. The other goal and most important is process goals which are not based on outcomes but focused on the process required towards the outcome. This is where most people fail to hit their mark or even know what that mark is because they are so focused on the bullseye way over there, that they lose sight of the process required to get there. This is where goal setting begins to become fun again and REAL!

So, now that we have a bit more of a basic working model let's tie it all together. Outcome goals are electricity or electrical waves seeking a touch point. In the Taoist medicine arts, they would liken this to 'Yang' which is the counter force to 'Yin'. Yang is a strong force which is direct and full of highly charged energy that can externalize itself naturally. Yin is a weaker force (not to be confused as weak or feeble) that is soft in nature and circulates life force throughout the body, nature, and the planet as a whole. Yin in other words could be accurately acquitted to the magnetic field that holds all else together. That is a profound thing to investigate for yourself and I have written extensively on this topic in prior books and online content. So, pulling this all together now begin to envision the outcome goals as electricity and the process goals as magnetism. Once we pair these two forces of creation together, we end up with electromagnetism and thus are ready to hold the electrified charge, create inner stability in order to stabilize the magnetic pulse(feelings/emotions), and execute from an inner resolve that is both fully surrendered and also fully capable of taking massive action.

Now, I know this all sounds like incredible philosophy sprinkled in with physics, Taoism, and some practical insights as well. The distillation point of this section is actually incredibly simple and clear. In order to maximize your goal setting potential, we need to have outcome goals and process goals. That part is stupid simple, which is why I am not giving that more focus than it needs right now. What is not simple though is the human condition and all of the inner workings that we all experience on our way from point a to point b, but we will make it simple and chart a new innovative path using these quantum principles. Let's keep going here.

The outcome may be to be fully recovered, in a harmonious love relationship, financially stable, and experiencing a body of incredible health. Now, what is the process to get there. Well, here's the trick, there is nowhere to get too actually. I can hear you already, here we go again, Ronnie's talking in parables and circles. Well, that is kind of by design because I really want you to exercise your innate faculties of critical thinking but trust me, this is going somewhere. The truth of the matter is there is nowhere to go as in setting a goal to get somewhere, to be something, to acquire something. Remember us talking about those seas of people going to seminars and never getting the results they came for? Remember, the 3% who were successful? What is the difference. The distinction here is that the 3% already were "it" ahead of time and that is what gave them the ability to make greater advancements in their progress.

Where this entire mental exercise is leading us is to the understanding that it's not who we think we are that is the problem but in truth it is who we think we are not that hurts us. Those 97% really do not know who they are, what they stand for, and in truth, and are not fully grounded in their bodies which means they are easily distracted, swayed by other's opinions, and are energetically unorganized within themselves. Now, this is not a judgement on anybody, I feel great sensitivity right here, but it is the honest truth. The majority of human beings walking this planet do not know who they are, what they really want, and are mentally fantasizing about who they could be instead of relishing in the fact of who they actually are. People project their unfulfilled desires and dreams onto externalized figures in our popular culture like a holographic movie screen and vicariously experience the sensations of a movie but are not themselves living in their own movie.

You want to ask me where true motivation, deep conviction, and an inexhaustible wellspring of energy comes from? It comes from being totally grounded in our own lives, taking absolute care of our physical bodies, stilling the mind through meditation, moving the body in a range of different ways, connecting our empathy receptors with the heart cells of other humans, making time to unplug from technology and plug in with the internet of nature, and to discover what is truly meaningful to our lives and what we are willing to lay our life on the line for. Once we know this inside of ourselves, we will then know exactly what we want to achieve and the process towards it will be fully supported via our own electromagnetic field effect that we create upon the force of inspirational nature our creator designed us to be. You cannot manufacture motivation or inspiration. It must be self-generated and if that is not the case then there are blockages and obstructions damping up the flow of energy. We cannot move forward until that flow is set free.

The way we set the flow of electrical current free (energy currency) is to focus almost exclusively on the process i.e., the moment-by-moment journey. In recovery of addiction that is the goal, and the process goal supersedes the outcome goal because the outcome itself will manifest as a result of sticking with the process. This is really the whole secret to achieving anything in life. Stick with the process, stay on the path, keep improving upon yourself, celebrate your successes, and keep on the journey. The results i.e., the outcome is never what we are after. Because after that then what? It's an illusion of the anxious mind trying to hold onto certainty. The only certainty is the process and who you become as a result of the process itself.

"A goal is not always meant to be reached; it often serves simply as something to aim at."

Bruce Lee

We need things to aim for in life, it helps keep our feet on the ground, and our vision allows for our consciousness to soar freely in the heavens. This is the unison of electromagnetism or the parabonding of the unstable and stable forces of our universe. We have all of these forces within us. We are an immaculate reflection of the physics and geometry of our world itself. When we learn to harness our own energy and stabilize it as we discussed in the previous chapter on dopamine, we become something extraordinary in a world that has succumbed to the common denominator of mediocrity. Someone who is able to hold themselves accountable, remain steadfast in their recovery, and who has actually freed themselves from the tentacles of addiction is so incredibly rare that it beckons us to pursue it with all of our energy and focus. But we do not chase it outside of us. We simply become it, right here, right now. We stabilize our urges, center our thoughts, and make one good decision after another and all of a sudden you discover that you are, in fact, recovered.

It all comes down to practice. Practice the process with the end outcome in mind. But stay focused on the process itself. This is how championship athletes are forged. This is how people pull themselves from the grips of despair and tragedy. This is how transformation happens. Who you become in pursuit of the outcome is really what you came for. Once you achieve your goal you will have already become a person who no longer needs that goal. You will then go on to set new milestones and repeat the same process.

Who you become is and has always been the goal itself. We simply got confused and complacent with the comfort zone trap our society has engineered for us and we rarely had to activate our primal instincts. We change all of that now. And with the power of this moment and the journey we have been traversing through it is time to integrate the final piece of this geometric puzzle, The Vision.

Vision

"We are pushed by pain until we are pulled by a vision."

Michael Bernard Beckwith

As we progress from the topics of purpose and goal setting, we now enter into the most important component that aligns it all together which is cultivating a powerful vision for our lives. In all of my pursuits, whether athletically or otherwise, the common denominator to any of my success has always been found in the clarity and profundity of my personal vision. In the same regard, the source of all of my shortcomings and failures have also been linked to the lack of vision as well. I have found this to be the single determining factor in whether somebody accomplishes their goals or not. It is also the determining factor in whether someone overcomes their addictive patterns or not. If we are simply chasing goals for the goal's sake, we will always fall short, even if we someone stumble upon our goals it will be without true fulfillment or longevity.

In the quote above Michael Beckwith presents a very important idea for us to meditate on. In life the common tendency is to be pushed by discomfort and pain. We can easily find ourselves getting caught up in familiar comfort zones and these comfort zones are a very dangerous trap. A comfort zone is the familiar territory we habituate into and what is so insidious about it is that it sneaks up on us, sometimes without us realizing it. It really is the illusion of comfort which can easily become complacency and stagnation. This is basically what all addiction patterns are; a comfortable situation that we adhere too but slowly and surely it weakens our resolve and stagnates our will power. The longer we sit in this comfort trap the harder it is to break out of it but break out of it we must, otherwise there is no possibility for growth and expansion to occur.

Just like in traditional goal setting we become entrained into incremental progress and when we are in this comfort zone abyss, we have to muster up a tremendous degree of will power in order to do simple actions to make incremental progress. This process is a painful one and in the withdrawal phase of any major habit change or life transition the pain is sometimes unavoidable. However, there is a way to transcend the painful pattern of pushing through the static field or stagnant energy in order to make a full recovery (whatever that means for you). If we are living in a daily experiential state of tension, anxiousness, and pain, then there is a monumental amount of life force that is not being made available to us. The painful process of incremental progress really comes down to our motivational impulse; are we motivated by pain or are we motivated by inspiration. Pain is like trudging up a muddy hill, slipping and falling back down, gripping our fingers in the dirt, and willing ourselves back up, only to get a bit further along than we were before but expending a significant amount of energy every time.

I know this pattern all too well, I have lived it for most of my life, and when it no longer felt good for me, I experienced years of continual challenges and suffered from bouts of terminal frustration. This is no way to live a life of purpose, in fact, truth be told, it is a sure-fire way to erode our purpose and diminish the spark of enthusiasm that we must protect and maintain, always. Instead of willing ourselves each step of the way, why don't we simply let go of the weights we are carrying i.e., the mental overload, the resentments, judgements, expectations, and disappointments of our prior short comings? What makes life so challenging is not the challenges themselves but feeling an inability to effectively handle what life has given us and before we know it the pressure stacks up on our shoulders until we can no longer bear the weight of our own frustration. So, then what allows us to release the pressure and weight? It is simple and clear; developing the visionary qualities that we were gifted with in this life.

When we are pulled by a vision as opposed to being pushed by pain our life becomes easier. It does not mean life is easy, it means life becomes easier. Bruce Lee told us all "do not pray for an easy life. Pray for the strength to endure a difficult one." If you are sincerely reading this book for the purposes imbedded in the title and the content as a whole, I am willing to bet you are a very strong person. Despite what people may have told you about those who struggle with addictions being weak, unmotivated, and lazy the real truth is you are one of the strongest people on the planet. For the simple fact that you are likely, like myself, have been in a struggle for most of your life or certainly a good deal of it anyways. The struggle creates immense depths of strength, discipline, and heroic

115

attributes, do not let anyone else tell you different! You are strong beyond comprehension and the fact that you have not succumbed to taking your own life, despite any suicidal ideations or fantasies you may have had, you are still here, and I urge you to acknowledge your strength right now!

Many of us, especially the men of this upside-down world, have had to be so incredibly strong our whole lives and likely received little to no acknowledgement for that. Now, knowing how incredible strong, discipline, and durable you really are you can begin to transition from having to be strong for survivals sake to being strengthened by an inexhaustible force that is based on compassion, equanimity, and love. Now, *wait a second,* you might be thinking to yourself. I really resonate with this, but you used a word I would never equate with myself which is discipline. Well, my friend, let me tell you something. You are far more disciplined than you realize. Think about it for a moment. How much discipline does it require to take on a new habit, rehearse that habit daily, multiple times a day, and carry it on for years beyond that? Now I know we do not usually think of addictive habits as a form of discipline but make no mistake, it does take discipline to carry out any habit, whether they are self-affirming or self-destructive. The only difference is in the level of presence, purpose, intention, and desired outcome we wish to receive from our disciplines.

This is where the magnetic power of inner vision comes into the equation. The only difference between a productive habit or unproductive habit is our level of awareness, our moment-by-moment presence, and whether it synchs up according to our vision or in most cases the lack of vision. I do not know anyone that is struggling with addiction that has a crystal clear, awe inspiring, and soul evoking vision for their life. Let me even say it this way, to the degree we do not have a powerful vision for our lives is the degree we will have self-destructive habits and addiction cycles in our lives. There it is! The master key insight to this whole discussion, right there for you. Vision is the space holder that allows for brilliance, beauty, magic, and miracles to naturally emerge in our life experience. When we refuse to craft a vision or even allow space for the vision to emerge within us, we will find other ways to fill in that space. The behavioral play book of childhood trauma is to fill in the empty spaces as quickly as they appear and with anything that would numb the pain. Most people are numbing themselves every day, at every opportunity they can, whether they realize it or not. And most people obviously do not know they are doing this, but this is what it is.

Where there is no vision, the people perish."

Proverbs 29:18

Let's bring together a few more elements of this overall discussion and tie together the symmetry of this entire chapter so we can begin to align our minds, hearts, and bodies using a holistic model towards recovery, rehabilitation, and reinvention of Self. I would like to bring up a concept called the wheel of samsara which is a Buddhist term used to describe the cycle of suffering that is built into the human condition and expands into reincarnation cycles i.e., birth and death, back to birth and death, and on and on it goes. The Buddhists have a famous saying which is: *life is suffering*. At first glance this seems like a pretty somber, melancholic, and depressing insight to receive. This is only true in the way that the human race has been entrained and indoctrinated throughout thousands of years of control, slavery, miseducation, and cultural misappropriation. We suffer because we do not know ourselves and we do not know ourselves because we do not know where we come from. We do not know where we come from because we have been dislocated from our source. We are disconnected from our source because we likely feel abandoned by our mother or father (literal or proverbial). And we feel abandoned by the mother (mother earth) and the father (heavenly father) because we do not know ourselves truly. What just happened there? That is a cyclical pattern of human conditioning that has played itself out throughout the ages and all the way back into our personalized experience of life.

So, the first key here to developing greater vision for our life is to get off of the wheel of samsara all together. In order to do this, we must go through a series of internal revolutions and the biggest one is to retrain our minds to operate outside of linear time and space and into the timelessness of what is known as the zero point or singularity point. The singularity point is a collapsing of all timelines, past, present, and future, into the sacred now point. This is where the forces of electricity and magnetism meet in synchrony and become electromagnetic wave fields.

117

Another way of saying this is this is how we create free energy generating technology and your human instrument i.e., your body is the most advanced Tesla modeled technology in all of existence. Rudolph Steiner, the great mystic and visionary, said that all external technology is an attempt to mimic what the human technology already does perfectly. Sit with that for a minute or two!

Let's touch on this birth and death cycle now. In the concept of chronological aging, it is a straight line from birth to death, from youth to elder, from timelessness to time, from cellular regeneration to cellular atrophy, and for some from unbridled magic to anticipated misery. This is the proposed timeline of the human experience we have all been brought up with and become accustomed too. It's a rapid ascension to descension, acceleration of life to deceleration of life. Our world view model is heavily based on the idea of entropy which is a scientific term that states that everything is subject to decay, deconstruction, disorder, and chaos. Well, there is a counter principle to entropy called negentropy which reverses entropy from chaos back into order, stability, structure, and geometric symmetry or simply put, back into greater organization. When our life force energy is in a state of entropy i.e., chaotic and scattered we are in an accelerating aging cycle. When our energy is in a state of negentropy i.e., order and organization we decelerate the aging cycle. This explains the counter principle to chronological aging which is biological aging. We do not have control of our chronological sequence of events, but we do have complete creative input into the biological factors which involves harnessing the power of our mind, our bodily health, and using our spiritual faculties to live our lives pulled by a vision.

You see, entropy happens when we are pushing through life, burdened by stress, frustrated with ourselves, or feeling powerless. The gravitational pressure placed upon us when we are living in an inner atmosphere of entropy is what actually ages us and locks us into linear time and space. This all comes about from living without a vision. Our inner vision enacts the magnetic pulse within our central core and once it is activated life begins to pull us higher instead of gravity weighing us down. The weight of linear and literal thinking is where we can get tangled up in the mine field of the reactive mind. This comes by way of placing far too much emphasis on the left brain and trying to navigate life from our head. We can easily find ourselves living from the neck up and lose all touch with the feedback intelligence of our body. Our purpose lives in our body. Our vision resides and comes alive from within the body. Left brain dominance is the most common condition I would use to diagnose the problems of this world and those who suffer the most. If we live neck up instead of neck down, we will find ourselves trying to solve problems in life with our mind when, in fact, our problems likely were caused or influenced by thinking too much. And every time we repeat this behavior we stumble up against the same truth; that we find ourselves exactly where we started. Wherever we go, there we are.

The left hemisphere of the brain accounts for at most 10% of the overall cognitive capacity and energy bandwidth of the brain. When they say we only use 10% of our overall brain power they are right and wrong. We actually use 100% of our overall brain capacity, functionally speaking, because the entire neo-cortex and various regions of the brain all turn on. It would be impossible, except in rare instances, for certain regions to be completely inert or not functioning. The truth is that we only access, at any given time, a fraction of the overall potential that is readily available. The secret to accessing our greater mental capabilities is by shifting energy and blood flow over into the right hemisphere of the brain. This is the source point for all of our creative genius, inspired insights, past life memories, and telepathy (Yes! You are telepathic!).

Here is what we first must understand about the right hemisphere and why it is so hard to adjust brain wave states. The right region of the brain houses all of the individual trauma's you've experienced in this lifetime, the ancestral traumas of your blood lineage via epigenetic transference, as well as all of your past life traumas. Yes, past lives are very real, and Dr. Ian Stevenson is the world's leading scientific authority on the subject. This helps explain why we have our own unique quirks, a spectrum of sub-personalities, and why some habits come naturally, or some addictions feel so natural despite the issues it may cause. The left brain is where our ego identity is housed, and the primary function of an undeveloped ego is to protect itself from threats or identity dissolution. Again, our right brain is where the stored trauma is held and as a way to preserve itself from perceived threats the left brain begins to overpower the right brain impulses. This is when we find ourselves in states of frustration, battling ourselves, feeling stuck, boxed in, or trapped. We cannot outthink our own mind. It knows everything about us, everything

119

we ignore, put off to the side, how we lie or negotiate with ourselves, and it also knows how to stimulate pleasure just as it does for stimulating pain.

Now it may sound as if I am saying that our left brain is inherently wrong or bad for us. Not exactly, what I am saying is that we have relied upon an aspect of our brain for solving life challenges but that is not what it is designed for, at all. In a way our biggest problem is simply we have become well-adjusted to a mismanagement of our imagination and creativity. The left brain only constitutes 10% of our overall cognitive functions because that is all it requires to fulfill its role. The ego is brilliant, beautiful, and is the distinction point between me and you, him and her, this and that, the one and the other. Contrast is built into the duality of our human experience in these bodies in this 3rd dimensional physical realm. It's all good but we simply need to understand it's role, how it best serves us, and how to set ourselves free from it. Once we let go of the need to protect ourselves from anything, anybody, or especially from ourselves then blood flow begins to circulate towards the right. Take 5 deep diaphragmatic breaths, hold for 5 seconds at the inhale, and slowly let out a big sigh of relief.

The left brain operates much like an electric circuit. Electricity is a transverse temporal wave meaning that it's potential is temporary and has a finite energy resource. The right brain operates under the principles of magnetism which is what allows for the genius of a Nikola Tesla, Rudolph Steiner, Walter Russell, and all the rest. They do not operate within time or space or go to sleep like a 'normal' person. They live outside of chronological time which causes them to live beyond gravity and thus their vitality is on a continual feedback loop with the divine. In other words, they are being magnetically pulled forward based on the resonance of their vision. In order to transcend left brain dominance, the first step is to begin feeling into a deeper and more profound vision of yourself. What do you really know about yourself? Underneath all of the density and degree of past life experiences, what can you find that is totally unique and special about you? Do you even know how special and unique you actually are?

The way to tap into your own inner magnetism is to first sit with yourself. Sit alone, quiet, and practice some rhythmic breathing as you begin to feel yourself more. As you feel into the layers of resistance i.e., tangled up energy in the body you can place your hand on that spot and breath directly into it. You can do this with any physical stagnation or pulled muscles even. The key is to breath into it while also releasing any holding pattern you may have such in the case of a tight muscle or cramp. As your body adheres the relaxation, ease, and safety what will begin to arise within you will be more clarity, more awareness, more compassion, more truth, more healing, more of you. The stress and resistance are in some ways static electricity that are no longer flowing easily in the system, or have an obstruction such as scar tissue, calcification deposits, tight muscles/ligaments/tendons, or inflammation. When the body is in a red alert state such as the pain of systemic inflammation, the right brain hemisphere kicks out because we may have a stored trauma that we are not ready to experience. That could also be the source code for why our bodies are tightened up and out of balance, in fact, in my experience it likely is also the prognosis if we track it back long enough.

The unfoldment and emergence of our true vision will come to the surface as we resolve our traumas, resentments, and judgements about ourselves and about others. In the upcoming chapter on **Plant Medicines,** we will dive deep into the ultimate pharmacopeia and ancient wisdom on accelerating the recovery path where this will all come back into play. For now, consider something as it relates to our self-identity and living into a greater vision for ourselves. First of all, you must develop a vision for yourself in order to live into a visionary life. You are the common denominator in your life, and everything will always come back down to you. So, knowing what we don't want helps us to better know what we do want. Experiencing the wheel of samsara and wrestling with our demons/addictions develops of type of inner resourcefulness that shapes us into who we are. It can be viewed as an initiation from adolescence into adulthood and we have truly become an adult once we no longer are riding the cycle of addiction. Experiencing the struggle of addiction can bear witness to the birth of an aspiration to experience life without addictions. Who you were does not have to be who you become. Your past does not define your future. One thing indeed leads into another.

What I want to leave you with in this chapter is the gnosis (knowing) of your own true greatness and potential. Your addiction cycles, just as mine, have informed you on what you do not want and created the necessary contrast to clarify perfectly what you truly desire. Once we honor our desires, act on our inspirations, and devote ourselves to the realization of a worthy ideal we no longer live in the wheel of suffering. We no longer live within the repetition cycle of birth and death. We no longer fear death because we are no longer protecting ourselves from fully living. This is the breakout of the matrix code right here. When we can fully accept ourselves, exactly as we are. With pride in who we are and how far we have come. Then, and only then, will our vision emerge and unfold into the moment-by-moment experience of our lives.

Now, our journey takes us onto the next frontier which is exploring, exposing, and revealing one of the biggest hang-ups we all find ourselves in, when it comes to addictive tendencies and how our society has made a population of drug addicts, high functional addicts at that. Some of the most dangerous and unassuming detriments to our health and our lives are some of the most well accepted, legal substances most people never bat an eye twice at.

Let's do this!

Section 2

Deprogramming the Culture of Addiction

Now that we have begun to unpack the subtle and the not-so-subtle elements relating to addiction we are ready to move into the next phase. This phase is about putting the magnifying glass upon the cultural value and exchange system we have all been accustomed to operating within. We are going to take a closer look into the appropriation of addiction within our culture and how it has placed anyone struggling with recovery at a significant disadvantage. It is important to consider that the cycle of addiction may not be solely an indication that something is wrong about the individual but perhaps that something is potentially wrong with the environment the individual has been raised in.

As we have discussed in the prior segment, our environment plays the most impactful role in the activation or deactivation of our genetic potential. Our bio-physiology is directly affected by the surrounding stimulus that we are exposed too, each and every day. This includes all of the messages we receive through our digital devices from media sources and other forms of virtual entertainment. Our minds adapt to the information we take in and it absorbs itself into our psyche which influences our state of consciousness, as well as alters the chemistry and structure of our brains. Until we learn how to detach from the virtual simulation of reality i.e., our reliance on digital devices, we will have a hard time reengaging with the whole of our actual reality. This form of addiction is hard to spot and less often even addressed in many discussions of addiction.

Our cultural influences have created a generic template for living that has homogenized the majority of the population into a kind of false reality. This shows itself in our chosen lifestyle patterns and habituated daily activities. We have been taught to consume instead of creating and give instead of receiving. The overwhelming statistics on addictions of all kinds are not a reflection of organic human nature or some kind of defective flaw within humanity. These are startling reflecting of the conditioning of the human mind through our cultural influences that we have followed for guidance and have allowed to play out, up until this point now.

Let's move forward…

Culturally Accepted Drugs

*"It's not the drug that makes you a drug addict. It's the
need to escape reality."*

Unknown

We have been raised and enculturated within a society that favors
high octane work ethic, perpetual stimulation, and has a serious problem
admitting when it is wrong or going off course. There is a great deal we,
as a technological society, have been very wrong about and virtually
everything to do with addiction and/or the usage of "drugs" is one of
them. In a recent statistic it was shown that up to 23.5 million Americans
are addicted to alcohol and "drugs". I find the usage of the term 'drugs'
interesting as it does not specify exactly what these substances are nor
does it bother to make any useful distinctions, other than including
alcohol as one of the obvious substances in question. Aside from that, we
are left in the dark as to what drugs are a problem and what constitutes a
drug in a society that uses a variety of natural and unnatural plant
compounds to elicit drug like effects.

One thing that is for sure is that when we have a strong attachment to
a certain substance that we use every day, we do not want to question
whether it is good for us or not. We would prefer to just let it be and go
about our business as usual, especially if this substance in question is
perfectly legal, socially accepted, and many more people are doing it also.
It is important to say that the use of the term 'drugs' does not discern
whether something is legal, illegal, popular, or unpopular. There are
plenty of substances we consider drugs that are extremely popular, illegal,
and are relatively easy to gain access too. We also see an overwhelmingly
booming industry of substances that produce drug like stimulation that
are both popular, legal, and highly celebrated. So much so to the point that
there are entire chains of store front gatherings where people can partake
socially. We call these establishments coffee houses/cafes, "medical"
cannabis stores, and/or bars.

It should go without question that we live in a society i.e., socially organized world that seems obsessed with altered states. An altered state simply means to alter our state of mind which also indicates an alteration in how we feel, how we think, and how we experience our own reality. This desire to create an altered state is the burning fuel that drives our economic climate and has an influential factor in virtually every decision someone makes in their personal, professional, and even relational lives. In the book *Stealing Fire*, the authors Steven Cotler and Jaime Wheel coined the term "the altered states economy" which indicates that there is an entire economy based in and around experiencing altered states. People work for money, save up money, and engage in transactions of money in order to alter their consciousness. In most cases, this transaction of money that was earned over weeks to months (in some cases years!) is to experience a very temporary and finite experience that creates little to no benefit in one's overall life. Why would this be the case?

First off, we could discuss the concept of the altered states economy much more in-depth and in the book Stealing Fire the authors did an exceptional job outlining this idea. What I wish to say about it is more about drawing the readers awareness away from the concept itself and bringing it home to where it plays out in the day to day. So, why would someone (or an entire population) place such a monumental emphasis (whether they know it or not) on altering their state of mind and their consistent felt experience. The simple answer goes back to the previous chapter where we discussed the disconnect that occurs in addiction between our sense of purpose, vision, goals and our day-to-day experience. Of course, if we are living out a life that feels mundane, without purpose, or we feel chronic bodily pain it is only natural we would want to phase shift from our normal experience to an altered experience. There is nothing inherently wrong with altering our human experience, let me make that point clear. But if we do not understand the desire behind it then we easily and unavoidable fall into addiction cycles with it, no matter what the drug or access point of choice may be.

There are perfectly healthy and productive access points or triggers for creating altered states just as there are clearly unhealthy and unproductive means to alter our consciousness. Much of it has to do with what is called the "set and setting" which is more of a shamanic perspective involving psychedelic plant substances (see chapter **Plant**

Medicines). The set is the mindset or psychological state we are in prior and into the substance or access point for the alteration of consciousness or another way of saying this is the adjustment to our brain wave state. The mentality we go into an experience with generally determines the tonality of the experience and whether it is a "good" or "bad" experience. In the world of psychedelics, they would term this having a "good trip" or having a "bad trip". Well, it is entirely possible to drink a cup of coffee and also experience either a "good high" or a "bad trip" because, coffee after all, is a plant that contains alkaloid compounds that illicit very mild psychotropic effects. Sit with that one for a moment before you reach out for your morning coffee.

The setting is the physical environment we engage with a substance or access point. Outside of substances you may see a training gym as a setting to engage in working out as a healthy and productive trigger for an altered brain state, for example. There is a certain type of environmental setting that resonates and vibrates differently for different people which is associated with a particular type of experience. When we go out and socialize, we tend to lean towards a specific environment that also facilitates certain state change agents whether it be food, drink, smoke, music, or entertainment. When you go to the movie theatre the obvious agent is the movie itself but what about the concession stand that happily caters to the indulgences of people who are looking to have an altered experience, which generally means they check out of their bodies for 2 hours or so and become fully engrossed in the movie that is being projected in front of them. This all goes into the conventional altered states economy we live in and the biggest businesses that facilitate these experiences understand this to a science and layer on the major access point as well as sub-alteration agents to stimulate the temporal experience so that someone will keep coming back for me.

With this understanding in mind, it is important to consider that the mentality and the environment are key pieces in whether a state change agent is helpful or harmful. Once we get that down, the next thing to really consider is whether an agent, regardless of mindset or setting is helpful or harmful. This is really where the truth of an addiction reveals itself because in order to arrive at the pure and undiluted truth of a potential addiction it requires us to strip away the attraction that is brought on, largely by the setting itself. For example, I remember when I used to really enjoy going to a coffee house to do my computer work. The setting felt very attractive to me and because of my desire to be around other people and experience the immediate stimulation of that butter coffee (which was a bad idea, only 98% of the time) I allowed my set or mindset to become easily malleable in order to convince myself that it was a smart move to go there. Wait, stop there for a moment! Did you just catch what I just said? Because I had a desire to go to a particular environment/setting I allowed my mindset to become altered in service to acting out the idea in my head in order to fulfill a temporary urge but the idea in my head was completely contrary to the reality of the act itself (again, only 98% of the time!) Re-read that paragraph if you did not catch what was just said here!

Many times, we will alter our own state/mind in anticipation for a desired experience and will rationalize why it is actually good for us when in actuality we know it is not. This is a perfect representation of an addiction cycle playing itself out in the hopes of experiencing that one altered state that will set all wrongs right and allow us to get through one more day. What is actually happening in this example is I was avoiding the reality of the moment and using logical fallacies i.e., this will help me get more work done and it will be fun instead of just being honest and sincere that I needed to stop trying to sugar coat the fact that I had a problematic habit. My need to alter my consciousness was greater than my need to heal my addiction, in that moment, and in all moments, I continued to play this sneaky little game with myself. What I am describing to you is the inner workings of how all addiction plays itself out in the mind and how we will use an environmental factor as a way to induce compliancy with our addiction. This is the story of our socially agreed upon altered states economy that has kept us in a perpetual looping cycle of chemical dependent drug usage and has slowly eroded the confidence and self-respect of countless individuals worldwide.

Now that we better inner stand the cultural entrapment system of the socially engineered drug addiction making machine and articulating it through the concept of set and setting, we can move into the culturally accepted drugs themselves. If we just led right into that it would have done little to no good for the simple fact that I am not alluding to anything anyone with a pulse does not actually know for themselves. There is no one I have ever encountered, in their right mind, on their best day, that would not admit that these substances below are nothing short of socially acceptable legalized drugs. Just because something is legal does not make it helpful, useful, or healthy. In fact, as history will happily reveal to us, this often times is an indication that it is opposite of good for us. That is another story for another time but important none the less. It is not as if this is some incredible conspiracy (although it might be) that is lurking in the shadows of society and designed to place limitation on people's potential for self-sovereignty, self-confidence, and experiencing optimal health. The fact of the matter is that these substances just so happens to have that side effect on everyone that develops a dependent relationship with them and that is a fact you can take all the way to the bank!

So, let's now discuss in detail the most common and socially agreed upon drugs within our legalized social drug culture which we are simply calling the altered states economy and taking this notion a bit further than the authors of Stealing Fire did and delivering a slightly different nuanced meaning to it. These, in my opinion, are the agents of the matrix control system. What I mean by that is they perfectly control someone's ability to act, think, and exist independent of the altered states economy i.e., the socially agreed upon drug dependency economy that fosters all the right ingredients for addictions and seems to remove the necessary guidance for true independence and spiritual recovery. I am holding no punches here and refuse to water down the sobering reality of this topic. The truth ultimately will set us free, even if it pisses us off or triggers us in the process. My prerogative is not to be a best-selling likable author. It is to help set you free!

So, here we go!

Coffee / Caffeine

"The drugs that a culture celebrates are the ones that helps it function most smoothly. Coffee and tea became popular during the industrial revolution because these were good drugs to take if you had to work a really long day if you were in a factory and needed to stay alert. They did not impede the wheels of capitalism. In fact, they lubricated the wheels of capitalism."

Michael Pollan, Author of Caffeine

Coffee is one of the biggest elephants in the proverbial room of our society when it comes to the basic maintenance of our work-based culture, the industrialized society, and also to a big effect the overall health community touting the supposed "benefits" of the world's most popular drug of choice. We live in a society where coffee is considered a health food and is promoted as a cognitive enhancement supplement among the "bio-hacking" community, which is a sub-culture of supplement and technology focused health enthusiasts seeking to optimize physical and mental performance. Over the last decade or more of being a professional health educator and practitioner I have watched the conversation swing from coffee being an unhealthy substance to an entire industry being born from the popularity (and excellent marketing) of the bullet proof concept proclaiming that coffee in combination with butter being a health "hack" or optimal tool for human performance. I have also witnessed in the last 6 years following this bullet proof movement the uncountable amount of people falls off of that bandwagon due to adrenal burn out, cognitive overwhelm, and simply expressing the downstream physiological results of that experiment gone to its ultimate conclusion.

Whether you think coffee is absolutely dreadful or you believe it is the greatest thing ever conceived by the human mind let's look at this topic objectively and from multiple angles. I know this will not exactly be the most popular thing I write in this book but once you realize what this substance does to the body you will either awaken to a greater truth or reject it for all the short term benefits you feel it has bestowed upon your daily experience. There should be no question, whatsoever, that coffee is a drug though, this is an established fact, and it ranks up there with the strongest natural drugs found in the pharmacopeia of nature. Does this inherently mean it is somehow bad or should be avoided at all costs? Not necessarily, because like everything we touch upon it is more to do with the individual's relationship to the habit itself and whether or not it creates a psycho-biological dependency. It just so happens, for more people than not, this bean that comes from the coffee fruit, once roasted and its chemical constituents are extracted into hot water, has an effect on one's mental state and emotional temperament unlike most others.

The first thing to understand is that the vast majority of commercial sold coffee beans contain an excessively high concentration of the plant alkaloid caffeine and that these beans are highly oxidized or rancidified. The oils that come from the coffee bean, like all plant oils, are delicate and once they are introduced to high heat treatment, they can easily become rancid which changes their chemical makeup. There are many different methodologies for processing and roasting coffee which you can explore and investigate if you choose to make coffee part of your ritual set. I am not here to judge you for anything but here to share information so you can make the best choices possible for yourself. Most of the coffee on the market, including organic brands, are heavily oxidized/rancid and also produce what are known as mycotoxins which are fungal byproducts in plants that can contribute to gut-dysbiosis otherwise known as a candida albicans fungal infection. This can lead to an auto-immune reaction and cause a systemic inflammatory response, similar to the effects of consuming foods that we are either allergic too or cause a digestive agitation.

The most basic estimates of caffeine content in an average cup of coffee around between 100 - 200 mg. How many cups of coffee do most people consume on a daily average? How many cups of coffee do you consume daily? This may not sound like a whole lot but in truth, it is a significant amount, especially when compounded each day, after day after day. The half-life of caffeine on average is between 3-5 hours. This means that it takes 3-5 hours for half of the overall amount of caffeine to be eliminated or metabolized in the body. This is why it is recommended by experts not to consume coffee after 2 pm for the average person. Every individual has a different propensity to metabolize the caffeine alkaloid different and each person has a different sensitivity to caffeine, as well as other plant compounds. Because of the metabolic issues that can come from drinking coffee straight the idea to introduce saturated fat in the form of butter, ghee, or coconut oil/butter was created to slow down the transmission of caffeine in the blood stream and produce a more consistent, long lasting source of viable energy.

This brings up another interesting point which is does coffee or caffeine actually give you energy? I believe, once we get to the bottom of the truth on this issue, we will be able to recognize a drug for what it really is. And what it really is a substitute for metabolic bodily energy. Coffee does not, in any way, shape or form, help your body produce mitochondrial/cellular energy. What it actually does is artificially stimulates our sympathetic nervous system by hyper producing the hormone cortisol and this creates the simulation of bodily energy. The central nervous system receives a rush of blood flow and increased activity. This signal specific regions of the overall nervous system to come online, not dissimilar to what can happen when someone goes into a fight or flight response in the face of perceived danger or stress. There is a very real stress response reaction that is happening, but it is covered up by the brain state alteration of dopamine and serotonin flooding in. You may notice the increased production of endorphins and the feel-good neuro-chemical cocktail that followed the first handful of sips. You may also notice, depending on varying health factors, the follow up of energy exhaustion, loss of mental focus, and jitteriness many people report.

Too much caffeine entering into the system up regulates the sympathetic stress response and immediately down regulates the parasympathetic (rest/recovery) system which can confuse the bodily feedback system on what is real or unreal. The bodies feedback mechanism can become easily confused as to what is happening when we hyper stimulate the stress response too frequently and do not know how to down regulate naturally and organically. Eventually, over time, someone develops a chemical dependency because the temporary hyper stimulatory altered state becomes that person's preferred new normal and thus begins the wheel of chemical samsara (wheel of suffering-karma). If someone needs coffee or any substance in order to feel 'normal' then what they have effectively done is inducted themselves into an artificial state of being and unless they continue to induce themselves, further and further, into this habitual routine they are not able to discern fact from fiction as it pertains to their daily inner experience. Does this sound like I am being a bit dramatic or stretching the point too much? Let's see if what I am saying is in fact true or not.

In traditional Chinese medicine there is a saying to describe the effects of caffeinated beverages such as many types of tea and especially coffee which is 'false fire'. In the Taoist Chinese medical system, practitioners work heavily with the elements which are earth, air, water, and fire for short. The element of fire in our health parlance represents digestion, metabolism, and cellular energy production. It is a clearly established fact, both scientifically and anecdotally, that coffee can seriously impede digestive function and lower the much-needed gastric stomach acid for digesting our fats and proteins. That aside, coffee/caffeine is considered a false fire agent and mimics bodily energy production but does not, in any way, help the body produce natural energy in of itself. If we are routinely consuming a substance with the intention or expectation that it will help us experience more energy but in fact it only simulates the experience of more energy, then what exactly is happening? Would it stand to reason we are participating in an artificial or false reality based on false metrics, false expectations based on a skewed understanding of fact from fiction?

"Truth is, depending on your own body chemistry, when the effects of the caffeine wear off, you can actually feel fatigued and depressed. So, you consume more caffeine to re-energize. Soon enough, you are hooked on the stuff – and it takes more and more to achieve that same feeling."

Dr. Daniel Amen

Let's explore this topic from a slightly more expansive and esoteric perspective. From a metaphysical point of view coffee reinforces the ego and has a tendency to close the heart chakra. Our entire society is running on a kind of coffee consciousness which can easily lead itself into candida consciousness because coffee acids have a damaging effect on the intestinal lining of our gastrointestinal tract. This is also due to the mycotoxin fungal infections that are similar to black mold toxicity laden in the poorly insulated walls of many people's buildings and homes.

It is true that coffee can temporarily increase blood flow(vasodilation), particularly to the brain and CNS (central nervous system), but what people fail to understand is that it pools the limited blood flow to the linear compartments of the brain which we commonly refer to as the egoic/reward based limbic brain. This tends to turn off critical thinking, objective reasoning, and to a more significant degree interrupt the empathy center of the brain causing one to become less patient, emotionally poised/centered, well rounded in their thinking, and less able to consider long term consequences of their short-term pleasures (addiction cycle looping). Coffee in this context is the ultimate representation of the pleasure/reward phenomena and is the quickest way to disrupt temporary pain/discomfort by replacing it with chemical gratification and dopamine sensation.

Coffee, like all 'socially accepted pain masking drugs', triggers the dopaminergic system which provides immediate pleasure, relief, and lights up the reward center of the brain as if to trigger the unhealed inner child that never received the love, attention, or recognition it deserved. This is how the chronic abuse cycle of this drug perpetuates itself through out many people's lives. If someone is dealing with trauma, PTSD, or any form of physical, mental, or emotional healing coffee is absolutely a detriment to their recovery and healing process. Well, here is the kicker to all of this. Every human being, in one shape or another, has experienced some form of trauma, may be a high functioning person with micro-PTSD in their nervous system, or is functional yet experiences bouts of depression and emotional disturbances. It is also important to include that these individuals and many more have repressed childhood wounding, have poorly functioning livers, kidney, and adrenal glands which would make consuming coffee an absolutely horrible idea, more so than it already is without these issues.

The dopamine release from coffee has been shown to be similar to amphetamines which sooth temporary discomfort but prolong bodily (or psychic) pain. When one drinks excessive amounts of coffee (2 cups or more) they begin to shut down their empathy circuits due to the stress response stimulation and become a bit more detached, psychologically compartmentalized, and increase the likelihood of repeating life experiences that force that person to wake up out of their caffeine induced medicated/numbed state in order to heal their trauma and learn their lessons that are being suppressed through this seemingly harmless beverage.

Caffeine is what is known as a methylxanthine molecule which is a chemical cousin of the molecule theobromine found mostly in cacao(chocolate) as well as theophylline. Caffeine is a unique compound in of itself within this grouping of similar but also dissimilar plant alkaloids. Theobromine and caffeine sometimes get lumped together as if they are the same thing, but they are actually very different. Theobromine, which is one of the key active components in cacao (cacao is where all chocolate comes from) and has a full spread of documentation showcasing its incredible pharmacological effects. Caffeine and theobromine,

134

although similar in their molecular structure, have very distinct patterns in the body. For example, theobromine is perhaps the most impressive smooth blood vessel relaxant of which the technical term for this effect would be vasodilation. Theobromine relaxes the arteries and dilates the blood vessels increasing oxygenation throughout the entire circulatory system. Caffeine has more of a vasoconstriction effect in higher dosages and can lead to muscle tightness, dehydration, and central nervous system imbalances which the general effects of theobromine are typically the opposite.

I am approaching completion of a book entitled The Hidden Messages in Chocolate and there is an entire chapter dedicated to this topic. Cacao has a long historical tradition amongst South American cultures dating thousands of years and is attributed to their longevity, quality of life, and is seen as a celebratory medicine. Coffee and cacao are fundamentally two different cocktails altogether, although mistakenly lumped up together as 'stimulants' and depending on someone's constitution and nervous system health this can be true, but they are very much different in most every way. In the early 1900's theobromine was used as an isolated compound where of which it was injected directly into the heart of heart attack patients in order to relax the arteries and revive someone in cardiac arrest. Imagine that, a chocolate extract was used to revive someone's heart. Caffeine, although not to demonize the compound, would not have such an effect and in all likelihood would stiffen someone's heart valves and arteries if it was injected in half the concentrations, it is regularly consumed. Good thing we were born with a liver to help us filter and reduce the toxic load of incoming compounds and chemicals.

To complete this section on coffee and caffeine I would like to say that coffee seems to work in a certain degree for some people better than many others. This is dependent on someone's unique metabolism otherwise known as their metabolic oxidation rate or in simple terms their metabolic type. I will spare you the lengthy explanation on metabolic types but suffice to say that your metabolic signature will determine how much of this substance (like other stimulatory substances) you can get away with, but it should be understood that I am not making a case for coffee being an overall benefit. I truly believe that everyone's bodies, nervous systems, and brain health would be far better served without it or in the case of using it making it a once-a-week kind of celebratory indulgence. If you find that you can enjoy a single cup of organic coffee once or maybe even twice a week (I am stretching big time now!) then perhaps you can enjoy it with little to no draw backs, but it is the rare (and I mean rare!) individual who can actually do that. The addictive tendency associated with coffee is one of the most extreme I have ever seen (and experienced) with any known drug (legal or illegal) and I will contend that most people are much better completely leaving it alone until they can control that urge or simply find they no longer need it for satisfaction, stimulation, or pleasure.

The Transition Process | Caffeine/Coffee

I felt it important to include a transition process for getting off caffeine dependency because it is one of the hardest common substances for people to ween off of. It can take some people only 7 days to get over a caffeine/coffee dependency but for others it can be more like 3-4 weeks, in some cases. Some people can do it easier, without headaches or generally lethargic symptoms, but for others they can experience headaches, lack of energy, and decreased motivation to do much of anything. Like transitioning from all chemical-based addictions, it is important to give yourself at least 5-7 days to be unproductive, move through the lack of energy, and place your focus on rest and sleep.

Following the **21 Dopamine Reset | Reboot | Recovery Method** will be a sure-fire way to exit out of caffeine dependency but below is a simple list of tools you should implement if you experience stronger withdrawal/reset symptoms. The brain itself needs to completely reset itself from the dopamine-serotonin feedback loop brought on by excessive caffeine/coffee usage. Especially if the coffee is used as a way to start your workday and "get things done". You'll have to let yourself take a break from being "productive" in the way you use coffee for and begin to be more productive when it comes to taking care of your health, your body, and your overall mental and emotional wellbeing.

- Magnesium

- Full Spectrum B-Vitamins

- Niacin

- L-Theanine

- Omega 3 Fatty Acids

- Green Powdered Superfoods or/and Green Vegetable Juices

- 1 Liter of Spring Water + 1/4 tsp Per Morning & Another Liter of Spring Water in Afternoon

Alcohol

"A man who drinks too much on occasion is still the same man as he was sober. An alcoholic, a real alcoholic, is not the same man at all. You can't predict anything about him for sure except that he will be someone you never met before."

Raymond Chandler, The Long Goodbye

Alcohol has been the kind of substance I never really understood why people around me growing up seemed to love so much. I mean, I don't think they actually loved it, but it was something all of the adults in my periphery seemed to enjoy and often indulge in. I remember sneaking into the refrigerator when I was four years old and somehow opening a beer can because I saw some adult in the house doing it. It was the absolute worst, most disgusting thing I had ever tasted and from that moment on I had zero attraction to it. Well, that is until I got into my later teenage years and alcohol made its return into my life experience due to the social influence of high school parties. When I think back on the recklessness of my youth it's astonishing that I made it through all of that with my health intact and in many instances that I survived at all. I think this is a common consideration for many who were exposed to the intoxication lifestyle that alcohol, smoking weed, and other substance experimentations provided.

Out of everything we discuss in this chapter I assume that this is the one topic the majority of readers will agree upon being the drug of society that has the least benefit to highest risk ratio. There are basically no perceivable or identifiable benefits that 'almost' all forms of alcohol provide in anyone's lifestyle. I say almost because there are some small nuances worth mentioning and types of alcohol that are actually therapeutic at the correct dosage, but we will get into that side of things a little later. The biggest consideration right now is that we have an entire socialized world population that has been raised around and even encouraged to make this substance a part of their common lives. I mean, it is highly discouraged amongst our youth as a brain and liver damaging substance that should be avoided at all costs and then there is the big milestone in our cultural rise from adolescence into adulthood which is our twenty first birthday and we all know what signifies that more than anything; admission into bars and legalized drinking. If that is not a confusing message to send to our impressionable (and often times bored) youth who are just trying to find themselves (by fitting in with others) then I don't know what is.

As with all substances we put into our body, our brains are subtly or profoundly affected by what we consume. Alcohol has immense effects on our brain and if we had begun drinking earlier in our youth before our brains had fully developed then maladaptive patterns may form. Alcohol (ethanol) produces a wide range of chemical effects involving our neurotransmitter systems which regulate our mood, emotions, mental clarity, motivation, sleep cycles, and sense of wellbeing. The pleasurable effect that the onset of inebriation can induce is due to the increase in dopamine and serotonin. This also includes the neurotransmitters Gaba and glutamate which we will discuss in detail. The brain is a vast chamber of neuronal networks that direct the flow of electrical conductivity that regulates the nervous system and influences our state of being, from moment to moment. Within this complex set of billions of neurons they can excitatory or inhibitory in function. Excitatory neurons stimulate other neurons to respond by sending electrical impulses wherever they need to go. Inhibitory neurons suppress electrical responses and buffer from excessive neuronal firing. The balance between excitation and inhibition is essential for normal brain function where of which alcohol disrupts this necessary balance.

Alcohol does not produce a stimulatory effect like many other common substances. It produces an inhibitory effect which is often cycled in and out alongside a day of stimulant usage. Alcohol is known as a depressant due to the pharmacological effects it has on our brains neurotransmitter systems. Alcohol increases Gaba production in the brain which is an inhibitory neurotransmitter which is responsible for relaxation of nerves. Alcohol is known to potentiate Gaba receptors causing an exaggeration of its inhibitory effect. This explains the sedative effect of alcohol. In tandem with this alcohol also inhibits the glutamate system which is an excitatory circuit of the brain. Gaba activation coupled with glutamate inhibition decreases overall brain function.

Frequent alcohol consumption shifts the normal regulatory flow of Gaba and glutamate causing an irregularity in how our brain neurons are performing. This could be called a neurotransmitter sea saw effect in the way that it can go from one extreme to the other in an extreme fashion. This disrupts our brains regulatory functions over time and creates a chemical chaos in higher alcohol consumptions without regular breaks from alcohol all together. This sea saw effect is the short-term consequence of frequent alcohol usage but over time that sea saw begins to tip over onto one side. Because the body is always seeking its homeostasis point (balance) it will send out other nutrients and minerals such as calcium (Ca2) in this case to regulate this imbalance. Due to this metabolic process the body will open up more calcium ion channels in order to send out this alkaline mineral to do its job. The longer-term effects of alcohol cause the sea saw to swing by decreasing Gaba inhibitory neurons and increasing glutamate excitatory functions as a way to compensate. This is how the brain adapts to the common place stimuli (ingestion of substances) and reroutes itself in order to acclimate to it.

This neurological adaptation process is the cause of increased tolerance to the same amount of alcohol that led to intoxication effects before. A new normal has been established within the brain. This is also what leads to over drinking and the result of going overboard where people can end up blacking out or having physiological reactions such as respiratory issues, for example. This creates a detrimental cycle of riding that chemical sea saw and also what makes withdrawing from alcohol usage so challenging for many people. When someone attempts to break away from long term alcohol usage the brain has to go into a completely new adaptation phase and a host of challenging symptoms can come due to this. It is important to have a basic grasping of what is happening during the break away phase which will allow you to put together a nutritional strategy to mitigate these effects. The lack of quality nutrition and supplemental knowledge is the reason why addiction withdrawal symptoms are so painful and can be buffered with correct knowledge.

Since alcohol increases Gaba production in the brain in the short term and then decreases Gaba production in the long term the brain produces an excess number of GABAergic receptors as a form of compensation. Because alcohol decreases glutamate production it will tend to produce more glutamate receptors as a signal that it wants more than it is receiving. So now we have an excess of receptors which act as satellite communication stations within the brain and without the chemical compound that fits into those receptors it registers an imbalance within the system. When the alcohol habit begins there is an excess of Gaba and because the brain does not need as much as is being produced it decreases the receptors. This is a short-term response by the brain to bring the system back into a state of balance. Eventually the Gaba to glutamate ratio becomes out of balance and glutamate production increases due to low Gaba production resulting in increased sympathetic overload symptoms such as anxiety, cognitive overwhelm, and even tremors. Over time the neurotransmitter receptors become overwhelmed and fatigued from this process and this is where heightened symptoms of alcoholism manifest.

The brain is being bombarded by a cascade of stimulatory neurotransmitters that it no longer has the receptors to metabolize properly and does not have the GABAergic support to buffer the increase of glutamate. This makes the withdrawal process particularly challenging without the right nutritional and supplemental support system in place. The liver takes on the brunt of the toxic by-products that alcohol introduces into the body and once the liver is too weak to buffer the load bigger challenges arise. It's important to understand that there is no safe amount of alcohol for the body or the brain. Alcohol is basically a poison to the body in its distilled form and our body simply does all it can to adapt to the substance it's interacting with, but it never has a net positive effect overall.

Now that we have covered some of the physiological aspects of alcohol lets discuss the most under acknowledged aspect of this cultural beverage which is the metaphysical side. You might be wondering what alcohol has to do with metaphysics or in other words with a spiritually orientated discussion. This is not so much about spirituality or a faith-based perspective as it is with pure energy. The word metaphysics basically means beyond physics or that which is beyond that which is physical or material. There is a very interesting term used to describe alcohol that we have all heard which is termed 'spirits'. The root of this term comes from Middle Eastern alchemy where alcohol was used in medicinal preparations to create organic therapeutics using alcohol as the medium because of its dissolving (solvent) qualities. There are dual meanings to this term because alcoholism also has been largely associated with phenomenon that can easily be described as paranormal but in the western medical reductionist perspective, they would use words such as hallucinations or sudden mood disorders to explain this kind of thing away.

Everyone who has spent a significant amount of time around alcoholics and/or in the general dive bar scene has had to have seen people who appeared to be one way before they drank and seemed to have a personality shape shift after drinking. I have witnessed this thing happen in one of my friends in my pre-adult years and the change around was truly astonishing (and alarming). One of my best friends at the time would literally go into a strange metamorphosis when he had a few drinks in him, and I am not talking about going from introverted into sociable and talkative. He literally became a completely different person. He became argumentative, triggering, and verbally abusive. I actually had to send him to the hospital one night because he became so immediately outraged and violent towards me as if a dark spirit had invaded his brain and hijacked his entire operating system. After that incident I had begun to look into this and see if this was simply an isolated case. Of course, it was not and was far more common than I expected.

Now, I think we all know that with an increase in blood alcohol levels there is a parallel increase in poor decision making, potential for emotional outburst, or causing injury to self or others. This seems logical and something many of us have observed in our lives. There is another side of this story though that is equally as important, and it pertains to the subtle nature of addiction as a whole. The phenomenon of addiction, regardless of the substance or habit, has its own kind of spirit or consciousness. We have discussed this but it's worth bring back up in this topic specifically.

Alcohol seems to have an effect on inhibiting someone's normal cognitive functions and self-control faculties where it is reasonable to assert that it can allow for a 'spirit', if you will, to enter into the psyche of the inebriated individual. Whether someone agrees with this concept or not, it is well worth strong consideration because the downward spiral of negative consequences that are synonymous with alcoholic behavior directly reflect the more shamanic understanding of all of this.

While digging deeper into the research I came across a term called alcoholic hallucinosis. This means alcohol-induced visual hallucinations. This is one of the reported symptoms that smaller amounts of people have reported while attempting to withdraw from alcohol or in some cases still had small blood alcohol levels but was 6-24 hours from their last drink. We could try to explain away this with a rigid reductionist scientific point of view, but I do not believe that would be of much use. It must be strongly considered that within the individual that has developed an alcoholic dependency for which such as phenomenon would manifest itself that it is a sign of a metaphysical occurrence. Other common symptoms associated with this are physical convulsions called seizures as well as memory loss and lack of motor coordination. Intensified mood swings and emotional instability are very common as well. These are all associated with a disruption of one's own consciousness in a state of inebriation but also can amplify during the withdrawal process due to the dependency that has been established.

When western "scientists" attempt to over identify the body as only a material physical instrument and exclude the spiritual component then we are grossly missing the mark. As a student of shamanism, traditional indigenous cultures, and having experienced many initiatory altered state ceremonies I can tell you firsthand that the physical symptoms brought about from all "drugs" are connected to a meta-physical reality. I will assert that alcohol, perhaps more than most others, has the strongest potential for opening our bio-field (auric field) to non-physical energies (spirits) that can influence our own consciousness and bodily state. In fact, when you think about it deeply a dive bar or crowded alcohol induced night club environment is simply a full-scale echo-system for invisible spirits. There is really nothing productive or healthy about alcohol related environments, particularly the night life fashion of our cultural trends. Just like all addictions function based on 'possession' principles, such as a tape worm or parasite, an alcoholic lifestyle works the same way. Alcohol consumption can 'possess' someone to say and do things they would never think of when they are sober or even high on cannabis.

With both the physiological and metaphysical understanding it becomes clearer why institutions such as alcoholic anonymous and others only work at a very small degree of "success." One of the primary teachings of AA is to admit and acknowledge that the user is an alcoholic. This is helpful if someone is in denial and needs a serious intervention back into reality. However, they, like most drug reform programs, insist that the user will always be an alcoholic and at best they are a recovering alcoholic who will always struggle with the temptation to return back to the old lifestyle. This kind of thing is absolutely inappropriate and functions along the same cult mind control principles of religiosity that teaches people to give away their power to some other entity or force outside of themselves because they essential are not worthy (they are a sinner) or they are helpless to help themselves. One of the common assertions is that the best someone can hope for is to be a recovered alcoholic and to simply never drink again. This is absolute nonsense, and I am calling this kind of disempowering (and possession based) "treatment" out because it is fundamentally untrue and certainly unhelpful.

In conclusion to this segment on alcohol I want to encourage anyone who has struggled or is in their own withdrawal process to understand that there are two forces at play here. The physical aspect involving our brains adaptation to alcohol, our liver and its adaptation to buffering the toxic metabolites that alcohol produces, and the metaphysical elements which can be distilled into mental attitude, emotional healing, and consciousness work. All of these things are detailed throughout the book and most specifically in section 3. The nutritional protocols for addiction recovery are provided and also focusing on the life you want to create beyond the life that alcohol has allowed for will be the anchor point for success.

The last thing to mention is that some forms of alcohol can be useful and even healthful. The disclaimer here is that if someone considers themselves to be an alcoholic or having a problem with alcohol it is recommended to not engage with these things for the most part. Good replacement drinks are things like kombucha and ciders that are now widely available and are produced from natural organic fruits using a fermentation process that can be useful for our gut bacteria. These are simply for entertainment when appropriate and not recommended as part of a daily lifestyle.

Also, there are herbal medicines called tinctures that traditionally use small amounts of organic grape ethanol or a pure alcohol to infuse with herbs. This is a long-tested modality for infusing the medicinal compounds in herbs, mushrooms, and animal medicines due to the alcohols solvent properties and concentrating the medicine. These are typically done in a 30-day cycle during the new moon and full moon. These can be very powerful and effective as the alcohol helps to drive in the herbal compounds into the blood stream in very small tincture sized amounts. These can also be put through what is called a dual extraction process which burns away the alcohol and leaves the medicine remaining.

Tobacco / Cigarettes

Out of all of the mentioned vices that our culture freely celebrates and promotes tobacco is possibly the most misunderstood and abused plant, with cannabis coming in at a close second. Tobacco, in of itself, is not as much of a problem as one may assume but when we talk about cigarettes however, that is a completely different story, entirely. You may ask yourself, what is the difference between tobacco and cigarettes? Aren't they basically the same thing? Well, not exactly. Cigarettes are the end product of a corporate corruption to what has always been a sacred and ceremonial plant which is natural tobacco. When I speak about natural and original tobacco, I am referring to the unadulterated version of it that is known as nicotiana which is the flowering tobacco from which the dried leaves come from.

There are over 60 species of nicotiana, according to the journal of the royal society of medicine, where of which most are indigenous varieties to the America's. Nicotiana tabacum is the variety currently grown and used for commercial cigarette production which is of North American origin. This is considered to be a weak variety of tobacco but also what makes it perfectly suitable for commercial high scale production for the cigarette industry. This variety is also much more habit forming and prone to addictive compulsion than the stronger forms of tobacco such as the nicotiana rustic variate used in South America in what is known as mopacho's. A mopacho is a high nicotine concentration (as high as 9% nicotine) cigarette/cigar that is used in ceremonial fashion with plant medicines or in prayer circles. It is also important to note that in traditional tobacco ceremonies it is not typically inhaled through the lungs but lightly puffed on and blown out to clear the energy externally.

Tobacco is also used in organic permaculture and bio-dynamic farming methods as a protective agent surround accompanying plants in the garden. Tobacco has insecticidal properties which make it a potent natural pesticide to ward off insects from invading and consuming nutritious plants from one's garden or farm. The energetic of tobacco is very 'masculine' in nature which includes a protective component and also a very grounding earthy element, which denotes its excessive use amongst people who feel very ungrounded, anxious, and/or have a hard time staying present in their own body. The draw for tobacco can be associated with a few basic nutritional and energetic needs that are not well known, even in sophisticated nutrition circles. Once one becomes aware of these biological needs of the body, they can access their tobacco usage and begin transitioning from excessive to moderate use and even releasing the attachment to it all together.

The alkaloid molecule found in tobacco that is associated with its habit-forming nature is nicotine. Nicotine has received a significant amount of research due to its purported health benefits yet the common administration of it through tobacco smoking has also been under heavy scrutiny, for obvious reasons. This has caused an emergent industry of nicotine products such as gums, patches, and vape pens to supplement users who do not want to smoke cigarettes/tobacco. Whether nicotine itself has health benefits or not, it has become obvious to me that nicotine itself can cause habit forming tendencies and lead to dependencies in those who are trying to withdrawal from tobacco usage all together. In my own experience and observing others withdrawing from this habit I have discovered that there is a much more effective way to do this without using nicotine whatsoever. Within the entire western population of cigarette smokers there is a clear and definitive b-vitamin deficiency syndrome and that is what needs to be addressed.

The draw for tobacco has a few nutritional considerations and one of them can be found in a nutrient called Vitamin B3, otherwise known as nicotinic acid, also known as niacin. Nicotinic acid is not exactly the same as nicotine, but it can have similar onset effects as nicotine such as elevated heart rate, immediate blood oxygenation, and even a flushing effect. In the supplement world there are two distinct forms of nicotinic acidic called niacin and niacinamide. Niacin is vitamin b3 and causes a flushing effect in the body which is part of a cellular detoxification process and increases metabolic activities. Niacinamide is also vitamin b3 but does not cause a flushing effect and is generally recommended for skin issues, as well as support for kidney and cognitive imbalances due to b-vitamin deficiencies. Persistent tobacco usage can elicit similar metabolic effects and provide temporary sensations that vitamin b3 is known to support with.

If someone is dealing with a tobacco addiction and is having trouble letting it go it is recommended to begin either supplementing with niacinamide or to begin what is known as a niacin flush. The niacin flush is of more interest to me, because I have a lot of personal experience with it and have seen tremendous benefits occur for people who are detoxing from all kinds of chemical addictions including cannabis, tobacco, alcohol, sugar, and even pharmaceutical/street drug withdrawals. The idea of a holistic niacin flush protocol was brought to my attention around the year 2011 by a urologist by the name of Dr. George W. Yu, MD who discovered it's benefits in helping people detox from chemical toxicity, including drugs of all kinds. Dr. Yu is the world authority on this methodology and recommending his advice to others I have seen incredible turn arounds in drug/addiction reversal, including going through a 30-day niacin flush myself.

The niacin flush protocol is a process that includes taking a specific amount of niacin (not niacinamide) geared towards a person's body weight and gender specific needs. An individual will take the niacin on an empty stomach in the morning and immediately begin a series of movement practices such as jumping jacks, jump rope, or whatever warm up patterns to get the lymphatic system moving. This also includes jumping in place for 15 minutes on a special type of trampoline called a cellerciser which mobilizes toxins from the cells and increases lymphatic circulation. Following this movement pattern, as the flushing effect begins to increase, an individual would go into an infrared sauna to sweat out all of the water-soluble toxins that are being released from the fat deposits surrounding the cells. Perspiration (sweating) is an essential component of this protocol as these toxins become stored in the fat cells and the niacin helps to break open the fat deposits, releasing the toxins into the circulator fluids, and out of the pores of the skin.

One of the most profound observations I have made over the years is that during the withdrawal period of any chemical addiction is a detoxification process. The withdrawal period can be especially difficult if the lymphatic system is sluggish due to food and lifestyle habits. The healthier someone is prior to the withdrawal determines how easy or difficult the release period tends to be. Sometimes our habit patterns (substance addictions) form and reinforce themselves due to the toxic nature of our internal bio-chemical inner-environment and making nutritional changes in our lifestyle can be the biggest difference maker. This also includes going into a sound cleanse and detoxification period to help eliminate these toxins which also tends to help eliminate the poor lifestyle habits we have picked up over time.

Another aspect to consider with tobacco is that it is what is known as a nightshade plant which many people are an allergic reaction or even an auto-immune reaction too. This presents an interesting idea that I have noticed over the years of studying health conditions and nutrition which is that many people can become addicted to foods/substances they have an immune reaction too i.e., have an allergic reaction too. The nightshade family of plants are a very common example and through the domestication of these plants the overtly toxic alkaloid compounds have been rendered less toxic but in copious amounts on a frequent basis can create a bio-accumulation effect that creates a white blood cell immune-reaction towards. This tends to make us feel a bit "energized" when we consume that food but shortly after we feel tired, weakened, and our nervous system can feel out of balance. The immediate energized feeling is not actually our body getting more energy, but it is our immune system being stimulated and the body can go into an adrenalized/cortisol state. This is the fight or flight sensation when the sympathetic nervous system is triggered, which is a stress response, and we can easily misinterpret that as a form of energy.

Again, this is why going cold turkey with most of our addictive habits is the absolute best approach because we can slow drip the chemical sedation we get from these things and not really experience the full effect of a detox process. This is also why I am not a fan or proponent of the nicotine supplements because they tend to mask the core issue instead of providing the bodily system a complete reset and reprieve from the tobacco habit itself. Once someone begins to completely remove tobacco from their routine and goes through the withdrawal process it should become quickly apparent the effect it has on our body's equilibrium. It should only take 2-3 days for the mucus build up (the tobacco tar) to rise up from the respiratory tract and begin to discharge in the form of coughing, excessive spitting, and mucus chunks depending on how much smoking someone has done. If someone goes 7-10 days without tobacco and decides to indulge again, they will likely experience the light headedness, frazzled/spaciness, elevate heart rate, and lung respiration decline that occurs because they no longer have the same tolerance they did before.

The last consideration to note around this habit is how it can assist in helping ground one's psycho-emotional energies in times of stress. This is likely the source point for the worldwide cigarette addiction phenomena that has become common place today. For people working in some kind of sheltered job environment that involves a lot of stress, having a cigarette break is likely the only time in that person's day where they get to reprieve and take a breather from their job environment. I saw this a lot when I worked in the emergency room of the HIV ward. Whether it was medical doctors, surgeons, security guards, nurses, ER techs, or patients alike, the same pattern seemed to play itself out like clockwork. The higher the stress, the more frequent the cigarette breaks would be. The neuro-association between stress and relief through a cigarette break was linked in direct ratio to each other. This seems to be a common theme in the work force of society and makes its way into the personal lives of cigarette/tobacco users due to its universal association for stress management.

So, with this broader understanding we can now see that excessive tobacco usage is linked to nutritional deficiencies, stress management, as well as the degree of 'toxicity' within someone's body. The research on the microbiome (the gut-brain connection) makes this aspect very clear. The microbial organisms (bacteria, fungi, virus's etc.) that exist inside our gut/stomach influence our food and substance habits, maybe more than anything else. This is why cleansing should be part of someone's regular routine and engaging in periodic detoxification protocols is essential for accelerating through addiction reversal. Now that we know the common associations to tobacco tendencies, we can choose to redirect our focus from the smoking habit itself and provide ourselves what we are really craving.

Like with all of these substance patterns refer back to the chapter of **The Dopamine Dilemma** on how to begin overriding the "itch" or impulse that leads to the dopamine trigger response. For more information on the nutritional and supplemental component you can find further information in the chapter **Mastering the Body and the 21 Day Dopamine Reset | Reboot | Recovery Protocol.**

Prescription Medications

> *"The person who takes medicine must recover twice, once from the disease, and once from the medicine."*
>
> *William Osler, M.D.*

In our pharmaceutical prescription medication driven "health care" society prescription drug abuse is one of the biggest and most under acknowledged areas of addiction in all developed societies. This is easily one of the single biggest issues plaguing so many who rely upon the allopathic medical model for guidance, support, and aid in their health issues, particularly in the area of physical and psychological pain management. In 2017 it was estimated that 18 million Americans have misused or abused medications at least once in that past year. Misuse of prescription medications seems to be highest amongst young adults between the ages of 18-25. According to the NIH (National Institute for Drug Abuse) prescription drugs rank the highest amongst 12th graders following alcohol, cannabis, and tobacco. I would also consider that this is likely the same basic spectrum for all adults who struggle with pharmaceutical drug addictions and their associated habits such as tobacco, alcohol, cannabis, coffee, pornography, and social media.

This is an extremely important area to explore because many people in our society do not consider prescription medications a "drug", although they are clearly labeled and defined as a drug by their manufacturers and marketers. In fact, think about where people tend to go to purchase their medications and pain killers from. A drug store! The store itself it called a "drug store" and the substances being purchased are often labeled as "pain killers" but they are also very clearly labeled as "drugs" themselves. This is a kind of cognitive dissonance where someone goes into the 'pharmacy' to purchase their 'medication' to numb their pain but does not make the cognitive link that what they are purchasing are 'drugs'. Therefore, the potential for 'drug abuse' and 'drug addiction' is not always factored into the buying decision or how much they choose to use these substances on a daily basis to numb whatever pain or discomfort they are contending with.

The underlining reason for the frequency of usage and the potential abuse of these medications is really just the same as it is for all of the other 'culturally accepted drugs' mentioned in this chapter. It seems that everyone that chooses to develop habitual patterns to one substances or activity or another (or two, or three, or four others) has their own pain medication of choice. Remember, all of these dopamine triggering medications are just that, a dopamine triggering medication. This could be a very accurate and simplified definition of what a 'pain killer' or medication is. A substance or habit that triggers dopamine in the brain and medicates i.e., numbs pain receptors that create the sensation of discomfort in the body and/or brain. So, the core reason for the usage of pain medication is to up regulate the pleasure receptors in the brain and down regulate pain receptors meaning to decrease the felt sensation of pain by increasing the felt sensation of pleasure or relief.

In my research I came across a few clinical descriptions of prescription medication and the role it can play in addiction. This is one such explanation from a clinical source.

Prescription painkillers i.e., opioids are derivatives of opium. Their role is to act on the nervous system to suppress the intensity of pain signals reaching the brain and simultaneously to stimulate areas of the brain associated with pleasure. In an addiction-susceptible person, the brain's reward system highjacks normal

thought processes to prioritize repetition of the
pleasurable activity, and eventually to perceive it as
essential to survival as breathing.

So, as we have discussed in prior chapters, the addicted brain effect is to create references points for heightened states of pleasure and eventually to regard the cause (substance) for the pleasure as an essential component for survival. This is extremely telling of the addictive nature of these substances and most telling of the addictive potency of pharmaceutical medications themselves. Now I want to share another description from the same source on the effects of these substances in addicts.

"Most people who take a prescription painkiller - even
those who occasionally misuse them for recreational
purposes can stop without much difficulty. Such is not the
case for the 5 percent to 10 percent of individuals with a
biological predisposition to addiction. Addiction is not a
matter of choice or a lack of will power. It's a chronic
disease affecting the brain's chemical makeup and
cognitive functioning that is characterized by irrational,
compulsive behavior, which continues despite increasingly
harmful consequences."

So, this is basically telling us that some people have a genetic predisposition to addictive tendencies based on their unique biochemistry and I would also add their psychological distortion or constitution. This is a fact that some people display more of a distortion for different forms of biological addiction based on many factors, I will not dispute that. What I will say though is addiction is actually a matter of choice. This statement is not entirely true, although I do understand that these individuals have a much harder time with addiction, and these smaller groups of people tend to stay addicted longer or over their entire lives. There is a reason for this, which we discuss all throughout the book, and it does not mean that some people are hopelessly surrendered to their opioid addictions or whatever else it may be they use for pain relief, etc.

There are two distinct prescription medication categories I want to highlight in this section over all others: opioids and anti-depressants. Opioids are the most regularly used and abused drugs available. According to the CDC over 191 million opioid prescriptions were dispensed to American patients in 2017. According to the Institute of Medicine about 100 million people in the US suffer from chronic pain, which is almost 1/3 of all Americans. So, it is not hard to see why opioid medications are so desirable to those who simply want to get out of pain and live relatively "normal". The problem is these medications cause other challenges to the individual who creates a bio-chemical dependency and does not deal with WHY they have the pain in the first place. This should be basic common sense but for 1/3 of the US population it simply is not, and many of these individuals have not received proper guidance or education by their health care professionals on how to effectively deal with their bodily pain.

According to the Institute of Medicine worldwide, somewhere between 26 and 34 million people are abusing opioids. More than 2 million of them are Americans who are abusing prescription opioids. It has also been shown that nearly half a million more Americans are abusing heroin, which has a very real association to opioid addiction. In parallel to the statistical rise in opioid abuse emergency room visits for abuse of prescription opioids went from 145,000 in 2004 to almost 306,000 just 4 years later according to the New England Journal of Medicine. By the year 2013 the numbers of drug overdose deaths by heroin increased to around 10,000 and 19,000 for prescription opioid drugs.

What most people do not realize is the thing that makes opioids so powerful for pain relief is also what makes them so addictive and dangerous. They act on the same part of the brain that heroin and morphine do. The constant "injection" whether by snorting or literally injecting into the blood stream can cause a heightened euphoria like state that can create an increased dependency to repeat the same experience. This is a classic effect of what we would consider a "drug", the intense pleasurable high which is followed by an intense low, and a biological addiction to repeating that high every time the low hits, and it always hits harder and quicker the more of the drug is used in consistent fashion. With repeated use, like all chemical substances, opioids lose potency, and therefore more of the same substance is required to elicits the same or similar effect on the brain state. This here in lies the spiral of addiction that has ruined so many people's lives and overall health due to prescription drug abuse.

Along my research into this subject, I came across one definition of addiction that fits perfectly into this section here. *"Addiction is defined as the compulsive using of drugs in spite of terrible consequences."* Unfortunately, when it comes to the abuse of pharmaceutical medications, the description of addiction is 100% guaranteed to become a reality, it just depends on the individual, and their cognitive and biological resilience to the substance itself. Eventually though, the result tends to be the same, it just looks different depending on the individual, and the weakest links in that person's life and/or physical health. You can only blunt the pain receptors for so long before the physiological needs of the body begin fighting back, and then more, and more of the pain killer is needed to medicate the pain that the body is feed backing to the brain. So, either someone breaks down due to the underlining pain that is not being addressed and/or they break down due to the harmful effects of the drugs themselves, and likely it is a combination of both in tandem with one another.

Now we are going to discuss the subject of anti-depressants which have 3 specific groups: SSRI's, MAOI's, and TCA's. SSRI stands for selective serotonin reuptake inhibitor which are the most commonly prescribed anti-depressants, specifically those with depression. The basic function of an SSRI is to increase serotonin levels in the brain by blocking out the reabsorption of serotonin into neurons thus making serotonin more available in the brain. MAOI stands for monoamine oxidase inhibitor which are also a class of medications used to treat depression. Dopamine, serotonin, and norepinephrine are neurotransmitters called monoamines. MAOI's inhibit the oxidation of these neurotransmitters and make them more available to the brain for neurotransmission i.e., cognitive function. TCA stands for tricyclic antidepressants which work on the neurotransmitter systems as well and are used for depression symptoms.

SSRI's are the chief focus when it comes to prescribed medications for psychological disorders and what our society simply calls depression or even anxiety disorders. These medications are entirely based on the idea that all psychological disorders are due to a chemical imbalance in the brain and a medication is needed in order to rebalance the neurotransmitter system. This concept is partially true, as chemical imbalances are very real, and must be addressed due to the amount of poor nutrition, lack of proper supplementation, chemical toxicity, and increased stress of daily living. The problem with this kind of medication is that, in more cases than not, they always have negative side effects to go along with their supposed benefits of the condition they claim to help. One of the most common long term side effects of SSRI's is, ironically increased depression and neurotransmitter dysregulation. This is also the case in issues with anxiety where a patient can become increasingly anxious after taking the medication that is supposed to decrease their symptoms.

In the case of antidepressant medication, it can appear to be a bit more complicated, and the 'side effects' being varied depending on the individual taking it. Some professionals say that the symptoms of feeling increased depression or increased anxiety are only temporary and will lessen the more you use it. Well, this is definitely not always the case as many people only get worse, and report feeling foggy headed, lethargy, unmotivated, and nothing really getting better. For some people these medications can actually make huge improvements in the beginning and even in the long term, but they have to stay on the medication, otherwise their symptoms get worse, and they cannot function very well without the 'drug'. This is always the risk when venturing into the realm of synthetic man-made drugs, either it makes things worse, or makes things better but the individual must keep using it for the rest of their life, otherwise they will then get worse, and they become an involuntary addict to the drug as a necessity to function normally.

I have studied this area of research for almost a decade in combination with all of my studies into nutrition and holistic health. There are clearly proven ways to improve brain chemistry and neurotransmitter balance without using synthetic medications or opioid molecules which result in biological dependencies. I cannot tell anyone whether they should take a prescribed medication or not. That is someone's own personal choice, and they should be informed of the potential benefits and known down sides before blindly taking anything that could affect their brain chemistry. What I will say is that before anyone chooses to go down the pharmaceutical chemical drug route, they should always try natural and organic means such as changing their dietary choices, proper supplementation, exercise and fitness, improving their sleep quality, moving away from long hours on computers and phone screens, and addressing any addictive patterns they have. Until all of these areas are addressed there is no medication that will prove curative in the long term, it will only mask the symptoms that can be corrected through a healthy lifestyle.

There is a tiered approach to weaning off prescription medications that is used in clinical settings as well as drug recovery centers worldwide. The first step is always detoxing from the chemical substances themselves so that the liver and kidneys can begin purging the residual compounds of any drug or substance that is creating a biological burden on the organs. Following the detox process there needs to be a human-to-human support system where individuals can confide in others to address the psycho-emotional causes for their drug use. After that there has to be an integration process that leads to full recovery and rehabilitation of an individual from addiction to wholeness and sobriety. I provide all of these ideas and strategies all throughout this book, and most practically provided in the **21 Day Dopamine Reset | Reboot | Recovery Method** in the back of this book.

"Exercise is the most potent and underutilized antidepressant and it's free."

Unknown

Processed Food / Food-like Products

Unknown to most people in organized society and within the entire field of addiction recovery, the most pervasive and under acknowledge substance addiction has been and remains the relationship we have with food. There are layers to the food addiction riddle which so many people in society secretly suffer from and do not even realize they have an addiction too at all. I could literally spend this entire chapter discussing the overall food addiction topic in its entirety, but I want to focus on the most important element which is processed foods and food-like products. Throughout my direct experience in the health food culture over the last decade I have explored virtually all known dietary ideas, food practices, and the benefit it has had on my life is beyond description. I am convinced that the most powerful adjustment anyone can make in their overall life (definitely their health!) is in how they choose to feed themselves. Our food is not only fuel for our body but can be (and should be!) medicine that heals our body.

Since the early 1900's, as the industrial revolution began to ramp up into the food and agriculture sector of society, we began to depart from organic farm grown (or raised) food and transition into a more chemical-based, industrialized version of food to sell to the masses. Speed up exactly 100 years later to now and what we have is a complete bifurcation between real food and processed, synthetic, packaged food-like products. What is even more alarming is that the general population cannot accurately tell the difference between what we could call real food or whole foods and processed foods. You may be reading this and thinking Yea Right! The distinction between the two is obvious! Of course, I know the difference between REAL FOOD and PROCESSED FOOD. Well, maybe you do but maybe you don't. We will explore the details of that inquiry but let's just elaborate on this point because it is one of the biggest misconceptions in our entire socio-economic world and it has the biggest impact on people's overall wellbeing, more than anything else, in my opinion.

In the early 1900's there was a famous health researcher by the name of Dr. Weston Price, who was a world-renowned dentist who wrote a seminal book called **Health & Physical Degeneration** outlining the overall health of indigenous native humans to the more modern industrialized humans in western society. He began to notice the dental degeneration of his patients who adopted a processed food diet based in white flour(bread), white rice, white salt (table salt), grains(cereal), pasteurized dairy products, and whatever people were eating at the time. The acceleration of aging he witnessed shocked him, and he began to travel around the world to see if he found any of the same aging markers in people who lived in their natural habitat, ate their natural diet, drank natural spring water, and basically lived outside of the industrialized city environment. He found that every indigenous tribe he studied has little to no indications of cavities, bone mineral density problems, infections, and

156

also generally reached beyond the age of 100 with a higher quality of health than those in society reaching into their 60's and 70's.

Dr. Price's work on holistic dentistry and health is a foundation for everyone in the wellness field to study. He made many other important discoveries, especially in terms of the dangers of root canals and mercury amalgam fillings but we will stick to this point about processed foods. What we know for sure is that since the advent of the industrial revolution and most specifically the early 1900's life extension "seems" to have gone up, but quality of life has certainly decreased. We have medical advancements and increases in basic sanitation which have helped in the perceived extension of overall life, population wide but it appears that the overall quality of health has progressively gone down in direct proportion to people's overall lifestyle and eating habits. This can be attributed to multiple factors, but the core factor is found in our eating habits and the industrialization of our entire food supply.

All foods we find in a store or even on a farm go through some form of "processing" in order to make them ready for consumption. There is technically a "process" with every variety of food we consume and the disconnection between the consumer who purchases their food and what goes on behind the scenes for them to receive their food is largely where the problem resides. If people could see through each stage of the food processing process, they would have a much different relationship to the food's they purchase and most likely would choose their foods based on what has the least amount of processing and where it comes from. The more processing procedures food products tend to go through, the less like food it becomes and the more of an artificial food substitute it becomes. In effect, what most people have been consuming as "regular food" is more likened to some form of processed human pet food than it is anything natural or healthful for the body.

When we look at the entire category of processed foods, we want to realize that these food-like products are designed to be addictive and to turn someone into a lifelong customer. This is just the same as for cigarettes or coffee, which are obviously highly addictive and habit forming. Big corporate food and chemical companies have "scientists" (chemists) who's sole purpose is to tinker around with chemical ingredients to figure out which combinations of chemicals have the most addictive qualities. The marketing machines associated with these major companies' sole purpose is to convince the consumer that their product is X, Y, & Z and ultimately to sell it to you through some kind of story. This is especially true in the case of marketing processed junk food to children and their parents. They make the product seem really 'cool', 'fun', or 'exciting' such as the cartoon commercials and cartoon box illustrations on hyper sugary, genetically modified, pesticide sprayed commercial cereal products. And do not forget about the 'happy meal' pitch when it comes to fast food, adding in a toy to appeal to small children and their unhealthy parents who are unable to think for themselves because they are eating the same stuff, they are feeding their kids.

The processed junk food addiction remains the biggest culprit underneath the massive health and degenerative disease epidemics worldwide. This is also largely responsible for the continual decline in growth hormones and genetic resilience amongst newer generations of children. Due to this addiction being so widespread amongst the western population (and worldwide) the genetics of our earlier generations have become weaker and less durable over time. The younger generations immune systems and brain function has decreased as a result of this epidemic and the only way to overturn it is to return back to basics, which in this case is back to REAL FOOD!

The obesity epidemic is linked directly to the processed food epidemic and obesity in of itself is the resulting manifestation of what we would call a junk food addiction.

The most important thing to take away from this section is that processed junk food made by chemical companies should be removed and avoided at all costs. The addiction to processed foods is merely an attempt to stuff down our emotions and subdue our bodies natural energy system. The attachment to our taste buds instead of how food makes us feel is an adolescent type of addiction and can easily be worked out once someone begins to prioritize their health over their immediate gratification of their pleasure/reward sensations. I highly recommend one who struggles with this issue to read the chapter **Mastering the Body** for more information on health and nutrition as well as participating in **the 21 Day Dopamine Reset Protocol** in the back of the book.

We are going to take this basic premise on processed foods and go into a bit more specifics to discuss the connection to sugar / refined carbohydrates. This is a huge source of food-based addictions/attachments people struggle with, even those who have been health focused for years.

Sugar / Refined Carbohydrates, & Food Allergies

When it comes to addictive cravings around foods the topic of refined or processed carbohydrates and sugar in general is a huge issue for many people. I want to begin this section off by clarifying that I never believed that 'sugar' or carbohydrates were somehow 'bad' or should be completely avoided in someone's diet. I actually battled against the anti-sugar/anti-carbohydrate diet gurus for years because we need a balance of all three major macronutrient groups in our dietary lifestyle. The focus of this section is more towards processed carbohydrates and excessive sugar which can easily create metabolic imbalances and lead to addictive tendencies, just like any other substance we have discussed thus far.

The positive note on carbohydrates is that when we are consuming water rich organic fruits, they can be very healthy for us and increase metabolic energy. This is also the case for certain types of concentrated sugar sources such as raw organic honey and organic maple syrup as well. Overall, of the years of being heavily involved in the holistic health industry I have seen all kinds of fads come and go. As I began to come into balance with my nutritional needs i.e., introducing more animal fats and proteins into my diet my desire for sugar began to minimize and some days I do not consume any sugar whatsoever simply because I do not desire it. There was a time when I consumed copious amounts of fruits of all kinds and included things like honey and maple syrup into my smoothies and herbal elixirs daily. This felt really good for a number of years but eventually I found that my body did not want so much sugar anymore, and as I began to minimize my sugar intake, I began to feel better consuming higher amounts of fats as my main energy source.

This is something everyone has to figure out for themselves. What works best for them at what time and make adjustments as needed. What we need to discuss here though is the very real sugar and carbohydrate

159

addictions that have become a serious problem for the majority of our overall population, not just in the Western developed countries, but worldwide as well. With the advent of industrial processing of our food supply people were introduced to processed forms of carbohydrates such as all kinds of breads, pasta's pizza, rice, bagels, breakfast cereals, white flour, pastries, and complex grains. These food products have been marketed as being 'heart healthy' and a necessary step towards a healthier lifestyle. Well, in some cases this could be true if someone is coming from a completely abysmal processed food, factory farmed processed animal food diet. But in the case of overall health, increased bodily performance, and especially addiction recovery I would argue that this is very far from the real truth.

There are plenty of books written on the problems with processed carbohydrates, gluten rich foods, and grains as a whole so I will not belabor the point here. What is essential to explain though is the connection between food allergies and food addictions. I was educated on this connection almost ten years when I was a 100% raw food vegan and only ate fruits, vegetables, nuts, seeds, sprouts, seaweeds (sea vegetables), super foods, and herbs. I did not eat any cooked foods for at least 3 years and due to this experience, I was able to see nuances within dietary approaches that most people never notice. I noticed that many people who had autoimmune reactions were also constantly eating foods they were allergic too and could not seem to get themselves to stop doing this, even if they had the knowledge about what was happening. Most people never make this connection which is why conditions such as candida, irritable bowel syndrome, constipation, and other digestive problems persist.

The fact of the matter is many people are addicted to foods they are also allergic too and thus perpetuates a devastating dietary cycle of struggle. The top five food allergies are cows' dairy, soy, wheat, corn, and sugar. These are the staple ingredients that make up the foundation of a standardized conventional diet, excluding meat products of course. When there is an allergenic reaction to a food or substance the immune system goes into an emergency reaction state and if the food habit is repeated every day, the body can go into an autoimmune reaction where the immune system itself is constantly in a state of reactivity and defense. Because of this phenomenon in the body, it can create the false sense of "energy" due to the immune system being constantly stimulated and thus set up a feedback response whenever a certain food is eaten. This is why people can develop an addiction to foods they are actually allergic too or have an immune reaction too.

In the case of sugar itself, many people are dealing with some form of digestive infections such as a bacterial infection or a fungal infection such as candida albicans. This in of itself is a pretty big topic, one of which I explain in great detail in my book **The Holistic Health Mastery Program** and online courses. Candida is essential part of the bodies recycling mechanism which is designed to consume dead necrotic material and byproducts left over from the digestive process. The idea that we need to kill candida or kill off bad bacteria is only partially true but not entirely true. The truth is instead of resorting to some kind of antibiotic or anti-fungal medication, what we need to do is change out the fuel supply i.e., our food choices that are feeding the microbes that cause a proliferation of candida in the digestive system. This is called 'terrain modification' where we identify the problematic foods/substances we are putting into the body and begin changing out the fuel supply in order to create a different result.

In the case of candida or any acute infection, one of the biggest culprits is sugar, and sugar in almost all forms. Many people that have long standing sugar cravings or even sugar addictions likely also have some form of candida which signals receptors on the brain to illicit pleasure sensations every time someone consumes sugar. Sugar tends to feed these microbial organisms thus we want to begin reducing the sugar content in our diet, and entirely remove refined sugar and processed carbohydrates altogether. Refined carbohydrates immediately break down into sugar into the blood stream. This is why the ketogenic higher fat movement has been so powerful for many people. It is a way of terrain modifying the microbiome of the body to produce energy from fat instead of always from sugar. In order to learn more on nutrition and the digestive process of food I would have you refer to the chapter **Mastering the Body** section **Nutrition & Biological Optimization.**

I wonder how many people realize that sugar has been a culturally appropriated drug of choice in pre-modern European societies for hundreds of years. Dating back to the 15th century the original drug of choice was refined sugar. It was added to everything in order to make it more palpable or simply as an indulgence. This has not changed in the last 500 years and to this day it is used exactly the same, except far more abused, and combined with every confection and processed food/drink you can imagine. This can be one of the harder habits for many to break but in truth it is also one of the easiest and simple habits to let go of. One simply has to choose their health and cognitive performance over the seductive temporary pleasures of sugar on their taste receptors which signal brain neurons that seek pleasure and immediate gratification.

In order to overcome the trappings of a sugar/carbohydrate addiction it is important to begin changing your overall diet all together. It is not simply about changing one or two foods and trying to just replace it with something else. It is necessary to do a form of terrain modification which can look like a short-term cleanse such as a parasite cleanse, liver gall bladder flush, or a green juice/super food cleanse, and then begin adopting a completely new lifestyle with food. One of the most incredible dietary changes we can make is moving closer to a whole food, raw food rich diet which often is either vegan or vegetarian in nature. This can work wonders for people, because you are retraining your taste buds and digestive fluids towards REAL FOOD instead of relying on false stimulation through sugar or the carbohydrate cravings that lead to lower energy and brain fog. Eventually including high quality animal foods such as grass fed, grass finished meats, organic free-range eggs, and fats such as pasture raised goat butter and/or ghee butter.

Virtual Simulated Reality

*"It has become appallingly obvious that our technology
has exceeded our humanity"*

Albert Einstein

"Technology is a useful servant but a dangerous master"

Christian Louis Lange

Within the generalized parameters of addiction and recovery conversations there are some hallmark themes and topics that are almost always discussed. The obvious addictions are so well known that it is almost unnecessary to mention them unless there is a brand-new perspective to share combined with new research and data. The challenge can be in the rehashing and recycling of the same old conversations of the past that may or likely may not relate to the times in which we find ourselves today. In today's day and age, we have a whole host of challenges we did not have only a few decades ago. The cultural landscape has done an entire 180-degree flip around and the formation of how addiction begins and reinforces itself through the usage of technology has snuck up on us in ways no one really expected. In ways no one was ever briefed on ahead of time. And certainly, in many ways none of us were ever prepared for.

The biggest epidemic of addiction in the 21st century is easily a hyper-inflated reliance and dependency of all forms of technology, the biggest culprits being mobile devices, which are almost tethered to us at this point in time. There has been a lot of discussion around the concept of trans-humanism in many futuristic circles over recent years, which is the merging of the human nervous system and technological devices of multiple forms. This conversation aside, what we should consider is that we have all been ushered into a micro-form of this techno roll out because of our dependency on gadgets and devices for our everyday needs and desires. There have been experiments and studies to demonstrate that human nervous system has already merged on one level with our smart phones and wearable gadgets.

You can run the same kind of experiment on yourself where you leave your phone (and your Apple watch) at home while you go out for the day. You may begin to notice you become uncomfortable without it around, as if you left your best friend at home or maybe more to the point; you left a limb of your body behind. Some people discover that they find themselves looking to check their phone and completely forgetting they intentionally left it behind. It's like a phantom limb, which we discussed before is one of the major symptoms of addiction withdrawal. Is it possible that we have developed an intense addiction to our technological devices such as our laptops, smart phones, wearable tracking gadgets, and you better throw video games into that mix, as well? It seems that our smart phones have outsmarted us as we have allowed our need for technology to outcompete our need for nature and self-reliance.

I will not take much time to balance this topic out by expanding on all of the benefits and innovations allowed through technology. That should be somewhat obvious and straight forward by anyone who has any conceptual understanding of history. We all understand that technology has allowed us incredible advantages and opportunities we would not enjoy without it. So, with that said, my purpose here is to have the hard conversation that is rarely ever had. Even some of the best-intentioned health experts and addiction specialists will skip over this topic, and for a simple reason. They, themselves are likely addicted to the very same thing we are unpacking in this chapter, and it's hard to speak out on a topic such as this if someone is entangled in it. I had to save the writing of this chapter towards the later part of developing out this book because I knew how much I would have to unpack within myself in order to do the topic justice for the readers. Even as I move through each paragraph, I notice the tendency to check my phone (which is on airplane mode) and the urge to minimize my writing screen to check my social media, browse the internet (for what?), or check on YouTube (as if anything has changed in the last hour or two).

I have found in my own experience that this techno-addiction has become the centralized addiction in which all others are either stemmed from or glued to, in some way or another. This is a very profound realization to reflect on because it can hold the codes for how to untangle from the rest of the spider's web of addiction and dissolve the silk webbing that is holding it all together. This would not have been as true 30 or 40 years ago as technology really did not possess much of an addictive developmental pattern to it. I mean, maybe you can get addicted to the rush of driving a fast sports car or some other hobby-based activity. Those are relatively mild in nature and it's not as if everyone had such easy access to these kinds of activities. Technology was still relegated to those who could afford it and furthermore the technology of its time was benign in its habit-forming potential. It could not hold a candle next to the thrill of the great outdoors, hiking in nature, bathing in the river, socializing with friends in middle and high school, playing sports, etc.

Nowadays the most habit forming, brain stimulating, addiction hard wiring technology is available to virtually anyone who wants it, and all of the organic pleasures of life cannot compete with the instant dopamine kicks that our gadgets produce instantaneously. In order to break free from this kind of addiction spell it is going to require a serious examination into the effects it is having on our brains, our minds, our attention spans, the reduction (or increase) in our intelligence, and our social development as well. There are many layers of this conversation to peel back and we will start, piece by piece by piece until we have struck it at the core. And the core of this issue is a very strange kind of grey zone we may end up finding ourselves in temporarily. It is neither black or white, neither here nor there, neither right nor wrong. It is something that is the stuff of sci-fi movies and futuristic predictions, but I want to remind us all that all technological inventions are released to the public at least 30-50 years beyond when the technology itself was developed. And many movies we watch strike a certain chord with us because they are depicting a theme that is already happening in our world but may not be entirely visible or obvious, yet.

It is going to be absolutely imperative, as a human species, and especially as individuals on a path of healing, that we learn to work with technology rather than be dependent or addicted to it. Our phones, computers, and other devices are merely tools that we use for our desired purposes. Just as our "vices" can also be used as tools or mediums for enjoyment, that does not mean we have to use them every day for dopaminergic stimulation or to create avoidance cycles in our lives. A tool is simply a tool until it eventually becomes a weapon and unless we know how to use it effectively and masterfully, we end up hurting ourselves or worse, others with it and that is the distinction between something being useful or it being destructive.

The misleading thing about our daily devices is that we rarely, if ever, associate them with being destructive or at the least damaging to our wellbeing. We have become so well accustomed to them in our lives and it being such an integral aspect of our reality that we easily take for granted what life was life without them. This puts us in a precarious situation that is not obvious at first but becomes clearer once we take a brief step back from our unconscious habits and observe how strongly tethered, we have become to our 'smart' gadgets. We will explore the multiple levels and layers that exist within our cultural conditioning towards dopamine triggering technologies and gaining a brand-new perspective towards it. There are a few layers that have to be unfolded in order to accurately access the role these things play in our own individual lives, our family lives, and whether they are steering us in a productive direction or possibly in a less than ideal trajectory. This, of course, is the same cognitive analysis we must take with all habitual patterns and addictive tendencies in our lives. Technology just is a very nuanced and unique kind of beast in of itself that we are now going to tackle.

I want to prepare you because the topics we are going to unwind in this chapter are far from the norm of our societies status quo. I imagine that should not come as a major shocker provided the subject matter of this book and the exploration we have already undergone to get to this point. The most important understanding underpinning this entire discussion is the realization that there has been a cult like cultural conditioning program, that has spanned many generations, in virtually all developed countries at this point, and has sought to create a centralized distribution of curated information to the vast majority of people on the planet. We have all been recipients of subliminal programming and suggestive marketing from various institutions and corporate entities in order to steer our minds, our emotions, and our consciousness in a particular direction that was not of our own choosing.

So, when we consider the depth and magnitude of the worldwide epidemic of addiction it is important to understand that it is not your (or our) fault. We have been raised within a system of addiction creation and this chapter simply represents the most accelerated means that have been used to tie an entire generation, along with all age groups, and cultures along into the spider's web of addiction cycling. Keep this in mind as we explore further into this and especially as we alter our perspective of the seemingly neutral or benign devices, we have become so well accustomed too in our everyday lives. This will be very illuminating without any doubt and we are absolutely ready for it. And, on some level, if not on every level, you already know what I am alluding too is absolutely true because our technology has made the worldwide spread of information readily available at all of our fingertips. You can research, cross reference, cross pollinate, and cross confirm anything mentioned in this book. And I suggest you do.

"Our culture has bred consumers and addicts. We eat too much, buy too much, and want too much. We set ourselves on the fruitless mission of filling the gaping hole within us with material things. Blindly, we consume more and more, believing we are hungry for more food, status, or money, yet really we are hungry for connection."

Veronica Tugaleva

The Virtual Reality Interface Network

What if I were to tell you that the vast majority of our upbringing was based in and around a carefully curated, artificial set of constructs that we have all been accustomed to, without a moment's notice or second guessing of any of it? This set of constructs can easily be simplified into our westernized culture and even more distilled down into the entertainment culture, the pop culture, and technological culture. More of this will be explained as we move forward in this chapter, but this section is going to be focused on the techno-culture and specifically on what I call the virtual reality interface network. The VRIN is simply the alternate reality that exists within our dominant reality i.e., our direct experiential lives based on our core senses of touch, taste, sight, smell, and hearing. We use this sensory system to distinct between things in the outside world (outside of our inner experience) and to navigate our way through it. One of the greatest skill sets is the continual development of our innate senses and fine tuning our sensory system because it is the only thing that we have to detect authentic threats in our environment, etc.

The VRIN poses a very real problem for us as human beings with innate sensitivities and sensibilities based on what appears to be real and true in our immediate environment. Over the last 20+ years, our innate sensibilities have been numbed out and dumbed down in a way that was never possible before in recorded history. We have been introduced into an alternative reality, other than the one our nervous systems have been acclimated too and one that does not play by the same rules as our physical senses have been trained for. Our nervous system is trained for tactile sensations from our environment and bridging the processes of the mind with the processes of the body. It should suffice to say that, as a human race, we have been completely unprepared and unequipped to properly integrate into a world so technologically focused, to the point that even within our own disadvantages to it we still rely upon it, for even the most basic tasks that our grandparents a generation ago did not.

Let's clarify what the VRIN means and what it is comprised of that would make more sense for us. In simple terms, it refers to the worldwide internet as its primary interface mechanism and by interface, I mean the way in which our consciousness engages with the virtual network itself. Keep in mind, this is a 'virtual' interface network which indicates it is a simulation of a real personal engagement or interaction. For example, think about one of our most common forms of communication that has become the norm in recent years due to our agreed upon adaptation to the VRIN, which is texting and instant messaging. There is nothing inherently wrong with this mode of communication and in fact it is extremely effective and useful to save time, send quick responses, ask for directions, etc. The problem here is one of overcompensating with this tool for quick messaging as a replacement for organic, authentic, and real human interaction. We will dive deeper into this particular example in our section on social media.

With the advent of social media platforms, online dating sites, expedited online shopping, online role play video games, pornography of varying extremes, media soundbites and click bait marketing advertisements, and an overwhelming breadth of noise on the internet it has become its own virtual universe and it especially appeals to the instant gratification, immediate dopamine hit mechanics of the addicted brain. In fact, it is not a stretch or even strange assertion to say that the virtual alternative reality I am calling the VRIN is likely the biggest addiction where all others pale in comparison in the 21st century. Think about it, we know how hard it can be to let go of our coffee, cigarettes, alcohol, junk food, and other more basic habits. As hard as these can be, people do it all the time in the countless numbers of individuals and they report feeling significantly better, more energy, more clarity, and more motivation for life. Well, how hard is it to apply the same approach to back peddling from our smart devices, our time on the internet, our compulsions to check social media, our urge to check or respond back to text messages, to break the spell of online pornography, or maybe even to check the status of our bank account via our online banking app. Whatever it looks like, it's all the same in the end and it is the single hardest thing to break free from because it's the single hardest to understand and accept.

All addictions have a way of lulling us to sleep with their opioid hits, dopamine stimulation, serotonin rollercoasters, and the dependency they form within our own psyche. The virtual world of the internet and technology is really no different, but it has an entirely different spell it casts upon us than the others. We are so tied to this alternative reality as a way to compensate for our true reality i.e., our actual lives outside of the online world. The online world in a lot of ways is like an entirely different realm in of itself where different rules apply, yet our physiology is directly impacted just the same. Our time and spatial awareness diminish when we find ourselves in a virtual vortex such as messaging with someone for hours, diving down a research rabbit hole, scrolling aimlessly on social media, etc. When we are operating in the 'real world' we have a more immediate sense of time (in terms of Gregorian time dynamics) and thus our time is much more measured, accounted for, and intentionally focused. When we are deep in the VRIN vortex we can easily lose track of time entirely and as a result it can feel like time has lost track of us, in terms of the days, weeks, months, or even years that can go by without us ever knowing what happened to them.

Addictions have a way of trapping our consciousness in a type of stasis which means in a suspended animation, which holds it in place, yet the outside world is going along as it always does. The VRIN is indeed a consciousness trap and there are countless hundreds of millions of souls on this planet right now who have succumbed to this trap of their own free will and volition. The reason this alternative reality simulation matrix (it really is a matrix) is so prone for problems in people's lives is due to a few key factors and these factors are prevalent in all addiction cases. The need to compensate for what otherwise feels plain, dull, ordinary, or boring. When compared to the hyper stimulation of dopaminergic hits and/or the entertainment value of Netflix, online videos, or whatever else people are into, the regularity of day-to-day life simply cannot compete. This obviously is not true in actuality but when someone is under the influence of an addicted brain this is the very real challenge and obstacle in the way.

We develop compensatory habits as a way to avoid things in our own personal lives that are uncomfortable, uninteresting, or challenge us in a variety of ways. If we are not aware of this then we can easily adopt avoidance patterns as a way to eject ourselves from our true reality. It has become increasingly easy to shift our focus into the virtual simulation of reality because it triggers all of the right emotions, brain chemicals, and short-lived sense of 'connection' that we are really craving in our lives. Again, like all addictive habits, the VRIN is a tool that helps us learn new skills, expand our understanding of the world, and to network with a vast amount of people that would not be possible otherwise. There is a fine line that must be drawn with this though because it can easily become a coping mechanism for avoidance and disassociation from the challenges in our real lives. This is where we learn how to create healthy boundaries with ourselves and to honestly track whether something is helping to make our lives better or is creating diminishing returns on our time and energy investments.

One of the healthiest things all of us can practice is intermittent internet and technology fasting. Abstaining from the 'plug-in drugs' of technological compliances that create convenance and ease in our daily flow is highly encouraged for long term wellbeing. One of the core reasons this is so important is because our brain wave states are highly influenced by technology and especially by heavily engaging on social networks for our primary form of human interaction. Generally speaking, the VRIN puts us in a beta-brain wave state which is the least desired state to be in and entrains our nervous system in a fight, flight, or freeze state. Think about how your body feels when you spend a significant amount of time on the computer, on your tablet, or on your phone. These technologies emit frequencies that do not support our overall health and wellbeing and put us into a state of mind that tends to be far more reactionary than it is responsive and creative. Setting intentional boundaries, based on our goals, is one of the most powerful tactics anyone can implement to regain brain state sovereignty and uses practices such as meditation, breath work, exercising, and reading physical books can help to retrain ourselves to become much more adapted to our lives outside of the virtual simulation.

Now that we have unpacked the VRIN a bit and discussed the concept of an alternative simulation of a reality outside of our own immediate life experience we can move into the next layers which include a deeper understanding the overall entertainment industry and how the artificial construct we call 'culture' has influenced us in ways that most people do not realize but are heavily affected by each and every day of their lives.

The Entertainment Industry

"We'll know our disinformation program is complete when everything the American public believes is false."

William J. Casey, Director of CIA - 1981

As we continue our theme of unpacking the dynamics of the virtual simulation that we are surrounded by and deeply woven into it is time to go a level or two deeper. This is a topic that is typically focused on by, what many would consider "conspiracy theorists" or fringe researchers who go against the status quo of society. It is important to consider that our entire society and the compensatory structures of the entertainment-based simulation i.e., simulating a manufactured culture that we all are influenced by is an addiction creating machine. We are familiar with the term 'consumer culture' and that is exactly what it is in essence. The nature of the consumer culture itself is to bombard people with suggestive messages, predatory marketing (preying upon insecurities), sub-conscious symbolism (dollar signs, corporate icons, etc.), and encourage people to consume whatever is being sold to them. Well, I do not know about you but to me that sounds a lot like the exact scientific formula for creating dependency, lower impulse control, and starting the subtle process of addiction.

It has taken me many years to decipher and decode the coordinated messages that have been coming at us through the various modalities of the entertainment industrial complex. This includes all of our favorite movies, children's cartoons, infomercials, media broadcasts, commercial billboards, professional sports, and all the rest. I had to become increasingly aware of how my own mind had become conditioned by the entertainment industry and all of the various actors assigned the role of planting subliminal messages into the impressionable minds of the youth. Now, I am not going to go too far into the conspiratorial side of this topic, but it should not be much of a taboo to say, in this day and age, that we have all been sold a bill of lies, false promises, and been strung along a narrativized program that we did not give consent or permission too. This is one of the most insidious and silent forms of addiction, the addiction to entertainment and idol worship.

When we watch a movie, we are participating in a completely scripted, curated, and surgical, precisely planned story that is artificial, unreal, and simulates the experience of the movie in our nervous system but we know it is not real. But do our bodies know that it is not real? That becomes a very important question, and I can assure you that the technology available to create these experiences has risen to a level where the distinction between what is real and what is not has become blurred. One of the traps of taking in too much external entertainment in the forms that are spoon fed to us through our "culture" is we can lose track of our own reality in favor for the one on the screen. We can even find ourselves living vicariously through the timeline of a movie or television show which then creates the desire to want more. This is how all of the most captivating movies, television shows, and musical performances are designed. It is not an accident. It is a scientific formulation with one intended effect; to capture an audience's attention and string them along a journey that makes them forget about their own lives for a short period of time but always wanting more.

There was absolutely a time when I found myself in a form of addiction to all my favorite movies. I cannot tell you how many times I have watched the same movie, knowing every detail of it, and yet wanting more of it so I could relive an emotional experience because I preferred that simulation over the actualization of my own life. This is what it means to binge watch movies, sports, online videos, news shows, musical performances, and whatever else. We are binging on an artificial reality simulation that we know is made up but elicits a cocktail of brain chemicals that allow us, in whatever degree, to experience the false reality as our own but of course this only lasts so long and drops off quickly. Most people feel this is very innocent and would not consider entertainment as an addiction but take a good look at the movie theaters themselves. We go in anticipation for an experience, they provide the concession stands of vices and junk food to enhance our experience, and by the end of the movie are we any better off than we were when we entered in? Of course not!

Now I am not saying that entertainment in of itself is evil or nefarious in of itself. Again, we live in a manufactured 'culture' that is based on consumerism and addict creation in order to sell ideas which are designed to sell a product. The question we have to ask ourselves is what are we being sold and why have we chosen to purchase the product? What is the motivation for the desire to be entertained? What is it about our own personal lives that we feel we need to escape from and seek out external entertainment? Do we truly enjoy what we have been sold and getting use value out of it? These are all questions worth asking because they are the same questions, we need to ask in regard to any addictive habit that we have formed and it all started by being sold an idea, which led to adopting a behavior, and that behavior was entertaining enough that it stuck with us.

The other aspect of this is very important and I really want you to sit with this for a moment. What does entertainment really mean? One definition of entertainment is 'the action of providing or being provided with amusement or enjoyment.' Another one is 'an event, performance, or activity designed to entertain others.' Ok, so this is very interesting once we break the word and its meaning down. The desire and seeking to be amused or to find enjoyment in an activity. Seems innocent enough, right? Well, that again, could be the exact definition we could insert into any form of addiction. All addictions are amusing or enjoyable in the beginning, when they do not have a downward negative effect on our lives but by the time, they do it usually has fully formed itself into our psyche that we either do not notice the effects or are too far gone to do anything about it.

The discussion on the entertainment industry is not just about movies or finding simple pleasure in what otherwise could be a very innocent temporary experience. This is all well and good to an extent. What we are really digging into here is the effects of socially manufactured cultural narrative that has imbedded itself into the mediums of entertainment and how that has shaped our brain state, our worldview, and only increased our dependency on the cultural agenda. Once again, the cultural agenda is to grow itself and it only does this by capturing the attention and energy of people who exist within the cultural norm. To be counterculture really means to take our energy, time, and resources away from the consumerism model of the status quo and redirect it into things that are truly authentic and organic to our own desires and motives. So, do we truly inner-stand what we are feeding or fueling by frequently seeking temporary amusement, fleeting entertainment, and following the scripted escapades of actors who are putting on a show in order to distract us from the greatest show that is going on all the time called our direct immediate felt experience.

The final point to make on this topic is the biggest underpinning to it all, which is the cultural indoctrination of idolization or in short, idol worship. Our culture props up its idols for all the world to witness and look up too. We literally look up to them when we are in a movie theatre or at a music concert or perhaps attending some kind of political rally. Interestingly career politicians have become modern day celebrities in their own right and have formed strange ties with the celebrity class of Hollywood, the music industry, and the sports world. That is a subject for another time, but it is an interesting point nonetheless when we consider that all of these factions of the entertainment machine all work in conjunction with one another and use their platforms (or are used by their platforms) to influence the minds, perceptions, and behaviors of the masses. It is about time all of us began to question the cultural architects that we call celebrities (or those who create celebrity) and break out of the hypnotic spell that perceived stardom has cast upon our world.

We must be careful about who we look up too and choose to admire and for what reasons we may have an admiration for someone, especially someone we have never met before. Celebrity culture has a way of influencing the impressionable minds of the youth more than anything else and these exalted individuals of the entertainment world often times are not who they appear to be on the screen. Many times, if not most of the time, these individuals are living a double life, which should be expected due to the fact that these are actors, performers, and professional entertainers in a thing called "show businesses". Their occupation is to put on a show and the big mistake we all have made in our lives is to assume the person playing a character in the show is in fact a representation of that person in reality. This is another example of how the virtual reality simulation plays a trick on our minds. These individuals are flawed human beings (just like all of us) behind the scenes and many of which, especially in the music industry, have a host of their own addictions to contend with and are using entertainment as a way to escape their problems of ordinary life away from the stage.

What I am attempting to point out here is a major distinction between what we see and what is truly real. The addiction to entertainment is one thing in and of itself, and the associations we form in our own minds relating to the idea of a person can set us up for major interpersonal challenges. It can cause us to compare ourselves to someone else which results in an impossible situation of self-limitation, self-doubt, and never ever feeling good enough. This can happen with anyone we may look up too but if we know someone personally then we also see they are not perfect themselves, which gives us a realistic sense of their own moral and ethical value system, which can actually help us improve our own lives. The main thing to take away from this portion of our exploration is the trap of idol worship that is the extreme of where idolization can lead us and has led a large portion of the consumer trained populace of our modern-day culture.

We should never worship another human being or any form of idols that are man-made in any way. All spiritual texts speak very clearly about this and the hidden booby traps built into what is often called false idol worship. This is not a religious cautionary warning, in fact, I am highly skeptical of any religious based worship as well unless its guiding principle is congregation for the sole purpose to spiritual devotion and to worship spirit or God. It is so important that we understand this and really get this at our core because faith, devotion, and spiritual belief are the foundation for recovering from addiction. In order to successfully recover ourselves in today's world we have to undo the conditioning of the false idols that have been appointed to us as replacements for authentic leadership and spiritual guidance. We have to seek within ourselves in order to untether from the false cultural values that have been taught and conditioned into us because, as I have stated, it is the culture itself that has provided all the opportunities for addiction, dependency, complacency, and a big dose of self-doubt which are all prerequisites for being a lifelong consumer instead of a lifelong creator.

I am urging you to become the master architect of your own life. Your REAL LIFE. And only consume what supports your goals, uplifts your spirit, enhances your creativity, and sets you on a path that brings all of your power and potential front row and center.

"We have to create culture, don't watch TV, don't read magazines, don't even listen to NPR. Create your own roadshow. The nexus of space and time where you are now is the most immediate sector of your universe, and if you're worrying about Michael Jackson or Bill Clinton or somebody else, then you are disempowered, you're giving it all away to icons, icons which are maintained by an electronic media so that you want to dress like X or have lips like Y. This is shit-brained, this kind of thinking. That is all cultural diversion, and what is real is you and your friends and your associations, your highs, your orgasms, your hopes, your plans, your fears. And we are told 'no', we're unimportant, we're peripheral. 'Get a degree, get a job, get a this, get a that.' And then you're a player, you

don't want to even play in that game. You want to reclaim
your mind and get it out of the hands of the cultural
engineers who want to turn you into a half-baked moron
consuming all this trash that's being manufactured out of
the bones of a dying world."

Terence McKenna

The Mainstream Media

"Television is by nature the dominator drug par excellence.
Control of content, uniformity of content, repeatability of
content makes it inevitably a tool of coercion,
brainwashing, and manipulation."

Terence McKenna, Food of the Gods: The Search for the
Original Tree of Knowledge

Now that we have moved on from the entertainment industry and its role in the addiction formation of consumer culture, we now take our attention to the mainstream media industrial complex. The MM is positioned as a platform to host a set of authorities on world events, politics, celebrity news, etc. within our socio-cultural world. These individuals we call media analysts, trusted journalists, and media pundits are the appointed bridge between all of us and the incoming news of current events in the world. We are expected to believe these characters at face value and/or with the "facts" they bring to us in order to stay up to date and informed about whatever information is being disseminated. The mainstream media platforms are the "trusted" communicators of 'breaking news' within our culture but trusted by whom exactly?

In the recent decade the polling for how much people actually trust the mainstream media has only gone done and at the time of writing this book they have hit an all-time rock bottom low. Growing up I had always had a strong skepticism about the media, in all of its forms, and never felt any kind of trust towards what they were broadcasting. Perhaps it just never felt relevant to my own personal life experience or I was simply not interested in so called world events. When I look back on my youth, I remember that I always had a strong intuitive sense about what felt true and what felt like a lie. This is something that was built into me at an early age and not something I really understood until I got a bit older. The media broadcasts always felt way too manufactured, scripted, and artificial for me. The pundits delivering the information also felt very off putting, as if they had an alternative motive other than simply providing the objective truth and it never sat very well for me. Now we come to discover that the entire media has had and still does have an alternative motive other than discriminating factual information, which is no different than the overall entertainment industry. They are actually one in the same and simply operating on different spectrums of the televised programming machine.

If we want to understand how our minds, beliefs, and perceptions have been conditioned for us than it's important to consider that the information we have been provided with, just like the entertainment networks themselves, is almost entirely fabricated and manufactured. It's been said that the best way to control people is to control their perceptions and beliefs. This way people will remain a consumer of whatever they are being sold, whether they realize it or not. This is how the biggest addictions in people's lives are insulated into their minds and grooved into the neuropathways of their physical brains. If you notice during these news broadcasts the commercials that sponsor their shows are almost always reverting to some false solution to fix a problem that they themselves have sold us. This is called problem - reaction - solution which means to propose that you have a serious problem in your life, next is to elicit a degree of fear or uncertainty surrounding this newly discovered problem, and finally to sell you the solution that only they possess to the exact problem they made you aware of. To qualify this point, think of how many pharmaceutical commercials are running during any given media show. It is well established that at least 70% of the MM's bulk sponsorship funding comes from the pharmaceutical industry. If that is not a conflict of interests, then I do not know what is.

The news itself is delivered in a particular way that runs on this problem - reaction - solution feedback pattern and only changes form depending on where they want our attention to go. There are far too many examples in the last 20 years to describe but you likely can already figure it out from reading this because it's all the same pattern in the end. A very good way of thinking about the MM is that they function as a legalized reality hacking machine that captures the attention of its country's citizens and strings them along into a world of half-truths, sound bite clips, click bait marketing, and deceptive salesmanship. The news itself is a series of cherry-picked clips and selectively chosen narratives designed to hack into our reality in order to sell us their product. And what exactly are they selling, aside from what companies sponsors them? The answer is they are in the business of selling us fear, doubt, uncertainty, and keeping us on a track of inner unrest in order to keep our attention. This is the essence of reality of hacking 101 but instead of us hacking our reality by our own design, our reality is being hacked into without our permission or knowledge.

When the television was introduced into the American household in 1925 it presented the world with a way to entertain themselves that was never possible before. This began to age of broadcasting entertainment in the household and eventually became a way to keep people in their homes much longer than they ever did before. Eventually, over the course of WW1 & WW2 new methodologies for covert warfare tactics were developed and implemented silently, under the radar of organized society. One of these methods was to utilize the television to broadcast imagery and messaging to people in order to influence their minds in highly specific ways. The television device ultimately became a form of transmitting subtle yet effective slow wave hypnotic messages and planting ideas into the impressionable sub-conscious of its country's citizens. Speeding up to the 2020's we see this assault on consciousness has taken a full-blown effect of monumental proportions and consequences. The generational programming that has been caused is overwhelming in scope yet is always very obvious to see once we unplug ourselves from the plug-in drug of media manufactured predictive programming.

The word television breaks down into tell-a-vision which means to tell a vision to the sub-conscious mind of the recipient on the other end. Once we have a clear-cut understanding of this basic concept and can see it clearly for what it is, we then begin to take our power back that we had

179

allowed to be taken from us, bit by bit. You see, the only way the media or the entertainment complex has any power or influence over us is if we give it away. We have to own a television set in order to turn it on and watch it. We also have to choose to watch what we are watching. It is always a choice on our part and once we have the knowledge, we can then make better choices.

The choice to revoke our attention from the entertainment industry and televised media broadcasting station is the access point of personal power in the 21st century. The addiction to needing to stay informed, updated, and also inundated is very real and one that lurks underneath the surface of more obvious addictive habits. This is all part of the virtual reality interface where we ascribe the holographic projections being put forth in front of us as part of our personal reality and allow them to take residency in the fertile soil of our minds. The mind is like a garden and can develop a host of weeds in the form of negative thoughts, distorted beliefs, and counterproductive ideas that only reinforce our addictive tendencies. When we cut the cords with the projection machine i.e., the TV set or online entertainment subscriptions, we plug back into our own inner innovative qualities and go from consumer to creator, almost in an instant but surely overnight.

"The question is not whether or not we have been sold a lie.

The question is: have we bought the lie."

Michael Tsarion

Social Media

"Social media is a dangerous place to seek affirmation, acceptance, identity, and security."

Cornelius Lindsey

"In a social media world, the danger is being overexposed and when something is overexposed it is no longer interesting, if ever it was."

Donna Lynn Hope

The final layer of this proverbial virtual reality onion is the biggest culprit for so many of the issues people face with technology addiction. Social media has become the most heavily used form of communication and engagement for the majority of our population across the board. This has allowed to us connect and communicate with more people, in a shorter period of time, than was every possible at any instance in human history. We can literally fit hundreds of thousands, if not millions, of contacts in the form of social media apps on our phones and carry that around in our pockets. It's really an unfathomable thing to consider prior to the advent of the digitized social economy that we now are deeply interwoven into and rely upon in our day to day lives.

On the surface social media platforms appear to be innocent enough and pose little to no negative effects but provide so much upside. The truth about SM however paints a much different picture and the research data collected on the impact of frequent SM use on psychological wellbeing and neurological health is conclusive. The effects of the digital social environments we frequent on a daily basis does, in fact have a significant impact on all aspects of our health and psycho-emotional stability. The tendency for SM to become addictive is astronomical and comparatively makes the other forms of virtual entertainment seem almost insignificant in their habit-forming potential. This also partly due to the fact that the entertainment industry, the mainstream media, and all forms of business marketing have interlaced themselves into the social media platforms which has only amplified their prior impact but now with much more leverage and ability to reach more people worldwide.

In recent years there has been a lot of discussion from leaders in the technology field of Silicon Valley and other sectors of industry regarding the negative effects of social media on a variety of factors. The work of Cal Newport is paramount in understanding the internal and external consequences that social media has caused on an entire generation who has become reliant on it. He wrote a book called **Deep Work** which explores this topic in relation to productivity, personal fulfillment, increasing long sustained focus, and doing better quality work over longer periods of time. One of the points he makes is that social media has helped to cause the epidemic of fragmented attention spans, lack of quality work produced in the world, and overall increased rates of depression and feelings of isolation. Cal has a virally popular TEDx talk which can be found on YouTube called "Quit Social Media" where he makes the 13:50 minute case for why we should all unplug ourselves from social media, what the consequences of staying on SM could be, and how all areas of life tend to get better with less and less time on these platforms. It is highly recommended to check out this presentation!

Now, let's begin to take a closer investigation into what social media platforms actually are and the scientifically verified effects they have on our health and our overall wellbeing. The first thing to understand is SM is not essential or indispensable to any of our lives as most people want to believe. SM has use value as any relevant tool would provide it is used with intention and thoughtfulness. It's one thing if you are running an online business, have an online influential platform, or simply use it to share information with an online audience. There is nothing wrong with any of this and in fact these are powerful uses for these platforms for most people. However, the way in which the vast majority of people use SM is more reflective of exactly what these platforms are designed for and that is for entertainment purposes. SM is a source of entertainment for most people and as we discussed previously in this chapter, entertainment is a culturally appropriated way to hide the need to distract and avoid from our personal lives.

The most accurate entertainment comparison I could use to explain what social media does to our brain is slot machines you would find in a casino. There is comparable research done to show that our smart phones and social media alike function almost identically to how slot machines are designed to persuade patrons in casinos to keep pulling the lever. Social media platforms are being engineered and redesigned constantly, every day, to speed up the algorithms in a way that siphons the end user's attention and causes them to frequent the SM app as much as possible. This works on the repeated dopamine hit principle we've discussed so much in this book thus far. Increased views on a video, likes on a post, or better yet comments signaling engagement on our posts trigger this spark of dopamine and serotonin and then drop back off again. When we see that these response signals (likes, views, comments) are repeated it creates a form of positive reinforcement, triggers the release of dopamine which activates the reward centers in the brain, and creates the desire for repeatable behavior in the near future. And when I say near future, I mean like in the next few minutes or less!

Slot machines are designed to gamify this exact experience based on random number selection generation and the principle of uncertainty, along with the possibility of a reward. This principle is called a 'variable schedule of reward'. This means if someone pulls the lever and gets a winning combination, they just received a reward and are happy. Following that is likely to be a losing round at the slot machine, followed by a feeling of either disappointment or possible anticipation which leads to wanting to try again, and again, until they get that winning turn. They will ultimately get another winning round because that keeps the patron engaged and putting coins in the machine, but it will be sporadic and seemingly random in order to create uncertainty and further anticipation. But this is anything but random or uncalculated. Slot machines are highly precise in their design and run on their own algorithmic response patterns just like social media platforms do.

In the context of social media, it functions almost identically. If someone makes a post on their SM platform and depending on the content, time of the post, and the size of their following it will generate a certain type of response. This response runs on a variable of outcomes based on different factors but those factors aside, what is important is that it operates in the fashion of the slot machine research. If you post something and it lands with an audience thus generating a big response in the form of likes, comments, or views on a video then it encourages the person who posted it to do it again. The same brain chemical cocktail secretions are produced as are in the casino example, which leads to a reliance on positive reinforcement. People will tend to try to repeat the same thing they did to get that positive dopamine producing result and chances are the next time or two it will not have the same result. This causes a drop in dopamine from a failed expectation and a need to receive more positive reinforcement / reward sensation thus leading to making another post, and another post, and another post until they get the winning response.

Also, the more people that engage with our posts the more significance we may feel about ourselves. This is one of the ways social media is leveraged the most in order to create significance, identity, and meaningfulness in our lives. Some people have become so good at playing this game that they incite a regularity of drama, conflict, and triggering content in order to drive traffic to their pages, create dualistic engagement in their comment section, and get as much attention on them as possible. This is the tell-tale sign of the influencer culture gone to its ultimate extremes and there really is no good that will come from that in the long run. Not only does this kind of digital playground environment create more dopamine stimulation but it also stimulates more of the left brain, false identity ego that thrives on OPA (other people's attention). This may be the biggest trapping of social media all together and a booby trap that has full blown addiction written all over it.

Returning back to our casino comparison there is an astounding discovery I found in my research when looking a bit deeper into SM platforms such as Facebook, and how a decade ago (2009) they released an online platform app called Big Fish Casino, which is a virtual casino game on the Facebook platform that people pay real money to play a slot machine on their tablet or phone. They give you the first round of "chips" for free but after you run out (and you will!) you have to purchase more of these chips to keep playing, but the catch is that the game does not pay out any real money back to the players. So, they are paying to play a virtual game as an extension of the Facebook platform but there is absolutely no monetary reward involved. The only reward involved is the dopamine driven center in the brain that temporarily light up during the escalation of the game.

A woman named Kelly was interviewed about how she got obsessed with playing this game on her iPad tablet and according to her "I just couldn't stop." According to the news story she was planning for retirement with her husband and got hooked on this Facebook game and within the first month of playing it she had spent $8,000.00! After 9 months of downloading the game, she had spent more than $40,000.00!! Remember, you cannot cash back your chips in exchange for real money. There is no real money involved other than what the person is spending to play the game! This, my friend, is what an online digital addiction looks like and how sneaky it can really be. It starts out as something subtle and innocent but very soon can become an obsession that one cannot turn away form or turn off, much like the regular social media platforms themselves. According to expert's social media engineered casino games are 5 times as addictive as physical casino's which helps to reinforce the addictive nature of the virtual reality interface network and the SM platforms that occupy it.

Before we move on in this discussion, let's just understand one fundamental distillation from the slot machine - social media analysis. Slot machines based in casinos are designed for one purpose and one purpose only; to make money. They are money making machines that weaponize human psychology to trigger the exact formula within someone's brain that activates a down regulated impulse control and increases the formation of addiction-based patterning. What is social media? SM platforms are mega corporations that have stock being sold on the national market and have financial partners, which means it has a fiduciary responsibility to be and remain profitable as its primary objective. The currency of the online world is ending user's attention span and the more attention they can garner the more energy they can harvest in the form of people's spending habits which hare trackable using AI (artificial intelligence) algorithm patterns and self-select sponsorship advertisements accordingly. Just like slot machines, social media platforms are money making machines and are designed to reduce impulse control, lessen attention span, and form hard to break addiction patterns.

185

There is also a very real cognitive consequence of frequenting social media and that is a serious cognitive decline due to lowered brain health. One of the most pernicious downfalls of the social media age is the hyper increase in rates of reported cases of depression, feeling of social isolation, increase in persistent anxiety, brain fog, sleep disorders, and even suicide rates. In the journal of abnormal psychology over the past decade (2010-2020) there has been a 52% increase in depression and a 56% increase in suicide rate. These increases were tracked in correlation to the 45% of teenagers that say they're online constantly, either on a cell phone or computer, and most likely social media being the primary form of engagement. This is alarming to consider but not very surprising when we understand how penetrable our emotional brains really are to the effects of how social media impacts our psychology.

Perhaps the biggest impact it can have on most people who find themselves getting caught in cycles of aimless scrolling is how it distorts our perception of what is real and what is not. This is the same distortion all rogue elements of the VRIN produce but social media takes it to a completely different level. SM is interactive, dynamic, always changing, and invites direct engagement, whereas the projections coming from the entertainment or media industry are unidirectional, meaning one way, but do not allow for us to engage back with them. Social media allows everyone to become their own public relations agent, and in our current influencer culture where everyone has a voice and can create their own platform, this has a few problematic potentials.

When our perception of reality is distorted by a virtual simulation (virtual community) dynamic our real life can easily get lost in the process of presenting a curated version of our lives to others. We may find ourselves editing out certain aspects of our normal life and editing in others along with a nice caption to only showcase an ideal version of ourselves to the digital world. Our day-to-day real life is no longer all that interesting or pleasurable on its own, so we become far more invested in the altered version than in the authentic version. We may not like certain things about ourselves so we change our profile information in order to fit an idealistic description of who we would prefer to be, instead of who we really are. We may not like certain things about our body, our face, our skin, or however else we look so we may proceed to doctor up our pictures with filters or frame cropping. We end up doctoring up our overall life experience in order to feel good enough and socially accepted because we no longer feel good enough in the normality of our daily life.

People are constantly playing the comparison game on social media in a way that has become overblown and incredible unhealthy. It is said that comparison is the thief of joy and that is so right on. This is likely one of the main reasons social media can be a sink hole for negativity, drama, and insecurity. We can edit our posts, alter our appearance, doctor up our photos, change and rearrange our profile bio's, and friend as many people as we like but to what ends does it make our real lives any better or more satisfying?

What also comes along with this series of events is the alteration in one's own sense of identity and how the internet landscape as a whole can allow for the creation of sub-identities that form in direct proportion to the variety of social media platforms one is exposed too. Each platform has its own type of digital culture, unsaid rules and guidelines, and standards for conduct. Different communities form differently on different SM platforms and this all has a very real impact on the self-identity of the individual who uses them. People are becoming more identified with the groups of people they associate with online in many cases than the one's they do in real life. This is where the lines of reality and virtual reality becomes blurred and unrecognizable.

In addition to this there is another knock-on effect that social media and other online platforms contribute too, which is the deconstruction of human empathy. Empathy is the ability to connect with our fellow human beings and feel the emotional resonance between ourselves and them. This is what allows us to feel how others are feeling and without it we lose all sense of connection to others and also to ourselves. The rise in depression, suicide cases, and social isolation are all byproducts of this internet age where we are able to 'connect' with vast amounts of people every day but on an emotional level more and more people feel disconnected and out of touch more than ever before. Social media has a unique way of providing the virtual impression of human connection but unless the instant messenger text translates into getting on the phone or meeting up with people in person, then we lose a fundamental component of what makes us human, which is empathy.

When we see people blatantly attacking one another on chat forums, video comments, or Facebook posts we are seeing a complete absence of empathy and emotional connection. Empathy runs on neuro-circuits in the brain and these circuits are connected to the sensory neurons in the heart. There is a heart-brain connection we are designed with in order to empathize with other sentient beings and as this capability slowly erodes due to lack of authentic and real connection, we lose sense of how other people feel in relation to our actions or words towards them. People can say whatever they want on the internet with very little, if any, real life or at least immediate consequences which creates a false sense of security, confidence, and bravado. If some of these people said what they say on the internet in real life the immediate consequences would be quick and without question. When there is a virtual buffer in the way of human connection then there is no emotional empathy for the other person but an intensification of emotion by the individual themselves.

The very last point to drive in is the fact that social media and spending a ton of time on internet as a whole tends to be a massive time waster. It's reported that the average person checks their smart phone at least every 15 minutes but I would guess it's actually a lot more in reality. Again, our smart phones, as well as social media networks are set up in identical fashion as casino slot machines and they run on an attention allocation currency model. The more attention we give to it the more sponsorship money they receive, and the slower drip dopamine hits we receive as our reward for being good consumers. Is this really the kind of exchange we want to receive from this digital relationship? Are we really getting a solid ROI (return on investment) for our time, energy, and our money? Is it possible that spending more time on SM platforms and scrolling the internet has a net negative effect on our daily motivation, self-esteem, and sense of individuality? Well, the answer is an emphatic yes and due to the unconscious abuse of these virtual networks we have now made wasting time one of the biggest addictions in our entire generation.

In the upcoming chapter, towards the end of the book, **The Dopamine Reset | Reboot | Recovery Protocol** we will go through a series of protocols and strategies to take back your power as a holistic human being. This will include mind set frame works for approaching the dopamine recovery plan and please believe that abstaining from social media, whether temporarily or long term, is a major part in the success of this process. You can skip over to that section now if you are feeling that this may be the most important part for you to implement now and for many people this will likely be the case.

Pornography | Sexuality

"Pornography, by its very nature, is an equal opportunity toxin. It damages the viewer, the performer, and the spouses and the children of the viewers and the performers. It is toxic miseducation about sex and relationships. It is more toxic the more you consume."

Dr. Mary Anne Layden

We are just about at the halfway point of our journey together and we have covered a significant amount of territory thus far. What we have uncovered in the previous sections has been nothing short of a miracle in regard to identifying what truly holds us back in our lives, our overall health and wellness, our emotional development, and also taking a sober look at the self-sabotaging infractions that can easily play out in our daily lives, holding us back from our potential, and keeping us hostage from the pathways of freedom and recovery. I want to honor you for making it this far and acknowledge you for the courage it takes to make it on the road to self-mastery and beyond!

So, this leads us to a topic among all topics in the rolodex of addictions, and one that tends to reside below the surface of our awareness, whereas the others tend to get the front row and center stage position. Pornography, for many men in particular, is the great elephant in the room and the single hardest addiction to crack, where all else is rather child's play in comparison and contrast. Pornography rides in parallel to the virtual reality stimulatory addiction of entertainment, mainstream media, and social media but has far more intensified effects on its user and has a far greater grip of control than any of these other platforms could ever hope to have. If you ask 100 men over the age of 18 and well into their 40's what their single biggest struggle is. Something that no one else knows about. Something they hold a lot of guilt or shame around and cannot seem to break free from, what do you think they would say? Would it be alcohol? How about a social media obsession? No, I know! What about their ongoing obsession with staying up all night playing online role-playing video games until the morning hours? That last one may actually be very close but the vast majority of what you would hear back is none of these. My strongest assertion is that the biggest struggle most men find themselves in is a secret undisclosed relationship with online pornography.

A recently updated 2020 set of statistics showed that around 12% of webpages are pornographic sites. Although this number may appear small in scope it is the ease and immediacy of access that poses the biggest cause of concern. Anyone of any age has the same availability of access to pornography as the next person and there is no legitimate gatekeeper ensuring that the end user is a consenting adult or a curious adolescent or even a pre-pubescent child. As most other addiction-based consumer habits and socially accepted drugs/substances in our manufactured culture, pornography has become a truly devastating weapon of mass distraction, of the likes that its effects on all forms of psychological development, brain health, intimacy and sexuality, and impulse regulation are only now being discovered. These scientific and anecdotal discoveries are not trivial by any means. In fact, they are truly alarming and pose a very real concern for the overall developmental progress of the human race, so long as high-speed pornography remains easily accessible, socially acceptable, and is the primary youth education for human sexuality.

Allow me to share some recent staggering statistics with you so we have a better grasp on a certain reality that is occurring underneath our veil of awareness. These stats were derived from an article called Pornography Facts and Statistics, by The Recovery Village, editor Megan Hull.

- 25% of search engine requests are related to sex
- 35% of downloads from the internet are pornographic
- 40 million Americans say they regularly visit porn sites
- 70% of men aged 18 to 24 visit a porn site at least once per month
- The largest consumer group of online porn is men between the ages of 35 and 49
- One-third of all internet porn users are women
- Sunday is the most popular day of the week for viewing porn
- Thanksgiving is the most popular day of the year for viewing porn

These are interesting statistics to say the least and there are plenty more we can drum up to make a certain point, but this is more than enough to gain a greater awareness of the situation. As we go deeper into this subject it will become more apparent what the conclusive effects of pornography are, whether someone is a periodic user or has a full-blown addiction, as some experts say, spends at least 11-12 hours each week viewing porn. Whether smaller amounts of exposure or frequent exposure, it is important to note that this is not one of those things any reasonable health inclined expert can recommend moderation where addiction is concerned. There is no moderate amount of pornography that is actually non-threatening to an individual's overall development as a functional human being. And there is certainly no amount that could ever be considered healthy or safe for exposure and I will proceed to explain why this is.

Some people may consider what I am saying a bit extreme or over dramatic. After all, we have all been exposed, in some degree, to internet pornography or video tapes growing up. For most teenage boys (and many women as I understand) pornography has become the primary sex education exposure they (we) have received and was the first model for what sexuality looked like and how it was supposed to be approached. We will wait to discuss the neurological consequences of porn exposure and further explore the effects it has on the developing brains of young boys and also the young girls who are affected by this as well. What I am explaining only appears to be an overreaching attempt to pose the extreme negatives of pornography, up until one see's the scientific proof of what someone's brain on porn looks like. When you see that porn, like all long-standing addictions, whether that be to our smart phones, our alcohol, our excessive caffeinated drinks, or pharmaceutical medications, have a very real and significant impact on the structure and functionality of our malleable brains.

I am not only communicating from the stance of a research educator and health expert here. I am first and foremost communicating from the position of a fully developed man who at one point had his own struggles and tussles with what could be described as a porn addiction, paired with a sex addiction. Whether or not I would personally describe my problem as a full-blown addiction is irrelevant because addiction lives on a spectrum and one person's moderation is another person's obsessive-compulsive disorder (OCD). Some of us may simply be higher functional addicts in some areas and complete train wrecks in others. In my case, I could consider myself, at this phase of my maturation into adulthood as a highly functional, highly intelligent, highly composed sexually obsessed, porn using individual. If, however, I had enough alcohol in me at this time in my life I would be a total mess, unable to operate in public, and basically just a disaster. The effects of alcohol in my case would have been very obvious, whereas the frequent use of pornography and the chronic over visualization of sex were not obvious to others but becoming more apparent to myself.

It took a while for the effects to become totally obvious but obvious they did become and by that time it had become such a powerful associative pattern that it was easier to ignore than it was to walk away from. I will share a very personal story of how this pornographic rabbit hole caused me to ruin the first real relationship I was in in the section **A Replacement for True Intimacy.** Moving aside from that for now what I would like to detail is the common manifestations of co-disorders that seem to accompany increased porn use. Each of these I have also experienced, whether directly or indirectly, in combination or as a byproduct of frequent pornography exposure. These include social anxiety, existential anxiety, depression, mood imbalances, obsession with sex, substance or drug abuse, memory problems (this is a big deal!), chronic tobacco smoking, and the most alarming for men which is erectile dysfunction. This last one is known as PIED which is short for Porn Induced Erectile Dysfunction. There is a tremendous amount of science and personal testimonial worldwide about the effects that porn has had on men's libido, sperm count quality, and ability to get it up. This is a by-product of both excessive ejaculation and over stimulation of porn inducted imagery via dopamine receptor burnout. This will be explained in more detail in the sections **Your Brain on Porn** and **Seminal Retention & Masturbation.**

Let's try to understand that internet-based pornography is an augmented virtual reality simulation of a hyper-sexualized experience arising from a holographic projection field. The hologram itself is the computer screen i.e., the virtual reality interface network we discussed in the prior chapter. The projection field is the imagery that is being received by the end user and projected outward from the holographic medium i.e., the computer, phone, or tablet. The experience that the end user is having is their own biological, psychological, and emotional interpretation based on the intensified stimulation of the imagery being projected forth. The neuroscience of this phenomena will be explained more in the section **Your Brain on Porn** but let's focus on the fact that what is being experienced is nothing more than an augmented interpretation of reality rather than an accurate version of reality. The most accurate interpretation of this scenario is that someone is on their computer, likely touching themselves, scrolling on a porn website, watching videos or viewing pictures, and is feeling a cascading effect of pleasure stimulation leading up to the climax of an intense yet solo sexual experience.

The reality is very different than the psycho-biological interpretation of the intensified experience itself. Because of the neurochemistry being activated in such an accelerated way and the heightened arousal state our body and brain cannot distinct fact from fiction. Our brain can interpret the experience as if we, ourselves are the one's having the sexual experience rather than simply watching other people on video recording being projected from a screen having it. This is what I mean when I say pornography is a form of augmented virtual reality because it places the end user into a chemical responsive position to initiate the same sensations of those in the video. This becomes a problem when our bodies become dependent on this kind of sensory input and although our conscious mind knows the difference, our unconscious mind (and biology) does not. If you thought a social media addiction, video game marathons, or binge-watching Netflix movies could become a problem, then internet pornography takes it to a whole other level.

The difference with pornography and sex addiction in general is that it is an intense spike in heightened states of arousal, sometimes very extreme highs but after a man ejaculates it's over and done, right? Wrong! This is the appearance of the cycle but in fact it remains long after the moment of completion and because it is so easily accessible it's easily repeatable and the next urge is only around the corner. What tends to follow the heightened sensations is a drop in self-esteem, self-respect, and feelings of either/or both guilt and shame begin creeping up. This is one of the most common reported feelings upon climaxing from pornography, especially if it has become a repetitive habit and the person feels they have a problem with it. I know for me I had experienced this repeatedly and knew I had a problem but for some reason I did not allow myself to feel the feelings of shame or guilt long enough to not repeat the behavior again. The immediate sensations of pleasure and gratification feel so good and so overwhelming that it's easy to push our moral or ethics to the side, because after all, we aren't hurting anybody. They are only actors on the screen playing an agreed upon part for our personal enjoyment, right?

I'll spare all of us a lecture on the morality or lack thereof when it comes to pornography or any addiction cycle for that matter. That is not my role here and it would be hypocritical to do so but what is important is to notice the self-critic that arises in moments where our moral compass has gone astray. This indicates that we are engaging in something that we know at our core is not in alignment with our values and goes against our true character. What many people do not take the time to inner stand about this whole thing is that pornography is not just watching other people having sex (at varying degrees of demoralizing the female usually) but it is also entraining the user to adopt the same patterns and begin seeing the opposite gender through the lenses of pornography. We can call this pornographic perception or having the porn goggles on too tight. This is where we begin to perceive those of the opposite sex as sexual objects rather than simply seeing them as human beings.

The well-known actor Terry Crews had gone public a number of years ago about an incident that had happened to him at a Hollywood party full of producers and staff. He was sexually assaulted by someone in a high position and was expected to laugh it off, as if nothing had happened. In Hollywood circles sexual harassment and assault is actually very common. It is actually more or less the norm as we have discovered with people like Harvey Weinstein and others who have been exposed for their abusive conduct. This caused Terry to go public about what was happening in the industry but in addition to this incident Terry also went public about a long-standing porn addiction that he had kept a secret from the world and from his wife. He has done a series of brilliant and transparent videos on his experience from porn addiction, how it almost cost him his family, how it affected his career, and how extreme this addiction could go without anyone else knowing it but him. In one of his videos, he said something so profound and so telling of how pornography can alter our perception of reality and mistreat others without us ever physically abusing anyone. Terry said "the problem with porn is that people become body parts. People become things to be used instead of people to be loved."

Porn uses people, just like all addictions do, and once someone is used up, they are disposable and it's off to the next one and the next one. We have to be very careful about how we are entraining our minds and the pattern recognition signaling that our brain is being normalized towards. Once a pattern begins to entrain itself in the neuropathways of our brain and synchronizes with the formation of dendritically connections it becomes extremely difficult to break that pattern and establish healthier brain connections. If this was not the case than it would not be difficult at all to reroute our ingrained behaviors and due to low resolution high intensification stimulation like the virtual pornography augmentation experience, we see an entire generation of boys in men's bodies suffering silently from over pleasuring themselves, to the point of losing all of their virility, motivation for growth, and masturbating all of their life potential away at the edge of a keyboard and computer screen.

This is a good place to pause on this stream of thought and allow it to take residency in your mind. This is one of the more important and urgent messages in this book among many others. We are now going to move into the deeper regions of this discussion by first exploring the neuroscience of pornography and how our brains are impacted, both in physical structure and the rewiring of chemical signaling. This will be very eye opening, if it has not been already and I hope it helps all of us awaken from the porn induced slumber our youth culture has been spell bound under for decades.

Your Brain on Porn

"In particular, a great deal of recent research suggests that the more that people's reward systems are tuned to forming social connections with others, the more likely they are to be both more physically healthy and more psychologically well balanced. This is what makes internet pornography addiction so troubling. It represents a tuning of the reward system from a very healthy type of reward,

*that of forming a genuine and intimate connection with
another, into a type of reward that removes the user from
social contact, and often leaves them feeling lonely and
ashamed rather than connected and supported."*

*Gary Wilson, Your Brain on Porn: Internet Pornography
and the Emerging Science of Addiction*

As mentioned previously, the effects of internet pornography are wide ranging but none so damaging as the consequences it has on the structural integrity and chemical signaling of our brains. Like all addictive patterns our brains tend to receive the brunt of the effects due to all of the hyper stimulation and excessive processing that takes place. The interpretation of the repeatability of a hyper-pleasurable experience in the brain is often times much different than the reality of the experience itself. This can cause the brain to become entrained into seeking to repeat that experience as much as it can in order to re-experience the quick burst of dopaminergic sensations. The associative patterning process begins to link the habit + the sensation of pleasure together and in order to experience another short burst of a dopaminergic wave the action is called upon immediately. This is when we feel the urge build up inside of us and when we try to suppress this urge, we experience tension thus an inner conflict arises and either the urge wins out or the discipline wins out. In most cases, we know which one tends to win out, especially when it comes to a stimulus as powerful as our sexual urge and as easily accessible as punching in a search engine and relieving ourselves on the spot.

All of these patterns we have played out have been recorded, synthesized, and grooved into the software programming of our central processor called our brain. The challenging thing about addressing an addictive pattern such as pornography that has been so well established in the transcription of our brain is that our brain knows our strengths and it knows our weaknesses. We try to exercise will power, discipline, and self-restraint to the best of our abilities. We may find ourselves successful in many cases, feeling more inspired, capable, and empowered. Eventually though, we might find ourselves relapsing in a moment of weakness, caving in on our commitment to recovery, and not really sure why we gave in so easily. This can be very frustrating to experience and feel like there's no way out of this addiction cycle.

This is why will power and discipline are only half of the equation. We also have to become more intelligent in regard to how our brains have been trained to want and need pornography (or any addiction) and have literally rewired themselves to seek out immediate pleasurable stimulation instead of postponing temporary pleasure for longer term fulfillment. The conscious mind understands this basic premise all too well, but the unconscious mind and the software formatting of the addicted brain are not working in accordance together and here lies the fundamental problem. We must use our power of will and discipline to retrain our brain patterns and the rest of the body will also follow along. Once people begin to get a better understanding of how the brain works, how it has been negatively affected by addiction, and are provided some tools to heal their brain or reroute the neuro-associative patterns they become empowered. Confidence comes from understanding and understanding leads to better results. So, let's begin to take a closer look at what happens when our brains are exposed to pornography and then how we can begin working our way back to cognitive recovery.

It is important to know that the human brain does not fully mature or develop until around the age of 25. It was commonly thought that our brains went through a period of explosive growth and development only in our juvenile (pre-adolescent) years and eventually balanced out becoming more or less fixed in place from there on out. As with most outdated scientific conceptions we are constantly learning new discoveries and putting old theories to rest. If this prior theory were correct that our brains remain fixed in place and do not alter much after a certain point than it's theoretically probable to say that porn exposure, after a certain age would not pose much threat or concern to the development of our cognitive faculties or overall health of our brain. This of course is not the case though and it is extremely well established that our brains are very malleable, flexible, and take on a plastic like adaptability which is known as neuroplasticity.

Neuroplasticity is the brains' ability to reorganize itself based on the exposure to new information, movement patterns, or external stimuli which allows for the formation of new neural connections over an entire lifetime. The brain has the ability to undergo biological changes and neuronal adaptations which can also significantly impact what is known as the brains cortical remapping process. A cortical map can be understood as a sensory mapping system that connects a part or parts of the brain to certain regions of the body and allows for the nerve-to-nerve communication from end to end to take place. The firing of our toes triggers the activation of another point in the body just as the firing of our fingers can trigger another. Through the activity of our lives and all of the information that is accumulated through our direct experience a cortical map is developed within the brain's processing station and this serves as the repository of stored data from brain to body and body to brain.

The brain's built-in mapping of the overall body system is constantly being updated through novel and unique patterns of behavior, thinking outside the box, and challenging old information. The challenge is when we get ourselves into familiar old comfort zones and stop challenging ourselves. This is when it appears that our brains do not have any more adaptable qualities left but this just means we are out of practice and need to begin exercising our innate neuroplastic abilities.

In order to overcome the old programming of pornographic addiction we must begin to develop a new sensory mapping sequence for the brain. This means we need to upgrade our brains entirely and do away with the outdated pre-programmed information that was based in reaction patterns to tension, stress, and overwhelm. This is what it means to upgrade the operating system of our brain to body (and body to brain) communication feedback loop. If we can upgrade our super processor (the brain) and retrain the signaling patterns of the neuron circuitry we can essentially become a brand-new version of ourselves.

When the brain has become well-adjusted to addiction it is operating in reactionary impulses instead of responsive solutions. This repeated pattern of operating, due to neuroplasticity, informs the cortical map i.e., the operating system and entrains the brain to react based on compulsive repetition. The brain is an organ but responds very much like a muscle. It will develop itself in whatever way it is exercised and utilized. So, with this understanding we can begin to see how the repetition of compulsive habits such as pornography create a neurological adaptation which eventually overloads the brain with pleasure and reward sensations thus creating the addicted brain condition. If neuroplasticity can alter our brain in ways that can become detrimental and lead to addiction through unconscious behavior, it can also be leveraged to improve our brain condition and to heal ourselves through conscious effort.

It is beyond a reasonable doubt that frequent exposure to porn can be compared to any other substance drug addiction. The neuroscience on this has become extremely clear and soberingly real. The long-term consequences of porn use are not as immediate or even obvious as something like excessive alcohol consumption, crack cocaine, heroin, excess caffeine, or even indulging in a junk food binge. These examples provide relatively immediate feedback as to the effects they are having on our body and brain. Pornography on the other hand does not provide this same kind of feedback and it's only when we begin to experience the loss of cognitive focus, short term memory loss, sleep instability, loss of vital energy, or the inability to form a consistent erection with a real-life partner, that it catches our full attention. This is why it has become a point of focus for alternative health care professionals and scientists to conduct brain imaging scans to identify what is actually happening in the porn addicted brain.

Dr. Valerie Voon, who is a top neuroscientist from Cambridge University, is one of the top researchers on the neuroscience of addiction. Her and her team conducted a breakthrough study using brain imaging scans to identify the effects on the brain of individuals who believed they had a serious problem with pornography. The study was conducted following a nationwide search of twenty men ages 19-34 who claimed that their lives were being controlled by porn which is why they volunteered to participate in the study. This group of men had their brain scans compared to another group of healthy men who did not report problems with pornography. The brain scan was done through an MRI screening to test for functional brain activity and to see what regions of the brain were affected abnormally.

During this MRI brain imaging scan, they exposed the test group to scenes from porn videos to see how their brains responded and if they showed identical signs to those of other drug addictions. An interesting finding in these tests where that although the group of healthy men had excitation (excitement) occur in their brains, as one may expect, the group

200

of heavily exposed men had twice as much excitation light up in the ventral striatum of their brain. This is the heart of the pleasure center in our brain, and it elicits the exact same response in these men as does in those heavily addicted to substances such as nicotine, alcohol, and cocaine. The reward networks in porn users seem to explicitly light up in anticipation to the porn through signaling cues, engaging in the porn, and also prioritizing the porn. Multiple aspects of the brains pleasure, reward, and anticipation networks were all hyper activated thus causing a tunnel vision prioritization of the experience being simulated by the stimulus in the brain.

This is a documented, empirical, scientific showcase of what happens when the pleasure/reward network of the brain becomes hijacked by porn and takes over the operating system of the body. According to Dr. Simone Kuhn, who is a neuroscientists and psychology from the Max Planck Institute for Human Development in Berlin, the grey matter held within the pleasure/reward centers of the brain is typically much smaller than that of individuals who do not have compulsive porn exposure. She stated in an interview you can find on the internet called **Experts Talk about the Effects of Porn on the Brain** that she expected the ventral striatum in the pleasure centers to be twice as big in porn users, but it is actually the exact opposite. Grey matter in the brain is a simply defined as unmyelinated neurons and other cells within the central nervous system. It is concentrated in the brain, brainstem, cerebellum, and throughout the spinal cord. This material contains most of the brains neuronal cells and is directly involved in motor function, muscle control, sensory perception (eyesight, hearing) as well as memory, emotional processing, speech patterns, executive decision making, and self-control/self-regulation.

We have already discussed in a myriad of ways how pornography addiction can detrimentally effect motor function and neuromuscular control via dopamine receptor depletion and adrenal exhaustion. There have always been suggestions that excessive ejaculation for men could lead to worsen eyesight, cognitive focus, short term memory, emotional instability, poor decision making, and problem self-regulating one's urges/compulsions. It seems all of this is true but it most likely is a dual effect of excessive ejaculation (we will discuss this in detail) as a byproduct of hyper-visual stimuli from highly frequent exposure to porn. If this is not an eye-opening discovery for us all, especially all men, then I do not know what else could be.

The shrinkage in the grey matter of the brain is also due to the fact that once someone has become normalized to their addiction, they require far more of it to enact the original effect. This means their biological tolerance to pornography has gone up and they need to amplify the stimulation in order to experience the same response they were getting from less of it or lesser intense versions of it. The increase in frequency of porn in combination with the more exaggerated or intensified versions of it (or more time spent on it) seems to have a neurodegenerative effect on the brain. The brain was once more adapted to the stimulus of porn but now it has developed a maladaptive condition where it is now in a chemical addiction loop that is destructive and has no upside to it. To drive this point one step further, these individuals are committing acts of violence onto themselves and killing off essential neurons (and other brain cells) that protect them from the effects of age associated neurodegenerative disease.

If this was not enough to take in let's also point out that brain imaging scans have also been conducted to show that there are changes within the structure of our delicate brain that can form due to pornography (and many other addictions). Remember, due to neuroplasticity everything we do each day has an effect on our brain chemistry, brain signaling, and brain structure. If we watch porn every day, we are training our brain in a specific way to process the pornography we are watching which will eventually exclude out other neurological processes leading to imbalances in the functionality of our brain itself.

Dr. Simone Kuhn, PHD conducted a study in Germany involving 64 men between the ages of 21-45 who watched an average of four hours of porn per week. Like in the previous study by Dr. Voon these men were put through MRI scans while being exposed to a mixture of sexual images and non-sexual images. Dr. Kuhn states, *"Our findings indicated that gray matter volume of the right caudate of the striatum is smaller with higher pornography use,"* The author of the article Fight the New Drug state in response to this finding; *"the researchers wrote in the journal article, referring to an area of the brain associated with reward processing and motivation. Men who watched more porn also showed less activity in another area of the striatum, called the left putamen, which usually lights up in response to sexual images."* It was also discovered that heavily exposed porn users had a noticeably weaker connectivity between the striatum and the prefrontal cortex, which is largely responsible for decision making and is known as the executive center of the brain.

This shows the neurological association to excessive porn use and the diminishment of personal motivation, will power, and increasingly poor decision making. This helps to explain the consistent reporting of memory loss, decline in focus, loss of motivation, and most specifically the combination of poor decision making and reduced impulse control. Many more studies have been done up to this point in similar fashion and all of them circle back around to the same basic premise. A porn users' brain can become and as shown in these studies often times is virtually identical to that of a more overt drug addict's brain. They work along all the same circuit boards of electrical activity and the reduction of executive function leading to the same slippery slope of cognitive decline and neurodegenerative risk.

Now we are going to discuss one of the most important topics, particularly for men, which is the necessity to begin mastering our sexual energy. The practices of seminal retention through abstaining from compulsive masturbation, whether porn induced or otherwise, is an essential act of self-discipline, self-respect, and self-development. It is also an essential part of rerouting the dopamine pleasure centers in the brain, establishing hormonal and adrenal balance, and overriding the hyper sexualized mind through pornographic programming.

Seminal Retention & Masturbation

> *"The reabsorption of the seminal fluid back into the blood is the best nutrition your body can ever get. So, control your lust and do not waste seminal fluid for short term pleasures."*
>
> *Prateek Kohli*

Now that we have thoroughly explored the short term and long-term effects of pornography, its time discuss the empowerment process of recovery. It is one thing to abstain from the visual exposure of pornographic entertainment, which in of itself has profound benefits in the healing process. The removal of pornography will allow the brain to reestablish the chemical balance and neurological signaling that it has been negatively impacted from. The pornographic programming has to also be addressed because the imagery and visual imprinting of porn has left its mark and must be cleared from the nervous system. However, just because we remove (or attempt to remove) the visual stimulus that signals the intense urge to engage in the activity does not mean we are fully freed up from the source of the addiction itself. This process requires a dual commitment. One of which is to remove the pornographic trigger itself and also to engage with the impulsivity that exists within the body as well.

This message is obviously geared towards men and as a man, I am writing with men who would read this in mind. We have discussed in detail the many damaging effects of short-term leading to long term pornography but that is only one side of this overall equation. The next part we must address is what we do as a reaction to the triggering in the body that porn provides. This may prove to be the most important chapter in this book for many men and this section may be the most useful for the simple fact that if we can master our sexual urges and practice what is known as 'sexual transmutation' than all other addictive tendencies lose their hold on us and we become far more empowered than ever before. As men, it is absolutely essential we learn to gain mastery over, not only our minds, but also over our sexuality. The ability to direct our life forces energy where we so choose is the power that births lives, creates worlds, and if uncontrolled it can also have the equivalent destructive counter force effect.

It is very important that I preface this with the understanding that in no way, shape or form is there any elements of shame involved in this conversation. Through our cultural conditioning sexuality has become distorted, exploited, monetized, and made to be something we both desire yet feel some degree of shame around. The only time one feels shame around their sexuality is when it has been perverted, such is the case with pornographic conditioning and the shame involved is what holds the addiction in place. When we are able to release all energies of shame, guilt, jealousy, and self judgement we begin to liberate ourselves to explore healthy forms of sexuality, with ourselves and especially with our partners. This segment is not so much about abstaining from doing something i.e., masturbation as much as it is about mastering the urge that leads to selling ourselves short in exchange for short term pleasure thus missing out on long term satisfaction and happiness.

With that said, let's be candid and straight forward about this topic. There is a plethora of reasons someone would choose to abstain from frivolous masturbation sessions. There is nothing wrong with 'self-pleasure' or even exercising any kind of tension or pressure that we may experience in this way. It really just depends on whether someone is in the recovery and healing process from excess exposure to porn and/or has developed an ongoing habit of masturbation that has weakened their health and wellbeing. When I was growing up, I was under the impression that there were no negative effects of frequent masturbation. In fact, it was heavily encouraged and just considered to be a very normal and natural part of "exploring" my body following the onset of puberty. This seems innocent enough but when I think back on those formative years, I realize that I never received any legitimate education on sexual development outside of teenage boys getting together to look at porn magazines and the one mediocre sex ed class I received from my gym teacher in seventh grade. I, like so many others, had to basically wing it and what was considered normal back then feels very unfulfilling and dissatisfying now as an adult man.

It was never explained or even considered that as men our seminal fluids had a significant source of concentrated nutrients, micronutrients, stem cells, immune cells, and other ingredients that play a major role in all biological functions of the body and directly aid in our longevity potential. In the Hindu Ayurvedic medicine system, it is said that it takes 40 drops of blood to make a drop of bone marrow and it takes 40 drops of bone marrow to make a drop of semen. I have seen some estimates that our sperm supply is replenished at least every 64 days. This is assumed that we are taking very good care of ourselves, eating right, exercising, and have a moderate to low stress lifestyle. As we go get older, say into our early thirties and early forties our bodies go through major changes hormonally and we can seem to lose some of the seeming "invincibility" we felt in our prime youth years. Because of the lack of awareness and education on this topic we tend to blow through our youth and have to pay for it once we get a bit older and are slowed down by the reality of time.

There are a lot of perspectives and pieces of information I could interweave into this discussion, but I want to focus primarily on the connection between addiction and total health recovery. What I will say is that there is a ton of great information on this topic for further exploration and research. Seminal retention as a lifestyle practice is taught in the Chinese Taoist healing arts where a man's seed(semen) is considered the apex of his life force potential and there are entire teachings around mastering sexuality in pursuit of maintaining our vital life force without wasting it or leaking what is known as our 'jing' which also is a loose translation of life force potential. The world's authority on this subject Mantak Chia wrote many books on sexual alchemy including **The Multi Orgasmic Man** which you may find fascinating and useful.

The thing to remember about this portion of our overall discussion is that it's not so much about whether someone chooses to masturbate or not. Again, there is no shame involved in this. This is really much more about rerouting the patterns and pathways that have been set up in our brain and regaining control over our urges. When pornography is involved it sends a wildfire of cascading chemicals throughout the nervous system and can make it virtually impossible to restrain self-control for most men who would otherwise be able to change their attention to something else. Once this hyper stimulus is removed then all we have left is the activity itself of releasing tension or inner pressure through ejaculation. The ejaculatory process itself is really where we need to develop a certain boundary or self-regulation around because that is where our weakness for quick pleasure is. Let me explain something you already know deep down inside.

The awkward feelings of shame and guilt that can arise on the back end of a masturbation session, most notably in combination with pornography, happens for a few reasons. There is the aspect of demoralizing and dehumanizing others which is what porn does to people. It is objectifying them, particularly the woman, and turning them into a pleasure-based object. There is also a much deeper reason for this, and it is a source point for the dramatic increase of low self-esteem, low confidence, low self-respect, and decline in motivation amongst men worldwide. What I am about to tell you is potentially uncomfortable to receive but if we are honest with ourselves, deep down inside we know it to be the truth. When we ejaculate in order to pass the time, distract ourselves from our problems, avoid issues in our lives, or simply to experience heightened states of momentary pleasure we are unknowingly exchanging our most valuable biological resources for the fleeting experience we receive from it.

The reason low self-worth and lowered self-respect are almost indispensable associations with long term porn users is because when we engage in this, we are literally giving ourselves away. We are allowing our most vital inner resources to be wasted and spent without ever receiving anything of any true worth in return. In a lot of ways this is the identical experience of all forms of addiction, but porn may be the most notorious and dangerous for how it alters our brain and psycho-emotional condition over time. Take porn out of the equation, the ejaculation practice becomes less about seeking short term pleasure sensations and more about building up the life force potential that is stored in our concentrated seminal fluids. I know we all learned this lesson in junior high but it's worth remembering that a man's semen is designed for one purpose and one purpose only; to create a baby. Think about that the next time you feel the impulsive urge to simply let it out because you are bored or do not want to deal with your emotions in that moment.

When we, as men, make it common place to ejaculate our seminal fluids what we are actually doing is releasing the life-giving force of nature that exists within us. In recent years an entire movement online has sparked up called the Nofap movement which basically means abstaining from masturbation. The accounts of countless men who have decided to take back their power by simply not giving into this urge and redirecting their energy into other focuses is astounding. The common reporting of men feeling more energized, more motivated, more confident, more focused, and more capable of pursuing their goals is worth anyone's investigation. Coupling this with the knowledge we now know about the health benefits of retaining our seed and resisting the urge to release shows us how powerful this practice can be. There is a direct and accurate correlation between excess ejaculation and loss of mental focus, memory retention, emotional instability, and physical energy production. There is also a direct correlation between abstaining from masturbation and increased physical stamina, endurance, cognitive function, and sustained happiness and confidence.

"The individuals of greatest achievement tend to be those who have highly developed sexual natures and who have learned the art of sex transmutation."

Napoleon Hill

As men we have become conditioned to seek out pleasure as a way to compensate for the inner tension, we experience daily and because we may not have been provided the tools to handle the pressure of life therefore, we rely upon ejaculation to take the edge off. The greatest tool we have for self-mastery can also be used to diminish our ability to master ourselves and that is the crux of what all addiction cycles are really about. In Napoleon Hill's classic book, **Think and Grow Rich** he discusses one of the most powerful attributes among highly successful men which is what we now know as 'sexual transmutation. Consider some of the wise words he shared in his investigations of the most accomplished individuals he studied which allowed him to arrive at his conclusions. *"One major reason why the majority of people who succeed do not begin to do so before the age of 40 or 50 is their tendency to dissipate their energies through overindulgence in the physical expression of the emotion of sex."* He is letting us know that success in life is not dependent on age but due to the excess of focusing on sex earlier in our lives we simply misdirect our most powerful force of energy and motivation until we no longer are being run by our base desires.

He also shares some brilliant perspectives on the power of our sexual energy and what is possible when we learn to harness it through self-mastery. *"Transmutation of sex energy calls for more willpower than the average person cares to use for this purpose. Though this requires willpower, the reward for the practice is more than worth the effect."* Transmutation is a term that derives from the ancient alchemical teachings which is the process of converting base metals into noble metals in terms of chemistry and mineralogy. This also means the ability to convert or transform lower energies into higher energies, negative thoughts into positive thoughts, and lower emotions such as shame or guilt into higher emotions such as appreciation and fulfillment. The transmutation of old patterns into new patterns is the core of all transformational work and the greatest force for change is in the procreative energies we possess that are often experienced as sexual attraction or sexual tension.

The inner tension that arises is not simply something we need to do away with or an unsettling feeling we need to remedy. It is a point of focus that we can use for our growth and to help us pour more energy into our goals. It becomes increasingly hard to maintain this kind of practice if we do not have anything we are striving towards and that is often times where the problem resides. We can easily use our sexual urges as a replacement for more worthwhile goals and aspirations for our life. When we become crystal clear on what we want to achieve and experience in our lives then it becomes increasingly easier to override these temporary impulses and redirect that energy into the pursuits that are most meaningful. This way we no longer find any desire to waste this precious energy on fleeting moments of discomfort or heightened stimulation. We now become more committed to utilizing this vital resource for what it is designed for which is maximizing life force energy, procreation, and sharing with our real-life partners (instead of the digital fantasies).

"So, I say, if you are burning, burn. If you can stand it, the shame will burn away and leave you shining, radiant, and righteously shameless."

Elizabeth Cunningham

A Replacement for Real Intimacy

"We can't fill up our eyes with our wives if our eyes have been previously filled with someone else. One of the many dangers of porn is that it neurologically trains us to find our wives less beautiful."

Gary Thomas

Alright friend, now that we have effectively traversed through the layers of the pornographic onion and its role in a much deeper addiction than is commonly on the surface, it's time to address what is really underneath it all. We have discussed the various damaging effects that porn can play in a human's life, including the effects it has on our psychology, our brain health, our overall physical health, and how it sets us back from being the kind of person we know we can be without it. Now, we have to go into the heart of the matter and explore what has been blocked up due to pornography and mismanagement of our sexual energies. We get to explore true intimacy, with ourselves, and with our partners.

In my research I stumbled across a website: (husbandhelphaven.com/porn-statistics/) that showcased a wide variety of statistics about porn. The first thing I saw when I went to this site was a statistic that said, "as you're reading this, there are 30,000 people watching porn right now in the US." Following that it said *"40 million US adults admit to regularly visiting mature websites. Only 200,000 of those, or 1 out of 200, believe they're addicted to porn."* I immediately thought to myself; I wonder how many of these people are married men or men in intimate monogamous relationships. I do not mean to inappropriately generalize men as the only people who visit pornography, because that's not true but there is a very real problem with infidelity in our culture and not all infidelity is physical sexual intercourse with another person. I would assume the vast majority of infidelity is done through way of pornographic fantasies or mental projections that go outside of the boundaries of the relationship.

As I continued my research, I came across a set of statistics regarding porn use in marriage and this is a real eye opener.

"How is porn use impacting otherwise healthy marriages? What happens in a relationship where one partner looks at porn?"

- When one spouse is using porn, 68% of couples report a decrease in their sex life.

- In 68% of divorces, one spouse has met a new lover over the Internet.

- In 56% of divorces, at least one spouse has an "obsessive interest in porn."

- 75% of the time, a spouse's porn viewing will be discovered on accident.

- 70% of wives who've discovered their husband's porn addiction display signs of Post-Traumatic Stress Disorder.

Without elaborating any deeper on any one statistic it should go without saying that there is a seriously underlining issue in our culture and there seems to be a lot of confusion about it. It is often assumed that now a day's monogamous relationships are outdated, and marriage is designed to fail due to the increase in divorce rates over the years. This is how the modern-day mindset has been trained to think. See a symptom, point fingers at the symptom, run all of the numbers regarding the symptom, and blame the symptom for the problem without investigating deeply into what caused the symptom and how did the symptom manifest itself in the first place. Are monogamous relationships really to blame or is there something really wrong with our culture itself that has influenced the outcomes of these relationships or marriages ending, in sometimes catastrophic separations.

I will let you think deeper on those questions, but one thing is for absolute sure and that is we have a serious issue with the one thing that ensures a healthy relationship which is transparent and connected intimacy. Pornography creates a situation where one partner is literally living a double life. They are the person they are when they are with their partner and then they are someone else when they are with themselves. When we are hiding secrets from our partner than we are planting seeds of destructivity within the relationship. We may think that we don't have a problem and it's not a big deal but trust me, that is only the wounded ego speaking. It is a problem and will become a very big deal, if it has not become one already. The entire point of being in a relationship is companionship, mutual respect, mutual trust, and devotion to supporting each other in this thing called life. If there is no transparency, then there will be little trust and if there is little trust involved then there will be little to no respect once the boiling point reaches its limit.

At the end of the day, an intimate relationship, where there is healthy sexual polarity, comes down to the vulnerability and trust. The word intimacy has commonly been translated into into-me-see. It is through our closest relationships that we are better able to see ourselves and through these reflections we can better navigate the inner journey, if we so choose, that is. If something like pornography is involved or even casual social media scrolling to check out other people, then we are subduing the quality of intimacy in our relationship as a way to avoid looking deeper into ourselves. If we cannot trust ourselves with ourselves, then how can we expect our partners to fully trust us either? We have to be willing to let go of the distractions and avoidance mechanism so we can begin to access our true vulnerability. Vulnerability is where true power resides, but we have to earn its power and the only way to do that is to let go of our defense patterns that block us from feeling and be felt.

I would like to share a personal story with you that has come up for me during this writing process. When I was in my early twenties, I met the first real love in my life and formed a 3-year relationship with her, along with her two children. We had an amazing relationship together for the better part of the three years and for the first time in my life I was starting to settle into the idea of settling down and starting a family. There were no conceivable issues on the surface of our relationship but at some point, in the relationship my imagination began to drift into the realms of periodic pornographic programming. I remember working in the emergency room of a large hospital and for whatever reason I found myself fantasizing about many of my female co-workers. This seemed natural enough, they were attractive and there was a fun kind of chemistry, but nothing ever happened nor did I have any intentions on making anything happen.

That was only the surface of it though, because I also allowed myself down time in my office at work to look at porn to pass the time. This was not something that happened a lot, but I can remember it happening a little bit and that little bit was enough to create a wedge between myself and my partner at the time. I found myself imagining some of my co-workers as sex partners in the porn scenes I had seen, and it became so vivid that I would sometimes go off to the bathroom to masturbate in order to come back down to reality. To make a long story short, eventually there was an emotional gap between me and my partner and with my lack of wisdom and experience I talked myself into breaking up with her. I thought that I needed to be single, was not ready for the commitment of family, and underneath all of that was the intensified desire to have sex with another woman. Woman other than the one I already had and sincerely loved.

This break up was an ego devastating moment for me because a month or so after leaving her it dawned on me like a pile of bricks that I had made a terrible mistake. I found myself breaking down into uncontrollable tears and feeling so ashamed that I would just walk out of the relationship. Especially because nothing really happened, other than the fact that I was not entirely honest and transparent with her in the first place. I did not tell her about the imaginings of other women and this intense sexual urge coming over me every day. Looking back, if I was honest with her and allowed myself to be vulnerable it would likely have been ok, and we could have talked our way through it. But I did not know how to do that, and I believed the fantastical stories in my head about needing to be with another woman. This of course, proved to not be true, and having sex with many women after that relationship in my life showed me that the answers were not in some sexual conquest or even in authentic sexual connection with others. This was just a surface level desire that was inflated due to porn exposure and one that cost me far more than it I was ready to pay at that time.

Porn and the propagation of psycho-sexual fantasies it promotes in the mind act as a replacement for true intimacy. If we are in a relationship with another person than it blocks total intimacy with that person and creates a substitute whenever it's convenient and easy. If we are not in a relationship, then it dampens our connection with ourselves and acts as a sedative for whatever emotional dependency it may serve in that moment. However, we spin it the truth is what we are seeking is deeper connection, authenticity, trust, and vulnerability, from ourselves and then from others. Porn creates an artificial projection of distorted sexuality but is completely void of connection and substance. Eventually this can leave us empty, hollowed out, and addicted to immediate dopamine pick me ups because we have exhausted the inner resources we were gifted as a human being with.

In order to create true intimacy with another we have to start with ourselves. It has been echoed all through this chapter about the deleterious effects of pornography and the messaging of sexual distortion upon our impressionable minds. I think that point has been effectively made but the other point to make is the effects this can have on our vulnerable hearts. Our minds are resilient and can bounce back. Our brain circuitry can reroute the electrical signaling with new information inputs and with commitment to the process it can be brought back to holistic balance and recovery. The heart though, is a bit more of a multi-layered process and the hurtful effects pornography has on the hearts of anyone involved is not well studied but is extremely well felt. There is no supplement or right eating pattern that can cure the hurt of a heart worn down by lack of trust due to something like this. It's a process of returning back to the truth and disposing of the habits i.e., pornography and self-gratification that either leaks the individual user and/or has broken trust with a significant other. This is where true intimacy is often born out of and it is the only way to heal forward.

I feel there is much more that can be said on this topic of intimacy and vulnerability regarding the effects of pornography and our sacred relationships. If this section is especially relevant to you then use the rest of this book as a manual for recovery and empowering yourself to be a better version of you. At the end of the day, it all comes down to being congruent with our values and living out our values as a matter of course. As a way of life. And in being transparent and honest about what is going on behind the curtains because what lives in the shadows will eventually reveal itself in the light. The energies we try to repress and suppress in private always have a way of coming out in public. It is far better to be honest with our partners and of course honest with ourselves before a problem builds up and feels insurmountable.

Remember, the fantasy projections or pornographic programmed desires are often times just that; programmed desires. Porn hijacks our brain chemistry, brain wave states, bodily sensations, and triggers our more basal carnal desires but that does not mean these are in any way natural or organic desires. I found being in a devotional relationship that

214

all of those old fantasies from porn scenes (and prior sexual experiences) are not even remotely appealing with my partner. What is the difference you might say? We have an amazing sexual chemistry, but the difference is that I love her with all of my heart. She is not an object for my gratification or to get me off when I so feel like it. Her pleasure is just as important as mine and sometimes that is more important than mine because she is a human being. You see, porn dehumanizes woman in a way where they really can become like objects and this causes our hearts to calcify and become numb.

Restoring Healthy & Whole Sexuality

"Originally and naturally, sexual pleasure was the good, the beautiful, the happy, that which united man with nature in general. When sexual feelings and religious feelings became separated from one another, that which is sexual was forced to become the bad, the internal, the diabolical."

Wilhelm Reich, The Mass Psychology of Fascism

Based on my own experience, I would have to assert that the most powerful force in life is that of pure and unadulterated love. This four-letter word has been so flipped upside down and imbued with so many different interpretations throughout our consumer culture that it has lost much of its potency, but the truth of what love is everlasting and is the singular reason we are here on this planet. The love between a man and a woman who are truly devoted to one another, through thick and thin, through health and illness, is a force that endures all obstacles and personal setbacks. The purity and potency of the love that a parent has for their offspring goes well beyond simple words and in many ways is simply indescribable. It is something that is universal and felt throughout the collective population as a nuanced but obvious fact of life. The love that is available within each of our hearts is the source code for all healing and is the very thing that breaks the cycle of addiction, no matter how strong the patterning has been solidified into an individual's behavior set.

Love allows for the most important principle of healing and recovery to take place. That principle is simply called grace.

We have explored the depths of what would easily be considered unhealthy sexual patterns based on the exploitation of societal consumerism that takes place in modern day pornography. All elements of love, vulnerability, and intimacy has been removed from the equation and what remains is a partially scripted scenario where two bodies are rubbing up against each other, leading to an excitatory climax before moving onto the next scene. This has been a living model of sexuality for the last few generations of young people to observe, engage with, and portray in their own sexual development. Where this has led to is anything other than a whole and healthy form of sexuality within our society because the love and intimacy has been replaced entirely for four play and physical pleasure.

I am not speaking as some kind of saint or standing on a mountain top here. I am speaking as someone who has experienced the effects of this firsthand, witnessed it in an entire culture, and I, as many others, are making my way back into a whole and healthy relationship with my own sexuality, as well as that which I share with a partner. This chapter, like much of this book, is just as much for me as it is for the readers. I am on my own path of restoring healthy and whole sexuality as a fully integrated masculine man and we are both taking a deep dive journey into the vulnerable layers of what that means.

The first thing for us to inner stand, if we have not already, is that our sexuality is where our life force resides. The sexual tension we experience in the midst of attraction is a life force spark rising to the surface and initiating a magnetic pulsation within our bodies. The true power of sacred sexuality is the ability to hold this magnetic pulse through our rhythmic breathing and allow is to charge the body like a battery. The common expression of sexual energy is to run it through the genitals like an electrical current and exert the energy out of the body as quickly as possible. There is nothing inherently wrong with this, but it is not optimal and can leave us feeling unfulfilled, depleted, and craving more quick bursts of excitement rather than feeling satisfied and content. When we allow the pulse of our sexual energy to slowly build and expand through the body like a magnetic field it has a restorative effect on the body and the mind. This is the desired consequences of mastering our sexual energy and the healing force it can have on each or both individuals involved.

Now, it's important to discuss briefly the distinction between what would be considered an unhealthy sexual repression and healthy sexual expression. Some may wonder what the fine line is here and where does impulsive restraint play into it. Well, I think it is just like anything we explore in this book. It is the ability to forgo immediate gratification in service of medium to longer term fulfillment and success in life. The real distinction here is who's in control? Are you in control of your sexual urges or are your urges in control of you? Has your sexuality been effectively integrated into the whole of your life so the entirety of it all makes for a harmonious and healthy balance? I think these are essential questions to consider and the answers to these will shine light as to what needs to be adjusted in order to create that harmonious equanimity between self-control and sexual expression.

In no way do I suggest we repress our sexuality because that is counterproductive and leads to further unhealthy patterns of addiction. What we want to establish is the balance point of impulse control and appropriate expression of self. The undercurrent to this discussion really comes down to the fact that the exchange of sexuality between two people brings with it a tremendous amount of responsibility which is not fully understood throughout our "sexually liberated" culture. The exchange of bodily fluids also contains the exchange of emotional content and the melding of two human beings, with two energy bodies has very real effects that go beyond just the possibility of pregnancy or transferring a sexually transmitted virus (those are pretty big one's in of themselves!)

The world-famous psychologist and philosopher Jordan Peterson has some brilliant perspectives on this topic which are worth mentioning. Jordan said that "I do not believe you can separate sex from its sociological consequences." He is alluding to the act that human sexuality is a major driving force in the entirety of society and must be considered. One of the biggest areas this plays out is in the workplace, for example. Having sex with our co-workers, our community members, or others within social circles has immediate and seemingly obvious consequences if not handled consciously and effectively. I think we have all seen this kind of thing play itself out and certainly the subject of many publicized blunders of

217

celebrities or corporate CEOs. Jordan also states very clearly that when we find ourselves in a loop of sleeping with multiple partners, as in "casual sex", "we corrupt our soul and hurt ourselves across time, as well as hurt others."

These are some powerful statements and should be enough for anyone to pause and consider the potentiality of what has become known as "casual" sex in our fast-paced society. This is not to demean or to say sex outside of partnership or marriage for that matter is wrong in any way. That would be extremely hypocritical for me (or most anyone) to assert but more so to emphasize the importance that our sexual relationships play and the effect they can have on one another and ourselves. Sexuality can be used for mere entertainment and to pass the time or it can be used for transformation and to increase one's vital life force. This is the ultimate distinction of all others when it comes to the use value of our sexual energy. It can be used to heal, or it can be used to harm. We have this choice in the palm of our hands every time we engage intimately with another human being, as well as ourselves. When we entangle ourselves with another person sexually, we are also creating a karmic link with that person and our bio-fields (energy fields) synch up together, exchanging information, and creating a shared experience that penetrates further beyond and far deeper than simply the physical body itself.

This is why bringing the 'sacred' back into our sexuality is essential for optimal wellbeing, harmonious relationships, and especially for recovering from any form of sex addiction. When sex becomes sacred again it releases all patterning of addiction because the energetics of grasping, taking, and satisfying carnal desires are no longer there. When we make something sacred it becomes much more about a ritual and ceremony then it is about the physical sensations of the act itself. It transcends the simple physicality of sexuality and evolves into a metaphysical alchemy between two individuated souls becoming one in the ceremony of co-creation. In all spiritual texts and teachings sexual alchemy was seen as the most rarified and potent process for manifesting one's dreams into reality. In more modern-day spiritualized connotations around sexuality and tantric practices this process is sometimes called 'sex magic'. Sex magic is basically the conscious intention of utilizing the amplified emotional and physical forces of sexual ecstasy (pleasure stimulation) to call forth one's desires. In simple terms this might look like one or both partners speaking into their desire during peak moments in intercourse and intensifying their conscious focus on it during climax.

I imagine this part just caught you interest and there is some level of intrigue about how to do this 'sex magic' thing. The truth is it is already encoded within you and it's a very natural thing to unfold into during intercourse, but it requires a certain ingredient. That ingredient is an emotional bond with the person you are involved with. If there is no emotional bond and it is purely a physical attraction, then it will lose the magnetic pulse charge that creates the 'magic' part of the sexual alchemy. When there is an emotional bond and love is the reason for the pull between two people, then there is a sense of magic that is palpable and long lasting. This is the secret ingredient in order to maximize the potency of shared sexuality and is the power that replenishes the organ and glandular system instead of depletes it. There are a ton of books and information online on the sacred tantric arts you can research to explore this concept more and discover practices you can undertake with yourself and/or with a partner.

"Aligning with yourself, then another and you both aligning yourselves together further in harmony will summon source energy in ways you couldn't imagine."

Shalom Melchizedek, Cosmic Sexuality

Section 3

The Initiation Phase

Welcome, my friend to the next phase in our ever-evolving journey together. We have crossed many bridges to get to this point and covered far more psychological terrain than most ever can imagine on the road to recovery. This is now where our journey together becomes less about an intellectual understanding of things but becomes more about a process of inner standing at a core level of our ancestral being. The warmup session has officially concluded and now is the moment for initiation. You see, behind every word of this book there is what I call 'a carrier wave of intention' which is designed to bring the reader i.e., YOU along for a ride. And up to this point we have been fastened inside the tour vehicle but now is the time to take off the safety belt, step outside the cage, and enter into the initiation of transformation.

In all indigenous and aboriginal cultures that were rooted to the earth there have been ceremonial rights of passages in order to mark important milestones in one's life. In traditional cultures there was always a rite of passage that was created to usher the youth into their maturation into adulthood. These ritualized practices are built into the ages of our history and that sacred process of maturation is stored in our cellular bodies. The artificial culture we have been raised within has systematically removed these critical junction points from the equation all together. This is the exacting reason for the widespread prevalence of addiction we see and is also the core intent for why this book was written in the first place. When a culture loses its mythology i.e., it's storied history and traditions, the following offspring lose their way which results in the loss of inner direction which manifests as outer chaos and loss of direction in life.

This entire section is about restoring what was once lost through the sacred sciences of whole human healing. We are going to explore four themes that all correlate back into the singular theme which is rites of passage and initiation. Without an initiation phase there is no coming out the other end phase. Without the crossing of the bridge, from light to dark (ignorance to awareness) and left to right (left brain to right brain), there can be no victory and the road to recovery is all about savoring the anticipating of victory. Victory of Self!

Let's Proceed…

Plant Medicines

"Psychedelics are illegal not because a loving government is concerned that you may jump out of a third story window. Psychedelics are illegal because they dissolve opinion structures and culturally laid down models of behavior and information processing. They open you up to the possibility that everything you know is wrong."

Terence McKenna

"We all have negative or contaminating energy in our bodies. That we are holding in our being. This is simply a process of disengaging that and letting it come out. It's part of a cleansing process."

Don Howard

Starting the third phase of our journey together we are going to enter into a new realm of discovery. This might be described as a bit more of a lucid experience than the prior sections but that will be for you to experience for yourself. We are definitely stepping outside of the consensus status quo and moving off of the reservation as far as addiction and whole human health is concerned. It felt both fitting and appropriate to begin this section diving deep into the world of plant medicines. There can be many categories to define something as a plant medicine. There are the medicinal plants used to help people heal and thrive in many plant-based diets. Food is medicine of course and you could easily consider organic fresh nutrient dense plant foods as plant medicines. You can also include the various types of plants we find in herbal medicines that are popularized by eastern medical system such as Chinese herbalism and Ayurvedic herbalism. This would all be appropriate but, in this context, we are going to explore the world of psychedelic/entheogenic plant medicines.

This could be considered a very taboo subject to discuss in any book but especially in a book on transcending addiction. For those who are either not personally initiated in this topic or have a particular perspective on it as party drugs or recreational escape toys, there is a much wider world to explore here. I feel a lot of confidence going into this though because there has been a tipping point in our world when it comes to the scientific research and clinical studies, the anecdotal research, the indigenous traditions using these medicines since antiquity, and also the emerging need for this topic to be talked about. The overwhelming research on what are known as psychedelics or entheogenic plants completely overturns all of the bad press and false assertions that these are dangerous toxic substances. The really dangerous drug like substances are the main source of what organized society offers in the form of alcohol, cigarettes, factory farmed animal products, processed foods, coffee, and especially the pills for every ill that big pharma tells us to our face that these prescriptions are in fact drugs!

It may be helpful to note that the meaning of the word psychedelic has nothing to do with any kind of drug or "high". Psychedelic translates into 'mind-manifest'. This is likely because in the altered state experience, between the highly physical and the lucid, it becomes clear that our minds are manifesting our experience. This is at least palpably true while undergoing these kinds of experiences. These impactful experiences can better teach us the true power of our mind when it is unlocking the memory banks of the human condition. We may have stumbled upon **The Power of Now** by Eckart Tolle or some other mindset/spiritual teacher, but those intellectual concepts take on a whole other meaning when we are able to see, taste, touch, and feel the sensations that arise from our mental patterns. So, in this way psychedelics are not so much about seeing wild, beautiful visual geometry but in actuality, they are best used to help reorganize the geometry of the mind itself.

Another term which I find incredibly important is 'entheogen". This has a more direct meaning which essentially means to generate the divine from within. Let's break it down. "En" means endogenous which means to produce a hormone/neurotransmitter/compound (dopamine for example) from within the body. Theo connects to the study of theology which is the study of the nature of God/the divine from a religious paradigm. Gen means to generate or produce. As an example, the word hydrogen (H2O - 2 hydrogen, 1 oxygen) means to generate hydration which chemically means structured water. So, this is a brand-new perspective on the sacred and ritualistic use of plant medicines entirely. When we better inner stand the true etymological meaning of the words we use the more accurately we can know their most effective use in our lives. After all, words are spells and through our language we are casting spells every day. These plant teachers simply help to illuminate the truth of this fact and show us how to better cast spells that empower us instead of disempowering us.

The clinical research that has been conducted using a variety of psychoactive and psychotropic compounds is immense and extremely well documented. Substances such as psilocybin mushrooms (magic mushrooms) and MDMA have a deep clinical use for those suffering from a range of psychological challenges such as PTDS, depression, mood disorders, trauma, and addiction recovery. Perhaps the most famous organization doing this clinical research is MAPS (multidisciplinary association for psychedelic studies). The biggest aspect of their work has been with MDMA assisted psychotherapy where the patient will take a dose of MDMA while being provided amenities and professional supervision. Some of the big issues they seek to help tackle through these therapies are individuals who have experienced sexual assault, trauma from war (veterans), domestic violence, and even those who deal with social anxiety or anxiety challenges relating to a life-threatening illness. Both the clinical research and anecdotal research in this context has been extremely powerful and encouraging, to say the least.

This is a good time for me to mention that I am not simply reporting 2nd hand or third hand information in regard to entheogenic usage of other people. I have a significant depth of personal experience with many of the most noted substances and certainly all of the individual plant medicines I will be describing in more detail below. I know first-hand the experience of going through multiple MDMA assisted psychotherapeutic sessions because I have used it to help put back pieces of my own puzzle that had gotten lost and scattered in the shuffle of life. I will be sharing my own personal testimonials with each of these sacred substances in the sections below. I just want you to know, as the reader, that this information is not just researched from my keyboard armchair but rather is deeply infused into every fiber of my being.

There is a lot more we could discuss in terms of the clinical research to build a rock-solid case for the efficacy of psychedelic and psychotropic plant medicines. That is not really my propagative in this moment though. I have a slightly different intention to bring through in this chapter and that is to help the reader gain a greater insight into the process that these substances can catalyze within one's own heart as the entry point for overcoming self-limitation, facing one's biggest fears, and transcending the cycle of addiction, once and for all. After all, that is why we are here together, right? To overcome self-inflicted limitations of the wounded mind and to discover those parts of ourselves that got left behind in the mad scramble to grow up, get of our adolescence, and be somebody in the world. Well, there is some retracing in the memory banks of our life that the psyche must explore, and I have found no more profound or immediately effective way to do just this than with the assistance of plant medicines.

Let's discuss a very important and somewhat subtle aspect of this topic that one should be aware of prior to engaging in any kind of altered consciousness experience. This subtle nuance is hard to describe but there are two questions that arise in this consideration. The first question is simply why someone would even consider doing an entheogenic ceremony in the first place. That is a very reasonable question to start with and the answer is unique to the individual, just as their fingerprint is. Obviously, I could not answer that for anyone else but what I have observed in others who report on their own psychedelic discoveries is that sometimes they don't even know why they did it but sometime during or sometime following the experience the answers came to them. They simply felt "called" towards the experience when it either made itself available or they felt an intuitive nudge to seek out an opportunity and it simply worked out for them.

There is a very important reason I am sharing this nuanced piece with you before moving on with the topic. Plant medicines, in fact all plants in general, have their own form of intelligence to them. The entheogenic psychedelic varieties seem to have an ultra-heightened kind of intelligence and many people report that they felt the experience called them in instead of them deliberately calling the experience in. People that are grasping for an altered state experience without it first calling to them can easily find themselves disappointed from the experience or even

225

experience what we call a 'bad trip'. It is not entirely clear why this is but suffice to say that your best bet is to be very intentional with your motives and not force an opportunity if it is not the right time or simply not right for you at all.

The second question that arises is how does one know if they are really ready to embark on such a journey? This one is a bit easier to answer for me. Judging from my own personal experiences when these medicines came into my life and when they helped me the most, I can say that it was simply when I was ready for it. I may not have known ahead of time if I was ready or even thought about it much prior to the opportunity arriving at my doorstep. Something in me knew I was ready and that something was my gut instinct encouraging me to move forward. The easiest way for me to answer this is simply to say that people tend to have the most transformative experiences when they are at a point in their life when they are ready to make a big change. We can easily get stuck in our own repetitive thought processes and cloud the clarity of our minds. These experiences can help to scrub off the windshields of our consciousness, reorganize our psyche, and remind us about the necessity to live life virtuously and morally. In a sense our moral compass gets put back in place when we had lost our way in life and need some extra support from nature.

"Psychedelics are to the study of the mind what the microscope is to biology and the telescope is to astronomy".

Dr. Stanislav Grof

Altered States of Consciousness

"A culture is what it eats, and a person's personality is often largely a reflection of their diet."

Terrence McKenna

As the subject of altered states of consciousness appears in conventional terms there is a strong tendency to oppose its validation or at the very least to raise defensive banners. This is often a misconstrued concept in civilization simply due to the fact that most lifestyle behaviors alter our consciousness in one form or another. Everything we put into our body stimulates a biological alteration due to blood sugar stimulation, metabolization, hormone secretions, and neurochemical enzyme reactions. A piece of fried chicken has a significantly different effect on one's conscious outlook than a green vegetable juice, for example. Watching the nightly news opposed to watching our children play will dramatically alter one's sense of well-being and perspective of reality. It is my opinion that society at large would benefit tremendously from altering their state of consciousness, both individually, and collectively since our personal and global problems have arisen due to a tightly regulated state of unconsciousness.

It is important to state that the achievement of an altered consciousness experience is not, and historically, has not always been conducted through the ingestion of a certain plant or animal-based products. Ancient people throughout recorded history would engage in various forms of ritual for heightening their state such as fasting, drum circles, chanting, breath work, meditation, sun gazing, reading, writing, painting, calligraphy, yoga, and martial art to name a few. The plant medicines can only open the doors of perception for us, but we are the ones who have to walk through. And the way we do this is by creating a lifestyle surrounding the visions we receive and integrate them into our everyday experiences.

The word entheogen means generating the divine from within, as I mentioned previously. The term entheogen is used to categorize psychedelic substances that have been traditionally used in religious, ceremonial, and spiritual practices. The word psychedelic carries with it dogmatic connotations but simply translates into "mind manifest", also as mentioned. The naturally occurring substances include peyote, psilocybin mushrooms, Huachuca, amanita muscaria mushroom, cannabis, salvia divinorum, iboga, ayahuasca, and bufo toad medicine(5-MEO-DMT) among many others. There is a mass cultural bias that prohibits the usage or consideration to use these medicines for fear that an altered state may cause one to question and ultimately alter their conservative value system. It is well correlated that every major form of religion and spiritual practice was inspired by the alteration of one's consciousness, we may call this an inner revelation. Many prominent psychedelic experts, researchers, historians, and alternative doctors worldwide believe the start of all religious teachings came from the inclusion of entheogenic plants found in nature. The well-established ethnobotanist and psycho-naught Terrence McKenna theorized that the evolutionary shift in human consciousness (enlargement of the human neocortex) may be attributed to the inclusion of wild psycho-active plants due to undergoing nutritional pressure, psilocybin for example, for bonding neurosynaptic-sequences and thus transmitting an expanded view of native's immediate environment, and their specific role in it.

There is a large body of research and evidence that certain entheogenic remedies are more effective in drug withdrawal treatments than any conventional psychiatric method available. This includes but is not limited to heroin, cocaine, alcohol, tobacco, and media formatted drugs such as television, pornography, and consumer driven attachments which appears to be why they are so politically opposed. Psychedelics threaten institutionalized culture by breaking down the accepted paradigms that rely upon consumerism and obedience. The role of the alchemist is to transmute the ills of the world into creative expressions of innovation in place of seeming destruction. This is often done through some type of medium used to bridge the tangibility of the material world with higher shades of intelligence that exists outside the comfort zone of the conscious mind. Entheogens have been used culturally in this way, and aside from the therapeutic uses they provide, is a core reason why many of the world's most successful artists, writers, speakers, and entrepreneurs have used, and to this day still practice psychedelic exploration.

In terms of altered states of consciousness, the pre-dominant reference western society uses as a measuring stick is casual and competitive drinking. This is greatly out of alignment from that of the shamanistic perspective which involves personal maturity, inner-courage, and spiritual growth. When approaching an altered state experience, it should be done with great intention, reverence, and an earnest desire for personal growth and spiritual insight.

It is important to consider the role of a shaman in world view as these noble teachers are considered the medicine men and woman of indigenous cultures. The shaman archetype is commonly viewed as mysteries, dark, and somewhat of a trickster by outside onlookers. This is not by accident or misinterpretation although when one comes a bit closer a new picture begins to develop. The shaman uses the tools that best serve the circumstance at hand, which in many times are humor, lightheartedness, and zaniness, yet in serious matters the shaman acts appropriately with laser focus and is highly functional. In this description we could say the iconic picture of Willy Wonka is a shaman of sorts. The shaman is playful, insightful, and highly non-dogmatic where in contrast the common physician is usually stiff, shallow, and locked into their way of thinking.

"The lack of culturally integrated altered-state initiation caused the egoic mental world-model which is based in only a single cognitive state to become completely predominant.

Michael Hoffman

Unearthing the Shadow Archetype

"The deeper the abyss, the brighter the light."

Jordan Peterson

This section is without a doubt the most importance part of this entire chapter. The overall information on plant medicines and their long-held lineage is important but not nearly as important as their role and function on the earth, specifically at this moment in our human timeline. In my mind there is no coincidence that the most powerful healing agents in the natural world resurrect themselves from the oppression of societal paradigms and arise front row and center into the mainstream lexicon. The parallel between the exact medicines that heal the exact ailments in our population is no coincidence but a very remarkable synchronicity in any case. The collective shadow of what has been repressed, suppressed,

229

and oppressed within the whole of our world, over many decades, generations, and centuries is all coming to a head. The boiling point has gone well past its tipping point and when the pressure has built up to a point of potential collapse, the right people (shamans) with the right tools (plant medicines) for the right job (healing) shows up at the nick of time.

As one begins to embark on a visionary quest using the assistance of plant medicines it should become quickly apparent that there is far more to this process than just the visual light show that many people become enamored by. There is an entire preparatory process that ensues once someone has made a sincere intention to do a ceremony and there can be a ruffling of the feathers, so to speak. The most important aspect of this kind of experience is unearthing the archetypal elements that have been laid below our conscious mind. In classical Jungian psychology these elements would be known as the shadow which is what runs our unconscious behaviors and most certainly runs our addictions. There is a monumental plethora of information on the shadow archetype from all ranges of developmental psychology, personal development philosophy, new age rhetoric, and certainly imbedded in the mystic teachings of spirituality. It's very important to grasp the psycho-intellectual concepts of the shadow, where does it come from, and how does it persist in our lives. It is entirely a different thing all together though to come face to face with it and be forced to confront our deepest fears, in real time.

This is really the gift that these plant medicines and psychotropic compounds can offer us, if we are ready for it. It does not necessarily mean that we are going to be confronted with harsh and heavy experiences. Sometimes our shadow elements are revealed to us in the most loving, healing, and clarifying ways that simply open our heart and allowing a deep sense of compassion to arise. And sometimes it can come to us in a way that is very challenging, humbling, uncomfortable, and forces us to take a 'sober' inventory of our past choices, mistakes, and trauma/wound patterns. What allows for someone to have the most graceful experience in any event is their willingness to simply surrender to whatever the experience chooses to be. If we hold onto our pain and resist the experience, we will likely plunge into a darker and more painful experience. That is ok too because sometimes we learn best through our own suffering but just know that it is entirely a choice. And the unearthing of the shadow side of our nature is a healing process to help us reorient our value system and integrate our shadow instead of pushing it away.

From a shamanic perspective what is happening in many of these experiences is we are unlocking memories that we may not remember that we remember. 'Gene keys' being woken back up from their dormant state of inactivity or repression. The internal safety switch that we use to keep us safe from disappointment, fear, or life itself is switched off and our receptivity towards life is switched back on. This can be a disorientating process (and often times is!) The passage from one phase of maturity into another requires some sort of ordeal or confrontation with the aspects of ourselves that do not support our future self. This is what the awakening process can feel like and having a context for what is happening can make it much easier to pass through the initiation portal without getting stuck or fixated on the bumps and bruises along the way.

It is true that this kind of transformational process can be done through means outside of psychedelic plant medicines. This initiatory experience is not for everyone but some people in our world are so stuck in the materialism of our society that they need an earth-shattering event such as entheogenic substances can provide to snap them out of their atheistic conditioning and bring them back to the dive spark of soul awareness. Unearthing the hidden aspects of our own psyche can be tough but the rewards and benefits of doing so followed by a healthy integration period are priceless. We are essentially opening up the subconscious gate ways of the mind complex and pulling back the veil to reveal what exists in the closest of the unconscious psyche. This requires a guided approach and a realistic integration timeline following the experience to allow the life changes to manifest naturally and in their own time.

The biggest issue many find following a powerful shamanic experience is in the transition back to their everyday waking life. The experience is so far from what they are used too, and it takes time for the conscious mind to assimilate exactly what just happened. The ego complex will try to reestablish its footing by pointing to all of the familiar surroundings, relationships, addictions, and patterns as a form of self-preservation. People can grossly underestimate the transition period because they had such a profound and immediately impactful experience, they assume that all the work is done. They assume that they are completely healed of their prior afflictions and can simply just go back to 'normal' but as a renewed version of themselves. Well, I am here to tell you it does not work exactly like that. In fact, it does not work like that at all.

The shadow experience is not just something that emerges in the altered state experience itself but something that has been with us all along. Just because we had a consciousness altering experience does not negate the reality that our addictions and the shadow aspects of our psyche that created them still must be confronted. The deep shamanic work allows one to face their fears head on and confront the dragon of their own mind. The tricky part is that if we do not make the immediate changes following the experience and make them with a strong conviction then the shadow always finds its way back into the mix. The real work is done following the ceremony or experience. The soul work is done in the ceremony or the experience itself. Once the soul has been cleansed and strengthened the human being is better equipped to go back out into his/her world and make the changes they need in order to embody the version of themselves they had experienced for a moment on the mountain top.

Remember, this is not about disassociating from our pain or trauma by using psychedelic drugs as some form of pain number/killer. It is quite the opposite, in fact. This is about integrating our wounds, our traumas, our unresolved pain points, and ultimately the shadow side of our human nature. This is part of a kind of timeline completion process where we stop carrying the unpacked pain of our past into our every waking moment forward. This entheogenic initiation practice is about resolution and whole human recovery. Which is why it is critical to ground into us, prior, during, and post psychedelic experience. The integration process begins the moment we decide to embark on the vision quest and continues months to even years following it, depending on how impactful it was. The idea is to take all that was experienced and reincorporate what was learned into the physical body i.e., one's physical patterns, habits, thoughts, emotions, and disciplines.

"There is a psychospiritual disease of the soul that originates within us and that has the potential to destroy our species or wake us up, depending on whether or not we recognize what it is revealing to us".

Paul Levy, Dispelling Wetiko

The shadow archetype/element is masterfully told through the lenses of what has been known in Native American shamanism as the 'wetiko virus'. The wetiko virus is the root cause of what we know as psychological or psychiatric conditions of the mind. It is a psychic parasite that infects one's psyche (psychological processes) and begins to implant negative, detrimental, addictive thoughts into their mind. It can be looked at as part of the ego complex, but it is also an entirely separate entity of sorts all together. The best book on the subject is called **Dispelling Wetiko: Breaking the Curse of Evil** by Paul Levy. The wetiko phenomena of the psyche is the repressed darkness that exists within the motherboard of humanity. Within the darkest regions of the human mind. Within the lonely dark places inside hearts that have not healed or carry resentment and judgement towards others and themselves. The wetiko is the manipulative, deceptive, and cunning side of the human intellect that can be extremely persuasive and convincing but misaligned and out of integrity with its motives.

It's that aspect of ourselves that likes to tell white lies, skims over the whole truth, and projects its own faults and shortcomings onto others as a means to take attention off of itself. You see, according to Paul Levy, who wrote the single best book that has ever attempted to approach this topic, the wetiko is the shadow projection of the psyche. What it does is to project one's attention onto dramas and distractions happening on the outside world as a way to hide out in the shadows, undetected by the mind of the person it has infected. It uses judgement, resentment, jealousy, anger, self-loathing, and despair as useful emotional states to feed off of. Wetiko feeds off of lower vibrational energies that we humans emit in states of addiction, emotional looping, and making unhealthy lifestyle choices. In a way it functions similar to an intestinal parasite which feeds on the waste products of our ingested food and whatever acidic matter that exists inside of us. They are like the recycling organisms in the intestinal echo-system and so long as there is junk for them to feed on, they will continue to show up. That is until we completely rid our bodies of junk, poor eating habits, and begin the practice of intestinal cleansing.

If we have a lot of negative energy and stagnation built up in our bodies, our minds, and our emotional body than are more susceptible to being influenced by what we are describing as the wetiko virus. Again, this is a mind virus that influences one's mental and emotional state. This is the spiritual roots of where addiction frequencies manifest and eventually builds up over time. For all intents and purposes, the wetiko is the great spell caster over a clouded and unclear mind. It can use whatever we may judge about ourselves and redirect it towards others, just as if we had those judgements about other people and not ourselves. Any emotion that is a byproduct of judgement towards others or towards ourselves is part of the shadow frequency spectrum. Judgement is the wetiko mind virus's favorite weapon of choice because it is so easy to judge others without taking responsibility for oneself, first and foremost.

The act of taking full responsibility for one's state of being, state of mind, state of emotion, state of health, and overall state of life is the only effective tool we have against this mind virus. Taking personal responsibility for one's own actions and the consequences of those actions create a spontaneous integration effect within the heart of that person. It is the negation of personal responsibility that inhibits one's healing process and this holds them back from integrating their shadow tendencies. If we have properly accounted for our mistakes and misfortunes in our life, then those shadow elements/archetypes of our human nature will not create addiction cycles anymore. The wetiko hides behind our shadows and utilizes the unintegrated aspects of our psyche/emotional body to perpetuate addiction because that is where it thrives, behind the shadows and in a state of total chaos. By taking radical responsibility and being soberingly honest with ourselves we can quickly step off the chaos wheel and out from behind the shadows of life.

The psychedelic and entheogenic experience have a unique way of creating the perfect storm of deeply moving emotional experiences, as well as bringing us dropping to our knees in weeping humility and repenting from ways we had hurt someone in the past, without ever knowing that we did or likely completely forgot about. When done correctly it has a way of bridging the cosmic forces of heaven and earth together in a way that is entirely palpable, directly experiential, and undeniably real. The wetiko mind virus uses the shadow aspects of our ego to manipulate and distort perceptions of what is real and what is not. The entheogenic plant medicines have a way of dissolving those shadow ego structures and breaking them down into a million pieces, sometimes in a matter of a few flashing moments.

I have certainly had my ego and my entire sense of reality smashed into thousands of pieces within a few moments upon ingesting certain plant medicines. It can seem traumatic at first, but the discomfort is really just like parachuting out of a plane for the first time. You anticipate it, you are aware it's going to happen, but once you are pulled out of the plane your entire sensory system is being hurled a hundred miles per hour through the windy sky's and it takes a few extended moments to reorient yourself to what is happening. That is what those kinds of experiences can feel like but it's a necessary trade off because it also does not give the 'ego complex' or 'wetiko' any time to prepare. It (the ego) ends up going down the portal into the next dimensional sensory experience too and out of that can produce the most glorious, awe inspiring, and deeply healing experiences that exist on this planet.

I want to share a quote from Paul Levy's book on wetiko that is particularly insightful. *"The wetiko collective psychosis is a field phenomenon and needs to be contemplated as such. The field itself is not a separately existing thing but a dynamically evolving living process in which we are all participating, simultaneously creating and being created by. The field has to do with relations per se, rather has the seemingly separate entities doing the relating. Instead of relating to any part of the field as an isolated entity, it's important to contemplate the entire interdependent field as the "medium" through which wetiko is articulating itself. The underlying field can only be perceived and felt when we step out of our habitual viewpoints of imagining that we exist as a fixed reference point, a center of volitional action, a "time-bound ego", and connect with our timeless, and nonlocal being, which ironically, can only be found in the present moment. This is to say that the doorway to seeing the field, and therefore wetiko, is to fully enter the present moment."*

This is a very deep insight into the nature of the shadow, and it's influence over our perspective of what we call 'reality'. I will let you derive your own insights from this passage by Paul Levy but what I will add to this is the emphasis on the 'field effect' as a direct experience I have had many times, both in psychedelic altered states and non-altered states. I have studied similar concepts relating to quantum physics, quantum biology, and what is called the unified field or morphogenetic field as the parapsychologist and scientist Rupert Sheldrake calls it. Whatever you choose to call it, it is an electromagnetic, geo-magnetic field that covers the circumference of our physical earth and is directly connected to all biological life forms, including human beings. We all have what is called a bio-field or commonly referred to as our 'aura'. This is a literal field of energy that emits out of us or perhaps is simply part of us. We are living energy fields and our energy interacts with the field of energy that surrounds us and connects us to the world as a whole.

I have had one ayahuasca plant medicine ceremony that was especially powerful in this regard. It was likely the most powerful shamanic experience I have ever had and has left an indelible mark upon me to this day. I had gone through every spectrum of my emotional bandwidth and was confronted by various elements of the shadow, or wetiko itself, perhaps. I was shown an entire rolodex of life experiences and was made to feel the heat of what living in my lower shadow tendencies would be like at the soul level. I was also brought through those experiences and dropped on the top of a high mountain, more like Mount Olympus from Greek mythology, look down upon the earth from what felt like a God's eye view of things. I remember shortly after this experience opening my eyes in a pitch-black dark room, no lights, no outside influences of any kind, outside of intense rainstorms in Kauai, HI. When I opened my eyes after 2 hours or so I closed eye meditation, the entire room was lit up like a holographic Christmas tree, except it was not anything like a lit-up tree, it was the entire room bathed in a golden light and it was in the shape of a 'chain-linked field'. It was a literal golden field of light and I know that for sure, because I was a bit disorientated, unable to move my legs very well, like a small child, and I used the light of the room (again, pitch black) to crawl towards the balcony sliding door.

I imagine this experience was likened to what it must feel to be fully optimized, fully integrated, and at peak energetic alignment as a human, in a human body. I felt that all distortions of the ego-mind complex were not only removed, but that they had been so thoroughly removed, that they were less of an afterthought, as much as they simply didn't to exist as an aspect of the psycho-emotional upgrade I was experiencing. As I write this, I am realizing that that experience was an entry point into a frame rate of reality that already exists and has always existed but is not readily detectable to the beta-brain wave state mind that is heavily conditioned with abstract belief programs, personal bias's, and is running addiction-based software programs as it's default operating system. This was more than just a glimpse into another realm of human possibility, this was a fully embodied state that has imprinted upgraded information into the cellular coding of my body but is still taking years to integrate (and remember to stop forgetting what was discovered).

"Addiction thinks in circles whereas invention thinks in spirals."

Richard Rudd, The Gene Keys

So, what do we make of all of this anyways? I imagine this is pretty interesting at the least and it may simply serve to help unlock the gene keys within your own mind, allowing for maybe a more detailed discovery of this theme. Remember though, that the antidote for chaos and disorder i.e., the wetiko fear virus is the very same antidote as recovering from addiction. It has to be addressed at multiple levels of the human experience. The mental body, the emotional body, the physical body, and then directly into the soul of the matter itself. As I have learned from my friendship and guidance from Richard Rudd, author of **The Gene Keys** (and who wrote the forward for this book) that addiction is a frequency pattern/signature that exists inside of the individual. If we get too caught up in pointing fingers outside of ourselves, obsessing over external circumstances, and struggling with external habits (addiction behaviors) we are caught up in the wetiko field. We have to address what is causing the addictive pattern to persist, otherwise we will continue to trade out one thing for another but remain addicted, none the less.

I am going to conclude this section by sharing another passage, this time from Richard Rudd in his legendary Gene Keys tome(book) on the subject of addiction. *"When repressive natures come across a gap in their awareness, the fear inside them causes them to freeze up. This freezing can manifest in many ways - physical as a complete lack of energy, emotionally as depression and mentally as a narrow-minded and guarded perception of reality. The secret to all addiction lies in how we respond to these gaps in the functioning of our awareness. The danger of addiction is that we seal our fate in these precious moments without realizing we are doing it. At the shadow frequency, we simply do not allow ourselves to experience the void that precedes a shift in awareness. The repressive nature shrinks from feeling that empty state of silence. If we were to face such times in our lives without either shrinking or reacting, something truly amazing would seed itself in us."*

Please take as much time as required to reread this and close your eyes to let it fully sink itself in. The gaps between thinking one thing and physically carrying it out is the pattern interrupt between an addictive frequency and it being acted upon. Often times we are doing the very thing we want to stop doing simply to avoid sitting in the proverbial gap. Resting into the in-between of the, this and the, that. This is the place where miracles are born and paradoxically it is also the place where fear resides. The wetiko phenomena (and the same thing of other names) seeds itself into those gaps when we are distracted by past pains or future projections. When we are fully present in our moment-by-moment life experience our attention becomes much clearer, and we are better able to detect any shadow patterns in our presence. And again, this is dependent on our ability to begin taking more responsibility for all aspects of our lives. The good and the bad, the easy and the hard. Dissolving the victim inside the mind as Richard calls it is the answer to the fear, paranoia, and addictive frequencies that hold us back from greatness.

"We are different facets of the same diamond. Different perspectives of the same being. I am you, living a different life."

Aubrey Marcus

Psycho-Emotional Healing Plant Teachers

In this section we are going to explore some of the seminal entheogenic plants and compounds I feel are of the utmost importance and have the greatest depth of both scientific and anecdotal research behind them. These are also the one's that I personally have the most direct experience with and have assisted me in my own psychotherapy sessions, whether it was in a traditional ceremony or in a self-facilitated process. Of course, there are many other plant teachers and unique psychotherapeutic compounds we could easily include in this list. Many of them deserve mention and can have a powerful role to play in someone's experience. Some of those include san Pedro cactus (Huachuca), iboga, peyote, LSD, ketamine, Syrian rue, among many others.

It is my feeling that the below listed plants and compounds represent what I would call the master teachers of the entheogenic realm. You may disagree with this list or feel others should be included. These are the teacher plants and compounds I have the most personal experience with, which is why I feel qualified enough to talk about them in detail. Regardless, this is the time in our human history that we all become far better aquatinted with the psycho-emotional therapeutic tools we have available to us. They have been oppressed, ridiculed, and judged by organized society for far too long. True healing is our natural birthright and to imprison a therapeutic tool for healing is to imprison our birthright and that simply will not stand any longer. The world is awakening to its own human potential and knowing what is available and for what purposes it may serve to assist us in this process becomes very important and necessary.

I am not going to provide a long dissertation on all of the nitty gritty scientific rhetoric on these substances. I certainly could do that but far too many books, articles, and research documents have already done this. It would be repetitive and only serve the intellectual mind in its quest for more and more information. I will provide the basic and necessary framework of what these substances are, where they come from, how they interact with our brain chemistry, considerations for using them, and my own personal experience with them. What you choose to do with this information is entirely up to you. I do not recommend using any psychedelic/psychotropic substance without further investigating it for yourself and using critical thinking to determine if this is beneficial for you or not. Nothing is for everyone and these experiences may not even be necessary for you at all. I will let you be the judge of that, for yourself.

Let's proceed...

Psychedelics are just tools, and whether their outcome is beneficial or harmful, depends on how they are used".

Rick Doblin, Ph.D.

5 - MEO DMT (Buffo Toad Medicine)

"When a person smokes 5-meo-dmt, there is an increased production and release of neurotransmitters and endorphins, such as serotonin and dopamine. They promote body regeneration, healing, and an enormous release of unconscious stress."

Dr. Gerardo Sandoval Isaac

One of the most unique altered state experiences I have personally experienced, as well as reporting of people worldwide, is that of the 5-meo DMT, which is secreted from the bufo alvarius toad, also known as the Sonoran Desert toad. This is an interesting compound (5-meo-dmt) that is extracted from the parotid glands of this most unusual toad that is found in northern Mexico and southwest of the US. This experience is unlike any other 'DMT' induced experience. This is due to the fact that 5-meo-dmt is a different molecule than the n,n-DMT molecule that is found in other psychoactive plants such as the chacruna leaf found in the ayahuasca brew. Unlike 'normal DMT' experiences, that also use a DMT enzyme inhibitor, such as the case with ayahuasca, 5-meo-dmt is not a long duration experience, but more so a 15–20-minute parachuting out of this dimension and into another kind of experience. Some people call this the working man's "drug" because someone could take an hour lunch break from work, go on a fast-tracked journey, and come right back in time. This is not recommended by the way!

There are countless stories on the internet of people's 5-meo-dmt experience and most of them are relatively similar in nature. There is a blast off effect, almost immediately where the individual's grasp of conscious reality falls away or dissolves and they are dropped into what is sometimes described as a pitch-black void. Suspended in the 'nothingness' of time and space. Many of these individuals also report to experiencing the most direct connection to what they interpret as God or an omni loving presence. The world-famous boxing icon Mike Tyson did an interview for ESPN that has gone viral where he discusses his personal experience of doing the toad medicine. I could not believe ESPN even did this interview but then again, it's Mike Tyson after all. He shared his colorful and inspiring experience of going on a full-blown odyssey, experiencing a mystical encounter, and feeling a sense of rebirth.

If you recall, Mike Tyson was not only the most famous and most formable boxing force in the last 4 decades or so, he also was someone who had suffered immense trauma, heart break, and fell into a deep spiral of addiction following his boxing career ending. If you take a case study of someone who has opened up to psychedelic medicines and have completely turned around their entire life, in a total 180-degree turn, that is definitely iron Mike. The famous success teacher Anthony Robbins also shared his experience of doing the toad medicine, alongside Mike Tyson ironically enough. Tony Robbins was looking to heal his own fear of death and could not seem to figure out how to resolve this, even though his own methods, which have been life changing for countless millions of people worldwide. He said that after doing the bufo toad medicine he felt a greater sense of peace and connectivity to life, to the creator, and his fear of death began to subside.

These are not isolated incidences; they are actually relatively common amongst those who experience them. My own 5-meo DMT experience was quite profound as well. I was visiting my favorite island in Hawaii, Kauai and one of my close friends happens to be a seasoned Shamanista (female shaman) who does ceremonial work with various therapeutic medicines, including the bufo toad secretion. We took an early afternoon to travel to the top of a sacred hilltop, overlooking the river of souls where legend says is the point on the island where souls incarnate into this world. It is a hidden away tarot (Hawaiian staple crop) patch and carriers a high spiritual-metaphysical activity to it. Anyways, we sat at the hilltop and she guided me into the ingestion of the bufo secretion. I was instructed to allow it to fill my lungs and into my entire body. I slowly blew it out and proceeded to take one more ingestion. As I was taking in the 2nd round my entire body began to lose its physicality and as I began to lay backwards, my mental framework began to dissolve without anything I could do to hold it together.

I laid on the dirt, breathing deeply into my heart, and feeling an emerging pulsation of electromagnetic energy waves coursing through out my body. It felt like a total bodily upgrade process, where energy circuits had become activated, and the electricity was moving all throughout my system. There was a specifically important part of this experience where my guide began fanning over me with a native American feather, clearing dense energetic blockages from my system. She then proceeded to chant what felt like invocations of clearing over my sacral center. She then began to assist me in physical moving out some kind of stuck energy from my sexual center, up through my stomach, up through my lungs, and out through my mouth. We both were tuned in together, working together to remove some kind of entity or stuck energy that had revealed itself through this open gateway of consciousness.

Following that session, I had felt incredibly light, liberated, and in a state of general gratitude. I ended up doing a second session and this time it was completely peaceful, serene, and calm the whole way through. It felt that I had gone through an energetic clearing and had done some energetic hygiene, similar to if someone smokes cigarettes for days on end, does not brush their teeth, and finally brushes their teeth. They will likely feel much more refreshed, clean, and even more positive about themselves. It had felt like whatever gunk I had picked up over time was moved out and cleared from my system. This was an incredibly positive experience and it only brought me closer to myself, my faith, and my connection to what we consider our 'creator' to be.

Dr. Octavio Ruttig is a specialist who has spent well over a decade of his life studying the use of bufo toad medicine to help others in all manner of healing and therapeutic measures. He is a medical surgeon from Guadalajara who has overseen more than 5,000 session, as mentioned in 2015 and likely far more by the start of 2021. He has also traveled all over the world giving talks at conferences on his discoveries. He even wrote a book on the subject called **The Toad of Dawn: 5-MeO-DMT and the Rising of Cosmic Consciousness**. He describes the 5-MeO-DMT molecule as a neurotransmitter chemical messenger that delivers the language of nature to one who ingests it. I feel this is the most appropriate description of this molecule because by all accounts it does seem to be just that. Remember, we have naturally occurring DMT inside our brain, which is produced during the tryptamine metabolic chain inside the pineal gland. DMT experiences may simply be reflecting or perhaps unlocking compartments inside of our brain that always exist but require an exogenous key (molecule) to fully open up.

Dr. Ruttig explains the user experience of 5-MeO-DMT as the individual losing all sense of "themselves" and going into the 'interconnectivity' of all life. He describes it as one being 'undone', in a sense, and after the experience, becoming reconfigured back together, coming back to themselves, but as a more evolved form of themselves. There is a great short documentary you can look up online called **Getting High with a Hallucinogenic Toad Prophet** that chronicles Dr. Ruttig's journey and taking a ride with him to procure the frog medicine, as well as exploring all that we discussed in this section. He also makes the point that the proper way to extract the 'toad venom' does not harm or hurt the toad in any way.

Another interesting point I picked up from watching this documentary is that Dr. Ruttig once lived on the street for 3 years, had a crack cocaine addiction, was begging and eating out of garbage cans sometimes. He states that "the only that helped me was the medicine from the bufo Alverius toad". This is a really powerful testimonial, amongst many others, that had changed this man's life so much that he then devoted his professional life to helping others heal through the same medicine that brought him back from poverty and addiction. Meditate on that!

Ayahuasca (banisteriopsis caapi)

"In truth, ayahuasca is the television of the forest."

Jeremy Narby

The treasured brew of the Amazon has been cherished and ritualized in visionary ceremonies for thousands of years with the sole purpose of deep physical and emotional healing, as well as spiritual insight. The practice of Ayahuasca has gained worldwide recognition and is protected in the Amazon by legal religious right. This act has been passed on through countless generations as a rite of passage, a symbol of environmental preservation, and acknowledged as a bridge between mother earth and mankind. This brew is often called "la purga" due to its liver and gall bladder detoxification effects on the body. Similar to a raw food cleanse, it initiates what is known as a short-term healing crisis in order to expel physical toxins so deep seeded emotions can surface. Some alternative psychiatrists who work with patients from a holistic view appreciate entheogenic medicine such as ayahuasca as it helps to reveal one's inner-conflicts where conventional medicine simply suppresses them. It has been stated that the psychoactive effects of this brew can offer ten years of psychotherapy in one night as the sub-conscious is opened up with no filters or restrictions. This comes as no surprise to the native people for this practice is deeply rooted in their culture and way of life.

Ayahuasca is highly anti-viral, anti-fungal, anti-microbial, and anti-parasitic. Mother ayahuasca as it is traditionally referred to as, is not commonly sought after frequently in recreational manner, due to its strong effects on the body, abhorrently bitter taste, and the transcendent effects it can bestow on one's life. More often than not, like many psychotropic plants, it is used as a steppingstone and put to the side for extended periods of time to integrate the lessons one receives or is left alone all together.

The traditional ayahuasca drink is a combination of the banisteriopsis caapi vine and the leaves of the chacruna (psychotic viridis) plant. Less often in non-traditional ceremonies chagranponga (*diplopterys cabrerana*) is used in place of chacruna. The b. Caapi vine is comprised of a complex chemical

psychopharmacology which varies in concentration depending on the plants set region. The activate agents are beta-carboline (*harmine, harmaline,*

tetrahydroharmine) MAOI (*monoamine oxidase inhibitors*) alkaloids. The Chacruna leaves contain the indole tryptamine n-dimethyltryptamine popularly known as DMT and referenced by author Dr. Rick Strassman as the spirit molecule. DMT is commonly administered through smoking in western recreational usage due to the monoamine oxidase enzyme present in the human digestive system, which deactivates DMT through oral ingestion. This is one of the key principles for why cacao, pharmacologically speaking, has been used to amplify an ayahuasca journey in the Amazon. DMT, although considered an illegal drug, is a natural byproduct of human metabolism and is fundamental to

245

neurotransmitter chemistry in the brain. The pineal gland secretes this neurotransmitter during euphoric states of ecstasy such as a conscious/religious awakening and when we fall asleep; it is the theorized chemical that is responsible for dreaming. Its full spectrum effects are not clearly understood by experts yet there is tremendous interest by scientists and researchers.

"To this day, the natives of the north-west Amazon in Brazil and Colombia use the Banisteriopsis drink for prophetic and divinatory purposes and also to fortify the bravery of male adolescents about to undergo the severely painful yurupari ceremony for initiation into manhood. The narcosis amongst these peoples, with whom I have taken caapi on many occasions, is usually pleasant, characterized by visual hallucinations in color, which initially is very often a shade of blue or purple. In excessive doses, it is said to bring on frighteningly nightmarish visions and a feeling of extremely reckless abandon, although consciousness is not lost nor is use of the limbs unduly affected".

Richard Evans Shultes

The very fact this sacred brew exists defies conventional logic. Out of the entire amazon rainforest where over 50,000 different plant species can be found, two distinct plants were identified. When they are left on their own, they are inactive, but when brought together, macerated, and spun through an extensive brewing process, they help to manufacture a psychedelic experience noted to alter one's pictorial outlook on reality and instill life enhancing insights unique to the user. This was uncovered by a seemingly uneducated, uncivilized band of tribal people living in the rainforest with only their intuition and instincts to direct them. There is a variety of legend and lore linked to the origins of ayahuasca. The shamans simply believe the forest is a network of intelligence that relayed the message to combine these plants for ritual ceremonies and purgatory healing.

It is important to note the discussion of ayahuasca and other entheogenic substances should be kept in their proper context. This is not a toy to entertain temporary rifts of boredom, such as cigarettes or alcohol are used in social gatherings. I only advocate the practice of plant medicines in a safe and sacred space designed for inner reflection of the user. Ayahuasca should be conducted by a trained and experienced shaman who knows how to guide others through the journey. There are numerous healing centers in the world that integrate these plant medicines with great success. The late Scott Peterson directed the Rufugio Altiplano retreat center in Peru who strongly advocated the medicinal use of mother ayahuasca and other associated healing plants. Scott explains the purpose of ayahuasca is to uproot suppressed emotional trauma, cleanse the digestive tract, the liver and gall bladder, as well as open up subconscious neuro-pathways and reprogram the neurological system at large.

The writer and public speaker Graham Handcock publicly states that his long-term addictive relationship with cannabis (marijuana) was pointed out and alleviated by ingesting ayahuasca. He had used marijuana as a crutch for creative writing for decades and it began to become abusive. Graham states in no uncertain terms that ayahuasca revealed this pattern of abuse and alerted him to stop smoking it immediately. This is just one of the examples that disprove common arguments that these substances create physical dependency and addiction. Ayahuasca centers, such as the Rufugio Altiplanao, are set up to help, not only with spiritual crisis and life direction, but very much to assist in breaking physical addictive patterns such as alcoholism, prescription drug use, and street drugs. These methods have proven to be highly effective and gives a clue to their current legality.

I shared briefly a personal story about my first ceremonial experience with ayahuasca that had a revolutionary effect on my personal life and awareness of reality itself. One of the central elements that makes this kind of experience so powerful is the usage of what is called 'icaros', which is a colloquialism in the indigenous South American medicine tribes. These are the songs that that the shaman sings during the medicine experience and they are always unique to the experience itself. I found myself being carried by the icaros while traveling through my inner landscape of highs, lows, and everything in-between. There is a real

247

therapeutic value to the icaros because the shaman is also operating within the thin veil between the physical and non-physical dimensions, which indicates they are with you the whole time, and helping to guide the energy of the ceremony through the vibration of sound and music. The research on what is known as 'cymatics' is the discovery that music/sound vibrations create geometrical patterns in physical matter, and thus having a physical effect on humans who are surrounded by the vibrational tones of the music/sound.

This, among other described reasons, is why conducting a plant medicine experience such as ayahuasca should be done in a traditional ceremonial setting. Every element is necessary to have the best experience that is perfect for the individual. Ayahuasca is the central medicine of the jungle and thus is codified with the energy of the jungle, which is a bit of a different dynamic than most people have experienced in the concrete jungle of organized, domesticated society. Plant medicines, and especially ayahuasca is anything other than domesticated, which is why some people can have such a challenging time letting go of their ego-identity constructs, until they are forced to shed their skin, and simply surrender into the experience taking place. This is a process of rewilding oneself from the shackles of domesticated patterning (addictions) and open themselves up to their dormant capabilities, and ancestral lineage that is often invoked during deep medicine work.

There are two exceptional documentaries on ayahuasca you can easily find on the internet to further explore. Aubrey Marcus released an excellent documentary called **Ayahuasca | Drinking the Jungle** which chronicles himself, our mutual friend Dr. Dan Engle, and a few others along their journey into the Peruvian jungle to conduct a weeklong ceremony with the retreat facilitator Don Howard. The other documentary I recommend is by Brain Rose and this one is a bit of a deeper, more personal, and full spectrum journey of Brian's life before, during, and after his weeklong experience. This documentary is called **Reconnect** and it also features notable public figures such as the ethnobotanist Dennis McKenna (brother of Terence McKenna), Jordan Peterson, Dorian Yates, and others. These both are the best documentaries I have seen that beautifully depicts the essence, the tradition, and the spiritual journey that this sacred plant medicine is all about.

Psilocybin Mushroom (Magic Mushrooms)

"Since all culture is a kind of con game, the most dangerous candy you can hand out is one which causes people to start questioning the rules of the game".

Terence Mekenna

In the world of psychedelic research, perhaps the most well studied and well-known substance is what our culture calls "magic mushrooms" or psilocybin cubensis mushrooms. The main point of interest in the clinical research on psilocybin mushrooms is for treating depression and other relative psycho-emotional disorders. At this point there is a tremendous amount of clinical research and anecdotal research on the efficacy of psilocybin for treating psychological conditions and helping people who have suffered regain balance and confidence in their lives. The fungi medicines have also been used for advanced stage cancer patients who struggle with anxiety as they are being confronted with the very real possibility of their own mortality. Like many of the entheogenic substances we have discussed in this chapter, psilocybin mushrooms are a proven and effective means for treating, both psychological disorders as well as spiritual disorders for the simple fact that they tend to be one in the same at the end of the day.

The active alkaloid molecule in psilocybin mushrooms is called psilocin, which is the metabolic byproduct of psilocybin once it is broken down by the liver after ingestion. This compound is what is responsible for the psychedelic effects. The experience is very unique amongst all other psychedelic substances and tends to last between 3-6 hours depending on the dosage and preparation which can include eating the mushrooms straight, making a tea out of them, or consuming them in some form of edible such as paired with chocolate or cacao. The combination of the mushrooms with cacao creates a very unique delivery because the pharmacology of cacao and magic mushrooms seems to synergize very well together. Pairing the cacao/chocolate edible with tonic herbs, nutritional super foods, and certain types of minerals such as magnesium, chromium, silica, and what is known as "ormus" minerals is a very unique experience in of itself, and very safe for the brain.

Psilocybin helps to stimulate the serotonin receptors in the brain and sometimes helping to produce an experience that serotonin by itself simply cannot do for some people. This is why it is so effective for helping people struggling with depression. In these individuals the serotonin receptors have become 'blunted' or 'short circuited', similar to how our dopamine receptors become blunted from sensory pleasure overload due to all forms of chemical addictions. It is now being widely discovered that consistent micro-dosing psilocybin can help to reset the brain in order to help manage treatment-resistant depression patients. This portion of the brain that is being reset is what is called the 'default mode network' which is the default psychological state we may find ourselves in due to our life experiences and how we have adapted or maladapted to stress and trauma. So, in this way it is literally unhooking the default mode network from its conditioned stress response and resetting it, in order to bring it back to a healthier baseline.

There is a very good documentary you can find online called **Magic Mushroom Medical Trial** which chronicles the real-life experience of three men who have suffered from depression and found no help from traditional medical interventions. Dr. Robin Carhart-Harris was the lead physician of the trial who helped to facilitate the experience for the patients. It was overseen by David Nutt, who is a professor of neuropsychopharmacology from Imperial College in London. This is a deeply touching movie that takes the 3 men through a multi-series of small to moderate dosages of psilocybin and films there before challenges, the actual induced sessions themselves, and the aftereffects of the clinical trials. It is one thing to read a trial result online intellectually and it is entirely another thing to witness the very real emotional journey of human beings who were stuck in their suffering, who then come out on the other end.

The common theme between these three men's experience is that the pain that had delt with in their lives was a result of what they had experienced in childhood. As they went through their therapeutic trials, they all recounted childhood trauma that had been buried inside of them. One of the men explained what he had received from the experience

250

following the trial. He explained that what the medicine did for him was to provide him a sort of psychological therapist. He felt as though he had a personal therapist onboard with him, inside of him to help him integrate his own healing process. This is actually not an uncommon kind of experience people have but not always so specifically articulated.

Perhaps the single most powerful function that these substances can elicit in the user is the psycho-somatic catharsis of unresolved pain, trauma, and accumulated stress. Psilocybin specifically has a unique way of helping to unlock the parts of the brain that have stored repressed trauma and help the body begin dumping the chemical memories through a somatic processing effect. Out of all of the psychedelic experiences I have undergone psilocybin mushrooms have always been the substance that unlocked emotional stagnation and long suppressed trauma. I have experienced the milder side of micro-dosing which brought me to tears in waves of passing emotions. I have also experienced much deeper surfacing of genetic trauma that was encoded in me from my genetic bloodline or perhaps even past lives (who really knows?). Those experiences were incredibly painful, profound, and absolutely necessary as there would have been no other way for me to have such a psycho-emotional release under any normal waking state interventions. It can help to unearth deep seeded trauma that we do not even realize we are carrying but are at the effect of each and every single day of our lives.

"People think the problem lies in taking too much but it lies in taking too little. Because if you take too little you can resist it. You can struggle with it. And then it can turn into a real mess because you're afraid of it. And you have, to some degree, the power to resist it. What you want to do is take sufficiently enough so that there is no escape and that the transition from ordinary reality to loaded is as quick as possible."

Terence McKenna

MDMA

In the book **Magic Medicine**, by Cody Johnson he provides a distinct classification set of different psychoactive and psychotropic plants, animal products, and chemical compounds to help the reader understand what each one is designed to assist with. There are 4 distinct groupings which are classic psychedelics, empathogenic psychedelics, dissociative psychedelics, and unique psychedelics. The classic group includes 5-meo-dmt, ayahuasca, DMT, LSD, peyote, san Pedro, psilocybin mushrooms, etc. The dissociative class includes ketamine, salvia, nitrous oxide, etc. The unique class includes biota, cannabis, amanita mascara, etc. And then there is the empathogenic class which only seems to include MDA and MDMA.

MDA is a chemical cousin of MDMA and precludes it as the original "love drug" which had a great appeal in the 1960's amongst the hippie and even progressive psychiatry communities. MDA had provided profound effects for opening the heart, increasing emotional empathy, and helping people feel more 'integrated' or 'whole'. It was associated with other psychedelics in that era and was banned as a counterculture drug. Speeding up a bit we arrive at what is much more commonly used and researched which is MDMA. These two compounds represent the entire category of empathogenic substances due to their direct effect on increasing empathy, emotional warmth, insightful realizations, and even in patients recovering from trauma, PTSD, and chronic stress conditions.

MDMA is often called 'ecstasy', which is most associated as a party drug and has carried a stigma simply as something people do recreationally to get high but with overt health consequences. It has been lumped together with substances such as LSD which carry a lot of societal baggage, and to the credit of those with serious concerns, poor quality MDMA or LSD is ill advised, and can result in negative consequences, both psychologically and biochemically. To simply chalk MDMA up to simply a recreational altered experience for partying or 'escaping' really does it a true disservice and misrepresents it's intended use by seasoned professionals in all domains of psychological healing and addiction recovery. In the early 2002's the FDA approved clinical trials using MDMA to treat post-traumatic stress disorder (PTSD) which have been well underway since 2004.

There is a great short documentary you can find online called **MDMA Therapy and Healing** which shares the testimonials of a few individuals including military veterans, an individual who struggled with cancer, and a rare survivor. There testimonies are profound and heartwarming. They all have similar experiences, of being able to process memories and life issues that they had repressed, or simply did not know how to talk about prior to the MDMA treatments. They felt increasingly clear, mentally functional, emotionally available, and were able to process their psychic patterns in real time, with no obstructions in the way. MDMA helps to break down the mental barriers that we develop through the trauma, stress, and hard experiences we go through in life. These walls that build up to protect us from feeling the pain are also the walls that block us from our healing. MDMA is one of the most powerful tools for effectively and safely removing those walls, gaining deep insight into one's challenges, and opening the heart in the process.

In this documentary, Rachel Hope, who is a rape survivor reportedly said that the MDMA assisted psychotherapy trial helped her *"go into my head and reprogram, like a computer, the story I told myself about what that traumatic event meant, why it happened, and learn the real truth, which is that some really horrible things happened, and they mean nothing about me as a human being"*. This is a profound testimonial of using a substance that was once, considered nothing more than a recreational party drug, and a way for people to escape their life problems. Following on in the film they stated that 83% of the subjects in the U.S. Phase 2 study no longer met the criteria for PTSD at their two-month follow-up.

Rick Doblin, PhD, Executive Director, Multidisciplinary Association for Psychedelic Studies (MAPS) is the leading proponent of

MDMA assisted psychotherapy and is spear heading the movement for clinical research to be conducted, and popularly accepted in mainstream culture. Rick speaks very passionately and eloquently about the beneficial use of psychedelics in a way that anyone can easily pick up on. In his TED talk on the future of psychedelic-assisted psychotherapy he had these words to say about it:

> *"Psychedelics reduce activity in what's known as the brain's default mode network. This is where we create our sense of self. It's our equivalent to the ego. And it filters all incoming information according to our personal needs and priorities. When activity is reduced in the default mode network, our ego shifts from the foreground to the background, and we see that it's just part of a larger field of awareness".*

This is the perfect articulation of my own MDMA-assisted psychotherapy experiences, where the stress and emotional charge from my daily circumstances began to shift into the background of my awareness, and a recapitulation of total clarity, and emotional stability rose into the foreground. These experiences were instrumental in helping me process vast amounts of life experiences, relationship challenges, as well as overcome psychic overwhelm due to all that had befallen me during the intensified year of 2020. If it had not been for utilizing MDMA I could not say that certain relationships would have survived, or my business, and especially the strength and conviction to continue writing this book every day. 2020 was the single most challenging year of my entire life and the assistance of MDMA was seminal in my own growth and healing process.

The pharmacological effect of MDMA is by way of its 'serotonin agonist' properties. A serotonin agonist helps to increase the amount of serotonin released into the synapses of the brain. It is a serotonin transporter and is carried into the terminals of the nerves. MDMA also helps to release copious amounts of dopamine as well, allowing for a harmonious balance between serotonin and dopamine. Oxytocin is also released which helps to curve out the effects of cortisol which is the bodies stress release hormone. These chemical molecules in perfect ratio to one another are responsible for the enhanced mental, emotional, and even physical state that user's experience, including increased confidence, inspiration, and creativity. Knowing this is important because the drawback of frequent MDMA usage is that it can cause someone to experience a serotonin/dopamine drop due to the brain needing to reproduce those neurotransmitters from scratch.

The way to avoid the serotonin/dopamine dump effect is by following the **21 Day Dopamine Reset I Reboot I I Recovery** protocol. It's helpful to be living a healthy lifestyle including exercise, organic food, spring water, super foods, and brain supporting supplements. When I did extended experiments with MDMA I took a significant amount of high quality fermented amino acids before, during, and following the experience. This helps the body to rebuild the neurotransmitters that supply the signal for the receptor sites such as for serotonin and dopamine. Without a well thought out lifestyle and supplement routine it can be very common to have the serotonin dump effect the next day and need to take a few days to fully recover. MDMA in micro-dose amounts can function like a highly advanced brain supplement in of itself, and in low but consistent dosages it can prove to be an effect supplement for psycho-emotional imbalances, cognitive challenges, and overall wellbeing.

Transcending the Addiction to Time

> *"Time is but an illusion created by beings with limited perception."*
>
> *Ken Poirot*

If there is one thing that the psychedelic experience can teach us with no uncertain clarity, it is that our entire perception of time is a total illusion. The entire framework of time we have become accustomed to is structured around basic principles of maintaining this illusion, which greatly supports institutions, socio-economic initiatives, and all other entities of organized society, but does not support the expansion, self-realization, or evolution of the human being him/herself. Our classical model of 'organized time' is based on the Gregorian and Julian calendric system. These, like so many of our agreed upon social constructs, are entirely based upon the ruminations of men, crafting concepts and structures in their mind, and then proposing them as universal facts that now set the template for how we all perceive life itself.

The primary function that an effective psychedelic experience will perform is releasing the individual from their conceptual framework of what they believe is absolute and real. An individual can (and often does) find themselves in a space where time, itself becomes very malleable, and impossible to track down. Impossible to lock down. Ungraspable by the mind itself because the mind is being reconditioned from its prior framework set and unwound from the constraints of linear time dynamics. Many people, including myself, have had the experience of multiple 'timelines' converging all together, bridging the past, the future, and the present together into a single moment. Where there is no split between past experiences, future anticipations, and the felt experience of the present moment. This is the 'zero point' where the timeless exists and pure potential without restrictions or borders can emerge.

Throughout our entire lives we have been taught many things around time and most of them have been less than empowering (or even factual). Have you ever heard the phrase 'time is money' or 'the only certainties in life are death and taxes?' First of all, what do time and money have to do with each other, as concepts? Well, in our economic driven society the idea of money i.e., financial currency is intertwined with our notion of time because we trade our time in order to receive money. Most people spend an enormous amount of time in the pursuit of money, all the way up into their final years, for retirement, security pensions, and cushioning the burden to their family from the expenses of their death and funeral. We have been taught to trade our most valuable resource (time) for the least valuable (and least scarce) resource called money. We are taught that 'money makes the world go round' but in actuality money does not make the world go round, it actually does nothing at all, except allows for the exchange of goods, services, and people's sense of security.

We have been trained to view money as the lifeline of our material existence and without it we feel insecure, unstable, and ill equipped to function in a consumer-based society. Time has become a linear concept, for which we organize our units of life force energy into a Gregorian calendar, as a measurement of the time we have spent, and the time we have left, whether in a day, in a week, a month, a series of years, and the remainder of our lives as a whole. The classical view on time i.e., the clock or calendar is a mental box that we place ourselves in and determine all other aspects of our lives in and around. When we adopt beliefs such as time is money or associate death and taxes together, we are creating a victimhood mentality within ourselves, which can only breed out scarcity, fear, and clinging onto the past, because we know that our time is steadily going away.

This is why there is such a 'death phobia' in our western culture, where people know they will eventually expire from their physical bodies, but rarely anyone wants to acknowledge it, and pick up all manner of addictions in order to avoid thinking about it. This creates a phenomenon called 'strauma' in the body and psyche. Strauma is the combination of stress + time which is a trauma that manifested itself due to too much stress compounded over many years of time. What is equally interesting about this is that many people report that doing a deep plant medicine ceremony was equal to doing 10 + years of intensive psychotherapy in one session. It stands to reason that this may be entirely due to the fact that the conceptual framework of time itself had become collapsed, and what was once compartmentalized in one's mind has now been released, expressed, and integrated together. The strauma that had been accumulated now became decompressed, perhaps entirely due to exiting out of the 'time box' and entering into a state of timelessness, where all things happen simultaneously, and all afflictions are healed automatically.

There are two concepts in the aging process called biological age and chronological age. Our biological age is how 'old' we are at the cellular level. Chronological age is how 'old' we are based on the number of years we have passed through. So, someone could be 50 years old chronologically but in their early 30's biologically. The paradigm of time-based aging has actually caused more people to accelerate in their aging process. If people did not have a negative connotation about their chronological age, in reference to their physical health, you would see far more people living well into their hundreds, as well as with excellent quality of life as well. This is proven by what are called 'the blue zones' in the world which is the longest living tribes and cultures in modern existence that all live well into their 90's and beyond 100 with good to excellent quality of health compared to most people in western society who are struggling to make it into their 70's with poor health. These individuals live outside of the structured calendric system and I imagine most of them have no idea how old they actually are, based on the years they have been alive.

Along the same line of thinking that we gain from the psychedelic experience regarding the notion of time being merely a man-made construct, we also begin to recognize that the world we have become accustomed too (organized society) functions similar to a consensus belief program. We all seem to agree that society is a certain way and that we all have an agreed upon set of moral and ethical principles that structure our behavior amongst one another. I would like to introduce the idea that what we know as our 'normal waking state' of reality is really just a 'dream spell' that functions according to the consensus agreements of everyone involved (which is all of us!). This includes our agreed upon perception of linear time, as well as the chronological aging process, and all that follows these kind of belief systems. Nothing becomes more overtly obvious during the psychedelic experience than the fact that we are waking up out of a 'dream spell' of linear structured time and beginning to explore what I call 'dream time'.

Now, I am going to share a little-known fact with you about our calendric system that very few modernist thinkers properly inner stand or have even considered due to their own 'dream spell' upbringing. The two calendric systems we use predominantly in organized society are the Gregorian & Julian calendars. I will omit the mathematical and technical details of these in order to punctuate the point of why I am writing on the subject of time in the first place. The Gregorian calendar was first introduced in 1582 by Pope Gregory XIII as an attempt to realign the calendar system to include the spring equinox and Easter together. The Julian calendar was brought forth by Julius Caesar in 45 BC in order to replace the Roman calendar which only consisted of 355 days per year. Both of these calendric systems operate using the same base linear mathematics and are attempts to "unitize" our notion of time, into fractions, in order to control time, or at the very least, as a way to 'manage' time. It should be made known that neither Julius Caesar or Pope Gregory (or any standing Pope for that matter!) were good hearted, caring individuals. The fact is these individuals, like so many revered figures of history were tyrannical, malevolent individuals who had one sole agenda during their reign in power; to control and use people as a resource for their own ends.

Would it stand to reason that these individuals would issue a linear calendric system as a way to control and manage the populations they sought to control? I will let you be the judge of that but due to my research on the subject, I am very clear as to the answer to the question. So, this simply furthers my original point, which is that our conceptual framework of time has put us in a kind of 'dream spell' which is the same 'spell' as being caught in the hypnotic wave form of addiction. We have become addicted to managing and controlling time, so much so that we may find ourselves struggling to hold it in our grasp, only to feel it slipping out from underneath us, and feeling powerless to hold onto it. This is all part of the 'program' itself, and in order to unhinge ourselves from the dream spell of scarcity, poverty, and lack that the addiction to time creates, we need to wake up out of this dream spell all together and embrace a brand-new dreamtime as our default reality. This default reality can be simply described as living within a space of the timeless mind and ageless body.

The timeless mind - ageless body concept is simply a state of being. It is an attitude adjustment from the obsessive focus on linear time and time management towards energy management as the focal point for how one lives their life. When we obsess over time, we minimize our energy reserves and initiate the chronological aging process which accelerates our biological aging process. By focusing obsessively on the concept of "time", we actually lose more of it, whereas when we stop focusing on managing time, we experience life in the present moment, and are able to maximize more of it as a result. The body responds to the focus of our mind and where we place our focus is exactly where our energy will be directed. The psychedelic experience helps to unwind the mental constraints we have around time and drops our consciousness directly into the state of 'timelessness', otherwise known as the omnipresent NOW.

Lastly on this topic, it would be important to consider that the addiction to time is really an aversion from the single biggest taboo fear in our culture, which of course is the fear of death. Why would we all be so focused on managing time if we were not concerned about time suddenly running out on us? Have you ever considered where this fear of time comes from? Where does it all start? Well, again, in our culture, we have a serious adverse reaction when it comes to discussing the single thing that no one has figured out how to escape from or bypass, which of course is the fact that our time in these physical bodies is finite and temporal. This insight can help bring about the realization that all of our human fears (and addictions) are all attempts to medicate our own existential fear of life and death. This is likely the most profound benefit many people can receive from plant medicines (and toad medicine) because it helps to rip off the ego-bandage of our fears, self-identity, stories, and holding patterns we use to compensate for the underlining sensation of our finite nature.

The construct of time is what we use to hold our perception of reality together in a way that makes sense, seems practical, and eases the deeper existential quandaries of life. Psychedelics have an interesting way of snapping us out of these manufactured constructs and exposing us to a deeper sense of reality, that resides beyond our 5 senses in the purely physical reality we all know and are familiar with. Funny enough, while there can be a healthy dose of trepidation prior to a plant medicine experience, many people discover that once they drop into it, they experience the most amount of peace, relief, and reassurance of safety they have ever felt in their lives. Often times the hardest part of a powerful entheogen experience is exiting from this space and returning back into the world of form. Often times the world we all consider to be absolutely real feels less real than the world of timelessness that we just experienced. The psychedelic experience tends to feel more real, more authentic, and more natural than the worldly reality we navigate each and every day.

So, with this all said, and explored, the idea itself is what is important here. Consider the consequences of being hyper focused on time. Notice when you are catching yourself constantly monitoring the dial of the clock and observe the reaction in your body as it clings on to the passing numbers on the screen. Observe how your mind begins to play tricks on you, telling you that you do not have enough time, or that time will run out unless you take ahold it, and try to control it. These are all illusions of the mind that has been conditioned into scarcity, poverty, and fear response patterns. All other addictions are simply attempting to ease the internal tension that manifests itself in the body as a feedback response based on a tightly bound mind that is obsessed with time, and committed to avoiding anything, at all costs, that would cause a confrontation (such as the topic of death) to the ego, and it's holding pattern to time itself.

Final Thoughts on Plant Medicines

This chapter is one of the more unique one's in this book because it goes against what many other experts in the fields of addiction and holistic health are comfortable discussing. Plant medicines and other psychedelic substances are becoming much more well known, and globally accepted, both in recreational circles of exploration, and in clinical research for their potent effects with psychotherapy. I could not imagine writing this entire book and not devoting an extensive chapter on this subject. It simply would not feel right to do so and in many ways would be inappropriate as well. This subject is far too important and is a necessary research exploration for anyone who is truly sincere about healing addiction, whether it is for their own personal benefit, or for educating others on the tools and resources they have available to them.

An important disclaimer is that these power plants and psychoactive compounds must be treated with reverence and respect. There are a lot of ways one can go about exploring these experiences, whether it is in the form of micro dosing certain compounds, or it is having a fully immersive ceremonial experience that is meant to help the user peal back the inner workings of their own mind. I recommend people do as much proper research prior to experimenting with anything they do not have direct experience with and also to seek out proper guidance from professionals or shamans that have many years of professional experience under their belt. These experiences are not meant to be recreational in nature but can be extremely powerful support tools for a variety of individual purposes. All of which should be thought out and with a clear intention to ensure one receives the most beneficial experience possible.

The set and setting principle are extremely important while entering into any medicine experience. It is advised to be cautious about doing plant medicines while in a city environment or any environment where there is a lot of outside noise, distractions, technology, or a lot of people outside of the medicine circle itself. The dark side (bad trips) of psychedelic experiences can often be attributed carelessness how one begins and finishes their experience, and also the lack of proper guidance by the facilitator. You only want to engage in this kind of experience with someone or someone's you can trust and feel safety around. If you feel any sense of lack of safety prior to entering into a ceremony I advise you consult with someone you trust or simply pass on it because emotional and physical safety is the absolute highest priority.

The other consideration is that the compounds you are using are of the highest possible quality. This goes hand in hand with knowing who you are being guided by and anyone else involved, if it is a group experience. This is why clinical setting are very useful for many people because it is a professionally monitored environment and the compounds used will only be of the highest quality. You have use your own discernment and do your own research in this area. It is important not to treat these things like some sort of recreational "drug" and that intention itself can help you bypass any qualitative issues with poor quality medicines.

262

Healing the Brain | Rehabbing the Mind

"Proactive interventions to increase the quality of life as well as prevention in psychiatry can be furthered through interpersonal education. This new kind of inner education will emphasize a conscious focus on the individual as a starting point for transformation towards sustainable lifestyles and society. To change one's internal functioning is the most positive step one can take to contribute towards increase for personal and world harmony."

Dr. Helena Lass

We have talked a lot about the role our psychology, cognition, and mental flexibility plays in all forms of addiction and recovery. Our mind is incredibly powerful and can be the most powerful tool we have in our arsenal. Unfortunately, it can also be a hinderance to our growth and progress when it is not being used correctly. For most people, I imagine, they are walking a thin tight rope between using their mind in a productive, and counterproductive way. It seems like at certain times in the day our mind feels clear, centered, and able to focus. At other times it can feel like our mind is cloudy, scattered, and hard to focus for extended periods of time. This oscillation back and forth can happen all throughout our day. If we are still engaged in the inner struggle with our addiction patterns, then it goes without saying that this is most likely the case.

This feeling of mental instability creates an experience of uncertainty and that can lead to further confusion. It is entirely healthy to feel waves of uncertainty so long as we also feel supported by life and experience a regularity of certainty. Certainty and uncertainty are merely two poles of the same magnetic. If one swings too far to one side, then it can create an imbalance. We need to feel periodic moments of mild uncertainty because that means we are in a growth point and are outside of our familiar comfort zone. We also need to feel certain of ourselves and our handle on our lives in order to make use of being outside the comfort zone, not simply overwhelmed by it and feeling defeated.

The mind is the most beautiful instrument for us to map out a new blueprint for our future, assess past mistakes or setbacks, and course correct a new path moving forward. Engaging with our mental faculties and exercising our minds in unique ways is fundamental to overcoming any obstacle we may face. The challenge is that most people were never taught how to use their mind to its potential or simply how it uses it at all. The compulsory repetitive public education system did little, to no good for us, in terms of learning how to exercise our minds. The rope repetition of absorbing irrelevant information, memorizing it to pass a pointless test, and dump the information quickly on our way to the next class, not only did not serve us, but it actually inhibited us in a major way. Most people do not know how their mind works or how to engage with it in a way that produces curiosity, excitement, and organic pleasure. Most people are addicted to pleasure, so they repeat habits that trigger the dopamine response in the brain which blunts out pain receptors and keeps our mind sedated by excessive comfort.

Our mind, just like our muscles, requires daily exercise and a conscious effort to learn new skills, increase blood flow to all regions of the brain, and to rehabilitate it from incorrect processing patterns. Relating the mind to our muscular systems, we pick up bad postural habits over time, incorrect exercise patterns, and can develop scar tissue or inflammation from unhealed injuries. If we have not corrected these patterns or healed the inflammatory triggers, then our body continues to weaken, and we experience chronic pain. This is no different when talking about the mind. We have developed bad habits of thinking, adopting false belief systems, constructing an identity and sub-personalities, and simply allowing the mind to atrophy due to inactivity. There is a rehabilitation process the mind (and brain) have to go through in order to fully recover from all it has had to endure. And trust me, all of our minds have taken a beating over time and some minds have simply gone offline and we need to turn them back on, fast!

Healing takes a full commitment, and it can take a seemingly gradual progression over longer periods of time. It may only seem gradual or incremental in the beginning but that is due to the neuropathways that have been formed and myelinated through the course of our lives. In neuroscience there is a term called neuroplasticity, which shows us that our physical brains are malleable, fluid, and can be reshaped. The dendrite connections spawn like spider webs of collected data that form our brains and the information traveling throughout the cerebral circuit processing station. What we put into our minds is exactly what is registered, insulated, and stored, just as what we practice with our bodies is what our muscles entrain into and normalize. How we become the way we are is only a series of habits and rehearsed routines. They do not have an iron clad grip on us, unless we resist them and try to fight them back as if we were in a Chinese finger trap with our own mind. Only when we bring both fingers together (both hemispheres together) do the tension subsist and we easily detach from the trap.

In this chapter we are going to discuss the mind and the brain from the perspective of recovery and rehabilitation. It's good to discern that the brain and the mind are two separate issues. The brain is a 2-pound organ that rests at the base of our skull and is very soft, delicate, and is encased around bony ridges in our skull. The brain is the central processor for the entire body and is fed electrical packets of information throughout all of our nerve endings. When we speak about the brain, we are speaking about the organic instrument itself. The mind is a different thing all together. The mind is its own multiverse, which has been called the noosphere. This is similar to the biosphere or the atmosphere but think of it as a biosphere of the inner human experience, the mental sphere. This is where consciousness exists, and we have complete creative input as to what goes on in the mental plane of our own experience.

The brain and the mind, as you can guess, work in parallel to each other. One is physical and the other is etheric. One is a full-scale computation mechanism and the other is the holographic out picturing of what is being transmitted and received. If we do not take excellent care of our brains than the mind slips into chaos and the transmission becomes altered or scrambled. Likewise, if we do not take excellent care of our minds our brains can atrophy, lose electrical potential, and become easily programmable. An addiction is merely a program operating within a brain that is wired for chemical indulgences and fixed patterns of thought. When people are trying to break out of this fixed pattern, they can experience mental fatigue, lethargy, lack of motivation, and brain fog.

These symptoms are showing us a more accurate representation of how our brains are functioning on their own, without the assistance of stimulatory substances or dopamine producing activities. This is very much part of the overall rehabilitation process.

We have to learn to train our minds and exercise critical thinking in order to regain ourselves and our lives. It is as simple as choosing something different than you normally would. Responding to an urge by breathing, shaking out the body, meditating, or turning on a nice cold shower. The mind has been conditioned towards comfort, passivity, and seeking pleasure. If the process produces temporary bouts of discomfort, pain, or resistance then you are doing it right. If that discomfort is so easily alleviated by seeking out the pleasure response patterns then our minds/consciousness does not strengthen, in fact it becomes more adolescent or dependent. Dependent on whatever it associates as the key to turn on the sensation it prefers in the moment. In this way we can start to understand how a poorly informed and trained mind can work against us and block our progress forward. This is merely the entrained ego mind or manufactured identity we have been accustomed to experiencing.

There is the lower mind and the higher mind. They are both components of the overall noosphere/mental-sphere and the whole is greater than the sum of its parts. So, when experiencing resistance and the booby traps of the conditioned, addicted lower mind, we can also command the power of our higher mind/higher nature to assist us. This is achieved by first developing discernment between the two, and mostly sensing what one feels like in contrast to the other. The lower mind deals with lower basal carnal desires such as security, safety, sex/procreation, and survival. Whereas the higher mind deals with elevated aspirational desires such as joy, fulfillment, pursuing dreams, helping others, protecting life, and making positive changes. When an urge arises and the mind kicks in, be aware of the mental images and the feeling tone they elicit in the body. Does it feel uplifting, expansive, inspiring, or does it feel selfish, contractive, or like a rush of lust (i.e., pornography) and desire to get a quick gratification/orgasm/pleasure.

This really comes down to which wolf do we feed at the end of the day. If we feed the wolf of immediate pleasure and distraction, we will experience more of what that creates in our lives. If we feed the wolf of commitment and devotion, we will also experience the benefits of that in our lives. The mind is incredibly fluid, adaptable, and able to reroute any programmed patterns into new patterns. It simply just takes practice, follow through, and repetition. The mind and the brain have a lot of circuits and mazes to unwind in order to return back to cognitive efficiency, inner stability, and harmony. Once we rehabilitate ourselves from the inside out, we can then rebuild a stronger, more integral foundation.

Let's now discuss the rehabilitation process moving forward.

"The greatest potential for opening our hearts lies in the opening of our minds."

Vironika Tugaleva

Rehabilitating the Addicted Mind

"Do not believe everything you think."

Unknown

"The soul always knows what to do to heal itself. The challenge is to silence the mind."

Caroline Myss

We have discussed in depth and unpacked many layers of how the mind works throughout this book, thus far. We have placed special focus on how the addicted mind becomes dependent on dopamine based chemical stimulation and habituates to repeating reward/pleasure-based activities. We have also explained in detail how one's life can become completely sidetracked and misdirected due to the neuropathways in the brain that are formed due to addiction and how this can hijack the mental processes that we all take for granted each day. We have gone very deep into all of these areas and now we are going to discuss something that is rarely ever mentioned in addiction and recovery education; how to rehabilitate the addicted mind.

Like with any rehab process, it is a gradual journey back to recovery and some people make a full recovery sooner than others. There is no cookie cutter approach to this process, especially because we are not dealing with something as mechanical as a knee, a hip, a strained quadricep, etc. We are dealing with something incredibly sophisticated and something that has the least amount of understanding amongst health professionals. The mind is not a body part you can easily pick apart based on motor functions, skeletal hinges, tendons or ligaments holding it in place. The mind is deeply personal, contains all information of an individual, and unique to each individual.

So, when approaching the idea of rehabbing or healing an addicted mind, we must first go into it with a fresh pair of eyes that do not contain the baggage of conventional perceptions. Those will not work here (and rarely ever work elsewhere for that matter). We, first begin by observing the patterns of our minds, tracking its habitual tendencies, and making course corrections accordingly. Once we become self-aware of our own addictions and the psycho-physical tendencies that reveal themselves we now begin to regain control over ourselves. Psycho-physical means the mental thought or image that illicit a physical response, such as a sexual image in our mind creating a chemical cascade of dopamine or "pleasure" in the body itself. We simply begin by becoming aware of this phenomenon and tracking it every time it arises so we can then engage in the healing process.

The interesting thing about healing/rehabbing the mind is that much of it depends on our own awareness of what is going on in our mental sphere. It is not just about "fixing" a pattern or "correcting" a thought process but simply to become aware of the pattern of thought itself and noticing the unconscious behaviors that routinely follow it. We are not so much defined by our thoughts or mental processes but more so by the actions and behaviors our mental patterns create. The combination of incessant thought loops and repeated actions to follow them up are what creates the addicted mind and reinforces the psycho-physical habit. Our patterns shape our minds, and our minds powerfully influence our habits. All we need to do is begin reshaping the mental image of ourselves, exchanging out who we thought we were for who we aspire to be, and then begin adapting our lifestyle habits to reinforce that new vision.

So, with all of this said, let's understand something very important about the mind and the easiest way all of us can fall into the mental booby traps of what I call the mine field of the mind. We can easily get ourselves into problems by overthinking a situation and then we try to think our way out of our issues. We try to outthink our own thoughts, yet we have not moved an inch away from where we started. The addiction of the mind is an addiction to existing mostly in our heads which disconnects us from the feedback of our body and heart. When we are connected to our body's innate intelligence, we are able to clearly think and process situations effectively. If we are too much in the mental sphere, i.e., our head, we can easily become trapped in this mental realm and lose touch with reality, as it is occurring outside of our inner experience. In short, we cannot outthink or outwit our addictions or thought loops. This way of being only reveals to us that we are using far too much energy yet going absolutely nowhere.

This does not mean that thinking in of itself is somehow bad, unproductive, or ill advised. In truth, true thinking is a powerful and necessary practice but when I use the term "in our head" or "outthinking" our thoughts, I am referring to a distinctly different process all together. Just because we have a bundle of thoughts at any given moment does not indicate we, ourselves, are participating in a conscious effort to critically think. You can discern the difference very quickly because one of these two approaches produces immediate results and the other prolongs the production of results, unless the result is mental constipation or cognitive overwhelm. If this sounds like a paradox, I understand and hope that the distinction becomes very clear and obvious here. Critical thinking is not just about "thinking" itself, it is more of an exercise into the inquiry of thought, for example, observing the threads of thought patterns and writing them down in a morning journal or simply watching them go by in a sitting meditation. This is a voluntary practice with the intent to unwind our thoughts and from there, reshuffle the cognitive deck, or dispense with the deck all together in order to upgrade our cognitive operating system.

What we often do, as in the case of an addicted mind, is resist our thoughts, battle against our thoughts, or become subservient to our thoughts, allowing them to have their way with us. The rehabilitation process for the mind requires us to take total responsibility for our thought process, feel the full range of emotions that arise when we sit with what is there, and install new actions/habits replacing the prior habits that were on autopilot. The tension or resistance that arises is the signal that our mind is seeking growth, expansion, and healing. Allow ample space for this tension to unwind in a space of breath work and/or meditation and watch how the thought loops begin to loosen up and detach by themselves. Critical thinking is a process of challenging the status quo of the conditioned mind but it does not happen by fighting the mind. It happens by observing the situation clearly and stacking all of the evidence that opposed the prior viewpoint, through research, and letting the truth do the work for you.

What does this all mean? Letting the truth do the work for you? Allow me to explain this idea. When we have a fixed perspective of something, let's say about ourselves and this perspective is based on an accumulation of evidence we have gained over the course of time. We may see ourselves as someone who is addicted to X, Y, & Z. So, in our minds we associate our self-identity with X, Y, & Z and through repetition of action we now see ourselves as someone who does/is addicted to X, Y, & Z. Now, in our minds there is a significant amount of evidence to support this perception of ourselves based on the clear-cut data. The process of critical thinking, in this example, is to dig up as much evidence/data that is contrary to this perception i.e., is in opposition with our viewpoint of ourselves as an addict of X, Y, & Z. We have already built a strong case that we are X, Y, & Z but now we have to balance the scales a bit and build a new case that we are not exactly who we had believed we were by default.

Once we place all of the evidence on the table and sort it all out, something interesting begins to happen. We discover a new and more broadened perspective of ourselves that encompasses far more than who we had believed we are. You may have felt you were unlovable, unlikable, and downright selfish. Because, after all, if someone has a drug problem, pornography problem, or any other addiction, that automatically means they are selfish and careless, right? Wrong! It does not mean that at all. All that it means is, in that dimension of someone's overall experience, at that

The beta brain wave state is best utilized like any good tool, for a specific purpose and function. Short bursts of beta activity which is channeled and harnessed for the potency it has would serve us best. Remaining in a beta brain wave state long term is like remaining in a sympathetic stress (fight or flight) state well beyond its expiration point where it is no longer helpful or useful. Learning how to down regulate the hyperactivity of the beta mind is essential.

Delta Wave

The delta brain wave state is the antithesis to the beta brain wave state. Delta is extremely slow and resides on the brain wave frequency of the loud drumming sensation if you were to consider all brain states like a musical spectrum. Delta state is generated in very deep meditation or in REM-less(dreamless) sleep cycles. This is where deep healing happens. This is also where our vast amount of stem cells is produced during deep sleep, which causes our body to regenerate itself and cells to replicate at a pace faster than they are breaking down. Delta is the natural counterbalance to the beta brain wave state and when one is having trouble getting out of beta, they can have a hard time getting deep restorative sleep.

Alpha Wave

The alpha brain wave state is one of the most heavily focused upon brain wave frequencies because of the emerging interest into the science of "flow states". Alpha represents the flow state in action whereas gamma and hyper gamma include internal flow but without external activity. When someone is in a dominant alpha brain wave state, they are fully fastened into the now i.e., engaged in the present moment. Learning how to tap into the alpha wave is an antidote to the dopamine dilemma because dopamine dependency tends to cause one to be in a beta brain wave state, fixating on the future, whereas alpha states cause one to be present in the moment. When we are totally present, we elicit more serotonin in the brain, which is the natural balance to too much dopamine arousal.

Alpha waves are extremely healing to the brain and help to synchronize all known functions between the brain, the nervous system, and the voluntary systems of the body. Alpha state increases mental coordination, steady mental processing, calm alertness, memory retention and deep learning. Alpha is the core resting state of the brain. This is the preferred brain wave state to spend the most amount of time in during the day, if and when possible.

Theta Wave

The theta wave state is sometimes called the twilight state. It is where the body begins to go offline but the mind is very much awake. Imagine being in the alpha state i.e., pure flow state and the body begins to slip out of waking state alertness and power down, but the mind exists in the in-between state between the body and conscious awareness. Brain scans conducted on long term meditators show that at some point in the meditation the brain will produce large amounts of theta-based chemicals the deeper into the meditation the person goes into. Another way to think of theta is as the transitional state between alpha and delta. REM (rapid eye movement) is produced in theta which is when we have colorful imaginative visions that are connected to our DMT production in the pineal gland during sleep or in some kind of visionary experience.

Gamma Wave

The gamma brain wave state is known as "super consciousness", meaning it is the brain state that allows one to be in total and absolute flow within their inner world. This state is connected to transcendental experiences described as 'oneness', 'altruism', 'higher love', or 'universal love'. In order for the brain to slip into the gamma state the mind has to be completely quiet and calm. This is why it is so challenging for many people in the beginning of meditation to achieve this and why many others never experience a moment of this in their entire lives. It is speculated that gamma state represents the brains doorway to 'higher consciousness'. I would have to agree with this assertion because we now know that gamma is the doorway to the higher brain waves states beyond this one which was discovered from doing brain imaging scans on lifelong meditators and Tibetan monks.

Rehabilitating the Addicted Brain

It is one thing to consider the intricacies of the mental body itself i.e., the expansive and multi-layered nature of the mind itself. This is generally the singular focus of most psychological discussions in personal development, clinical psychiatry, and various other modalities involving the repression of our psycho-emotional faculties and prior life experiences which may have led to unresolved trauma. The mind is a vast dimensional territory that can take us on an infinite odyssey into the nature of the human condition and for some, it is an incredible ecstatic experience, and for others, it can be like navigating their way out of a confusing labyrinth. This theme has arisen in multiple chapters throughout this book and the best attempts were made to tie it all together in this chapter, so we could discuss the often-overlooked aspect of psychological recovery, healing the addicted brain.

Perhaps this is somewhat obvious to the reader, that there is a dual repair or rehab process necessary to overcome the slippery slope of addiction and psycho-physiological dependency. What we need to understand is that the brain itself is the master processing agent/mechanism that allows for all other bodily functions. This also includes the possibility of expanding one's consciousness, emotional development, and spiritual awareness. It is not enough to simply state the paramount importance of having a spiritual practice that increases one's faith in a higher power. In order for this to move from a simple concept into a felt experience the central processor of the body technology must be working accordingly and if not, well, we lose conduction in the system and our minds are not able to hold the feeling experience for lack of processing power.

I know you have heard me say this same idea in a multitude of ways and it cannot be overstated because it simply is the truth. A truth which very few, if any of us were taught growing up and must reinforce into our understanding so we can get the results we want and deserve out of life.

The brain is the central processing unit, the nervous system, skeletal system, muscular system, and overall bodily structure is the hardware (think of a stand-up computer), and the mind is composed of all of the software programs and information from our life experiences. The brain's role is in processing all of the accrued data/information, organizing it into mental folders, prioritizing it based on relevancy and usefulness, and showcasing a roadmap/blueprint of sorts, in order to effectively execute towards a probable set of outcomes/goals. This is a major undertaking, but the brain is highly capable of doing all of this and much more, so long as it remains uninhibited by the distractibility of temporary dopamine hits, chronic systemic inflammation in the body, and is structurally as healthy as possible.

In the last two decades or so, there have been some astonishing scientific discoveries in the fields of neuroscience, cognitive development, and brain health, which all translate into higher quality of life and overall increased longevity potential. There are brain scan imaging technologies that have been developed in order to safely scan the state of someone's brain and how healthy or unhealthy it is depending on their lifestyle factors. I have personally studied this aspect of neuroscience for almost a decade myself and the discoveries that have been made in relation to the effects of an 'addicted brain' vs an 'non-addicted brain' are remarkable and sobering. The thing about our brain is that it tends to exist within the principle of "out of sight, out of mind." The brain is not constantly registered in our immediate awareness such as say our hands, arms, legs, stomach, or facial features are. We do not witness our brains in the mirror or can touch our brains like we can our forehead, skin, nails, or hair. Our brains are the single most important organ in the body and are absolutely indispensable on all levels, yet they receive little to no regard by the average person.

The most common way someone develops a sensitivity to the state of their brain is usually when they feel discomfort such as a headache, brain fog, cognitive disarray, or other brain-based performance symptoms. These are the major tell-tale signs of an unhealthy brain that is likely afflicted by inflammation of one form or another. The danger in this scenario is that once the brain has become malfunctioned or there is an inflammatory agent involved it becomes very difficult to know how to work our way back to equilibrium, simply because we were not fully present from the process of a healthy brain to an unhealthy brain. The conscious mind has been set to autopilot and things were going along as normal, yet the state of our delicate brain was progressively becoming abnormal, and we only took notice once the symptoms became unbearable.

This is a hard pill to swallow once we become conscious and alert to the fact that we may not have treated our most important organ with the love, respect, and care it needs from us. I know this might be hard to receive but I also know that in order to heal our precious brains, we must acknowledge the afflictions that have been done (conscious or unconscious), take responsibility for our actions (or inactions), and pledge ourselves to being better caretakers for our bodies and brains. It is remarkable how adaptable, flexible, and resilient our brains truly are. It's almost as if they are like little children in a sense, that they are full of innocence, wonder, and love but can become easily manipulated, wounded, and filled with so many false theories and concepts, that they lose the spark of divinity they came into this world with. Well, I want to help you understand that your brain carries the codes for regeneration, reparation, and absolute healing. The first step in the process of brain rehabilitation is to begin lovingly communicating to ourselves the thoughts, affirmations, dreams, and inspirational feelings that you would associate with a truly healthy and infinitely capable brain and mind.

Brain imaging scans have demonstrated exactly what is happening in the brain when there is an addiction cycle fully rooted over the course of months or years. Every substance is unique in of itself but the commonalities and similarities amongst all addictions are well documented. The reward system involving dopamine is involved in every addictive tendency and the brain itself loves the immediate flooding of dopamine, or at least it seems to love it because it feels really good, until it doesn't. The problem the brain has with overstimulation and frequent hyper-dopamine production is that the dopamine receptors become overused and wear out due to an unnatural and far too frequent usage of them. Once the dopamine receptors wear down it takes a significant increase in dosage of the habit itself in order to experience the familiar baseline effect and we all know where this cycle leads us in the end. It can only lead us to massive depletion of dopamine receptors which are linked to our endocrine system (hormone production) and translate into our adrenal/kidney system and thyroid metabolism system.

Since the brain is the central processor for the rest of the body the imaging scans depicted of the brain are a snapshot representation of what is likely occurring in the remainder of the body and to what degree it is able to function optimally or not. Because of the pleasure/reward feedback loop set up in the brain, we are literally training ourselves to repeat habits that produce a similar or identical effect i.e., the sensation of pleasure, which causes us to feel rewarded in some way. The mechanism responsible for this effect is the dopamine d2 receptors which are located in the prefrontal cortex of the brain and allow us to exercise self-control, restraint, long held discipline, and delayed gratification. As long as this mechanism is healthy and functional then we will be able to exercise these necessary qualities with relative ease. When these dopamine receptors become overused and are not sufficiently restored with chemical building blocks (such as amino acids) or the usage rate is much faster than the replacement rate it becomes increasingly harder to carry out basic tasks, exercise discipline or self-restraint, and this is how the brain becomes feverish for repeated experiences of immediate pleasure.

What is really happening in this scenario is that the brain is going into a kind of panic state, which also triggers the central nervous system to initiate a sympathetic stress response. The pleasure/reward drive is simply a way to provide a sensation of relief and reprieve from what is, otherwise, a red alert emergency. This can happen for a variety of health reasons such as chronic inflammation (cellular damage), heavy metals (mercury amalgam fillings), digestive infection (microbiome imbalance), toxicity (substance or environmental), nutrient deficiency (poor diet or incorrect body type diet), or in the downstream effects of dopamine depletion leading to a lack of vital life force in the system and the brain literally starving and/or under distress. So, in order to rebalance and repair the addicted brain we have to treat it exactly like it is, which is a brain that has fallen under addiction, just as the human him/herself (as we understand it) can become addicted. The chemistry set of the brain has become hijacked and is running on a binary set of linear codes and patterns that all are based on dopaminergic stimulation i.e., short term relief. We must reroute these coded patterns to become more diverse,

278

more advanced, and to lead in the direction of fulfillment, satisfaction, and self-discipline.

How the Brain Forms Habitual Patterns

"Take up one idea. Make that one idea your life - think of it, dream of it, live on that idea. Let the brain, muscles, nerves, every part of your body, be full of that idea, and just leave every other idea alone. This is the way to success."

Swami Vivekananda

Perhaps the single most fascinating area of brain research is on how the brain and nervous system reforms its software set according to the inputs we give to it through out each day, and over the course of time. The brain is without a doubt the most complex and sophisticated biotechnology that exists. Even with all of the man-made technologies that surround us today, nothing even comes close to the technological capacity of the human brain. The brain can be programmed for optimal performance, hyper processing capabilities, and can even regenerate its own neuronal cells for enhanced longevity. The brain can also be programmed for sluggish performance, increased cognitive lag time, and atrophy, causing apoptosis of its own cells (cell death). The brain could be likened to a sponge in this regard but that would be a very crude example to describe how the brain functions.

The entire neurochemical and neuromuscular system of the body adheres and adapts to the most frequent patterns we reinforce each day. Our brain chemistry adheres by stimulating the glands and organs to secrete a spectrum of hormones based on what is needed to carry out the inputs we are giving it (thoughts, emotions, physical movement). The brain then adapts itself by organizing the electrical current to flow into areas of the neuromuscular system as a process of what is known as 'myelination'. The more habitual a pattern is, the more rooted in the entire body it becomes. The more rooted a behavior has become, the harder it is to uproot it. The brain itself needs to be retrained in a way that it easily

279

begins to loosen the neuromuscular and chemical bonding it had in order to form a brand new 'neurosynaptic dendritic bond'. Healing the addicted brain is entirely a process of three key factors: Myelination, Neuroplasticity, and Neurogenesis.

We have discussed briefly the concept of neuroplasticity in different regions of this book, but it deserves a more in-depth explanation in this chapter. The idea behind this discovery is that our physical brain is highly adaptable, malleable, and changeable based on the information it receives. The brain itself shapes our model of reality and to a greater degree, our model of ourselves. We are largely shaped by the behavioral patterns and the health of our brain. The word 'neuro' translates into the overall nervous system including the brain, the spinal cord, and the nerve bundles that exist in the body. The word 'plasticity' is derived from the Greek word plastos which means moldable. Neuroplasticity means to mold and shape the brain. This concept was introduced in 1906 by an Italian psychiatrist by the name of Ernesto Lugaro who was interested in how the brain could adapt, learn, and even recover from neurological injuries. This idea goes back even further to 1904 during the famous Pavlovian experiments by Ivan Pavlov using the ringing of a bell to cause dogs to salivate thus creating a repetitive pattern to elicit a predictable response.

There are two things that are especially important about this phenomenon which is the ability to accelerate learning potential and also the ability to accelerate regeneration of a healthy brain. We will discuss the second aspect further down in this section on neurogenesis. As it pertains to the framework on addiction recovery the concept of accelerated learning becomes incredibly powerful because all that is happening here is the switching from one reinforced pattern (addiction habits) into brand new rehearsed patterns (new habits). The discomfort we feel in the withdrawal and habit transition phase is a byproduct of neuroplasticity at work. Neurons that have bonded together through synaptic wiring are disassociating from each other in order for new bonds to be created. The brain is still accustomed to the prior behavioral patterns, which simply means it's treading outside of its default comfort zone.

In order for neuroplasticity to take full effect it requires a consistent stimulus to trigger a response in the brain. Following this 'trigger', there is an opening that occurs and with enough repetition coupled with emotional engagement (energy/passion) the brain begins to 'rewire' itself to adapt to the new stimulus. If the brain has developed an addiction, it has been neuroplastically wired for, the heightened dopamine stimulus that elicits sensations of pleasure, relief, or signaling the reward centers in the brain. The repetition of the addictive habit/pattern creates the grooves i.e., neuropathways in the brain, which insulate the behavior into the body. The reason why change can become so difficult is simply because there is not enough emotional 'intensity' to change from the old pattern into a new pattern. Our brain was comfortable in the old pattern, even if it was harming the brain. It gets lulled to sleep in a way and can begin to atrophy as a result. The brain, although technically an organ, functions almost identical to a muscle, which needs to be exercised and stimulated in order to work at optimal capacity.

Just like riding a bike, learning martial arts, or going for a swim, engaging with the brain is very much a physical process and requires the entire body to be fully engaged. Movement practices tend to be the most immediate way to stimulate the brain into making brand new neuronal connections and disbanding from synaptic bonds that do not serve the activity at hand. When we engage our respiratory system(lungs) and our cardiovascular system(heart) we pump more oxygen into our blood cells, which reaches into the brain. I have found that without a solid exercise or physical movement practice, breaking away from sedentary addictions is near impossible to fully do. The entire nervous system is wired and primed for the activities the body has been accustomed towards. Once we begin to engage our full bodily intelligence the brain begins to recondition itself due to the fact that it needs to adjust to the immediate demands being placed upon it.

Mediation and breath work practices are also very powerful for this process. Deep diaphragmatic breathing can create a 'pattern interrupt' when our nervous system has become sluggish or stuck in a comfort state. Like exercise, this drives oxygen throughout the entire system and into the brain, which helps the brain come alive. When the brain is depleted of oxygen it begins to atrophy and this is the start of many widely known neurodegenerative conditions many in their older years suffer from. The combination of breath work and meditation helps to unwind the old, bonded neurons and open the mind so that neuroplasticity can more easily take effect. If you recall in our prior section on brain wave states, this is like tapping into the alpha and theta brain wave patterns which is the source point for heightened neuroplasticity and what is known as myelination.

Piggy backing on the concept of neuroplasticity is one of the most fascinating ideas for me, which is myelination or the myeline sheath that surrounds our delicate nerve fibers. I came across this emerging discovery in brain science around the year 2011 (10 years ago) when I stumbled on a book called **The Talent Code** by Daniel Coyle. More on the book in a moment. I was especially interested in the idea that the brain can regenerate itself, even from environmental toxicity, chronic inflammation, or impact injuries. It appears that myelination is one of the answers to this inquiry. The myeline sheath is a fatty material that insulates itself around our nerve fibers and helps link the axons together, particularly in the peripheral nervous system. The myeline material is formed through what is known as glial cells and this is the key element for information processing in the brain. The function of myeline is to insulate the nerve bundles in order to allow for speedy processing of information throughout the entire body, which is carried out along the electrical highway of the spinal cord and gut-brain axis.

In his book Daniel Coyle shares many stories of some of the most talented athletes and performers/learners he came across in what he calls 'talent hotbeds'. He discovered remarkable talent in these quadrants in his studies and determined that talent is not something someone is born with but rather something that is grown and developed. A deduction he made in his research is that all human skill resides in the wires (neuronal networking) of the brain. He reminds us that the concept of muscle memory sounds nice, but it is inaccurate. Our muscles do not actually have any memory in of themselves. It is actually neuromuscular memory that this concept is referring too and that is a big distinction. From a purely mechanical perspective, all of our talent and skill resides in the neuro-circuitry of the brain. It turns out that this circuitry grows and developed in a very particular pattern based on how we practice our habits and the intrinsic motivation behind it.

This is exactly what he discovered in these 'talent hotbeds. The big discovery from this was that it was the myeline sheathing in the brain that seemed to be responsible for people's ability to learn, master, and execute on their developed skill sets. Myeline is like the rubber insulator around electrical wires and whatever neurons are firing in sequence together in the brain, the myelination effect takes place, wrapping those synaptic bonds together. This creates a kind of mental map or cognitive blueprint for executing the behaviors associated with the myelinated neuronal associations. This is how electrical information flows through out the nervous system, which is why I draw the distinction between the idea of muscle memory and neuromuscular memory. We can lose a limb due to an amputation but still retain the memory signature of it in the brain. This is called the phantom limb phenomena.

The purpose of myeline is to make sure the electrical signal does not 'leak' out i.e., miss its destination in the physiology of the body. When myeline has been damaged this can cause motor function imbalances in the body and increase cognitive decline, muscular atrophy, and other potential health problems. The key with this is to comprehend the role of myeline and how to use this concept to repattern new habits by displacing the old ones through practice and repetition. The other is to realize that myeline, like any part of the body, can be subject to wear and tear, inflammation, and damage. Correct nutrition, supplementation, cleansing, and sleep are important areas to focus on for repairing any damage done to our myeline sheath in our lives. If we have been exposed to environmental toxicity, heavy metals (especially mercury/thimerosal), fluoride in tap water, pesticides of all kinds, and/or chronic stress we can be assured that our myeline could use some repair. In the **21 Day Dopamine Reset | Reboot | Recovery** protocol there is a solid map for helping the brain recovery from any form of decline, including demyelination.

Concluding the topic of myeline I want to explain that the difference between a well-developed brain and an undeveloped brain is the difference between a high-speed internet carrier vs a dial up broad band carrier. We can all upgrade our operating system to function like a high speed, quick processing network and the way this is done is through deep practice. The brain becomes very comfortable if we leave it up to its own devices. It has no need to keep growing and making new neurosynaptic connections if we leave it where it is at. The motivational force behind our actions is a huge factor in the myelination equation. It's not just going through the motions. It's a fully immersive experience that disassociates (breaks apart) old neuron bonds and then forces new synaptic connections to form. This is also why it is so hard in the beginning to adopt a brand-new habit and leave alone an old one. If your motivation behind it is strong enough that will signal a message to the brain that this is do or die. Once the brain realizes that there is no counter option for growth, it automatically begins to grow and force a cognitive change.

We are going to complete our dissertation on the brain by discussing the concept of neurogenesis. This is the perfect way to tie a bow on this entire chapter and lock the myelinated brain neurons firing in this moment together. Around a decade ago I became incredible interested in all things to do with the brain, as you likely could tell by now. The first major breakthrough concept I learned was that of neurogenesis and how the brain is literally designed to regenerate brain neurons. It has taken many decades for this simple and seemingly undeniable aspect of neuroscience to reach the fore front of mainstream academia. This is due to the long held and outdated paradigms relating to how the brain operates and that of genetic determinism. Genetic determinism comes from its own outdated scientific paradigm of the human genome. It was once believed that our genome is fixed in place and what you are born with is what you can expect over your entire life. We explored this in more detail in the chapter **The Dopamine Dilemma** in the section on epigenetics. This same paradigm was founded in neuroscience claiming that whatever amount of brain cells/neurons you are born with is all that you get, and you can expect age associated cognitive decline to manifest if you live long enough.

This is not exactly an inspiring or particularly motivating concept for an entire population of people to buy into but nonetheless this is the basic framework people have built into their belief model of life. Thankfully the updated and unbiased scientific discoveries of the last 2-3 decades have blown these antiquated paradigms into the wind. The truth is your brain is also repairing and regenerating neurons, just as fast as it is deleting or 'pruning' out old ones. The brain has a weeding out process calling 'synaptic pruning', which is a cancel and deletion process of neuronal connections that no longer serve someone's consistent behaviors. Think of this like a detoxification process for the old wiring of the brain as it makes way for new connections to form. The problem arises when one becomes sedentary in their life, reverts into their default comfort zone, continues to participate in unhealthy habits, and refuses to outgrow old identities. It is only when we choose to grow as a human being and adopt the necessary habitual patterns that reflect our inner growth that the brain engages in a combination of neuroplasticity, neurogenesis, synaptogenesis, and synaptic pruning.

Neurogenesis takes a huge effect when an embryo in the womb is going through its spontaneous growth cycle. This also happens in a rapid fashion during the formative years of a baby's development and into the following years, assuming the child is actively engaged in frequent learning. It is well established that this phenomenon also takes place throughout an entire lifespan but steadily declines in proportion to the activity and development of the adult themselves. Neurogenesis signals growth factors in the nervous system by way of what are called neuronal stem cells. Stem cells are molecular packets of information that cause a big growth spurt or influence the healing/regeneration of various parts of the body. Stem cell therapies have become extremely popular all throughout the world but are still under scrutiny by the allopathic corporate medical system, simply because anything that actually works is under scrutiny by the conventional health care (sick care) management establishment.

These concepts I have shared with you here are source codes for radically empowering your cognitive capacities and regaining total control over your life. Addictions can only take hold if the brain itself has developed a co-dependency to the chemistry and wiring of that behavior. By focusing on creating and maintaining a healthy brain you can easily maintain a healthy life. Use these ideas to explore a wider concept of your own human potential. Put them into action right away. Begin picking up a new habit you have neglected. Begin exercising in new ways you may be uncomfortable with. Read a book you really want to but are intimated by. Mediate for longer than you are accustomed too. Keep stretching the boundaries of what feels comfortable and push your comfort zone to next heights. This is the formula for human potential and transcending the limitations of addiction and the dopamine dilemma.

Mastering the Body | Physical Health

"I have come to the conclusion that human beings are born with an innate capacity to triumph over trauma. I believe not only that trauma is curable, but that the healing process can be a catalyst for profound awakening—a portal opening to emotional and genuine spiritual transformation. I have little doubt that as individuals, families, communities, and even nations, we have the capacity to learn how to heal and prevent much of the damage done by trauma. In so doing, we will significantly increase our ability to achieve both our individual and collective dreams."

Peter A. Levine,

Healing Trauma: A Pioneering Program for Restoring the Wisdom of Your Body

It has been brought up numerous times throughout this book that the hidden component in healing our addictions stems from both, the healing of our minds, and more to the source of it all, in the healing of our bodies. There is no addiction that exists in someone's life that does not exist in someone's physical body. The mind and the body operate very much as a singular unit in many respects and must be addressed from a holistic approach in order for any significant and long-lasting results to occur. In fact, I would venture so far as to say that the mind is a mirror reflection of our body, thus making the point that the mind may, in fact be the body itself. Allow me to expand upon this thought.

As we have explored in the previous chapter on healing the brain and healing the mind, you will now have a much better comprehension of what exactly the mind is, in distinction from the brain. The brain is technically a part of the physiological system of the body, as we understand what the body is in its totality, and how it functions and operates. So, the brain is the central processing station of the physical body, but what if I told you that we actually had multiple "bodies", other than the one we are most familiar with, and these other bodies were other than physical or physiological. We have what is known as an emotional body, a spiritual or ethereal body and we also have what is commonly referred to as a mental body. This expanded understanding allows us to think about ourselves (and our addictive tendencies) in a far more expanded and enlightening way.

We will explore this concept much further in the sections following this, but let's stick to the mind as the body idea for now. The mind is constantly tracking every physiological function, electrical impulse, enzyme interaction, muscular contraction, and chemical reaction that happens in our body. When we begin to track through our conscious awareness what is happening in our mental sphere (or mental body), we then become much more aware and alert as to what is happening in our physical body. The mind is basically reflecting what is going on in the body. If the body is tense, contracted, or out of balance the mind tends to be very much the same way. This is also true in the opposite scenario, which indicates there is a direct and accurate feedback response between what we call the mind and what we understand as the body. You cannot have one without the other and you cannot heal one without healing the other. When the mind reaches its balance and equilibrium point, the body begins to find its equilibrium point as well and vice versa.

Now, you may be wondering why I am bringing all of this up. What is the point of elaborating on this concept any further than has been, all throughout the book already? Simple answer: this is the access point to all of our inherent and infinite potential in life, which also includes the understanding of how to heal ourselves, heal our prior conditioning, reverse long held patterning, and transcend the stronghold of any and all addiction cycles. It is only through the body that we truly access our potential for healing and transformation. All of our genetic information, from past lives, our blood lineage, ancestral wisdom, and all that we gained in this life is stored in the repository warehouse of our most incredible technology, the human body. In order to access the full utility of our body technology, we have to also unlock the constraints imposed upon our mind or mental body, which we explored in the past chapter in great length. Now we must merge the two topics together in a way that is practical, tangible, and REAL!

287

There are a few important dimensions built into this conversation that we all must understand and practice in order for this subject to go from being a very interesting idea, to producing immediate results in our life. This chapter may prove to be the most important in the entire book because the fine tuning of the body and developing a mastery of this instrument really is the crux of the matter at hand. Understanding what true health really is becomes something of a positive obsession once we begin to experience the benefits of a health-based lifestyle. Once we begin to feel better, we tend to want to do things that make us feel better. When we feel better, we do better. When we do better, we produce better results. This is the positive swing to contrast the negative addiction loop which has a downward spiraling vortex and only brings us down in all facets of our lives.

The truth is people don't do well because they don't feel well. They don't feel well because they do not treat themselves well. And they tend not to treat themselves well because they tend not to think well. When we upgrade our thinking i.e., our mental body health, we automatically upgrade our feeling state i.e., our emotional body health and the physical body responds accordingly. The combination of a thoughtful approach to natural health, whole food nutrition, cleansing and detoxification protocols, hydrating with pristine water, improving our sleep cycles, and incorporating daily meditative practices all have a compounding effect that build on each other. This helps to create exponential rewards in our life as a whole, as the compounding interest we accrue from stacking one healthy habit on top of another.

We are going to explore some very nuanced and unique aspects of holistic health as it relates to maximizing body intelligence and transcending traumatic imprints encoded into our nervous system. This will be a fascinating deep dive into regions of the human experience I doubt any book on addiction or even overall health book addresses in detail or if at all. There is both a purely physical component to this, as well as a deeply metaphysical component and we will explore both so that you may fully inner stand the process and protocol for holistic healing and human optimization. Once you become passionate and committed to the path of optimizing yourself as a human being, then all addictions and lower-level habits begin to fall away naturally and effortlessly. This becomes the hyper positive obsession and an obsession you can only feel absolutely great about, which will only produce positive, productive, long lasting effects in your life.

Let's dive in!

The Trauma Based Pain Body

"Although humans rarely die from trauma, if we do not resolve it, our lives can be severely diminished by its effects. Some people have even described this situation as a "living death."

Peter A. Levine,

Healing Trauma: A Pioneering Program for Restoring the Wisdom of Your Body

From my earliest years as a martial artist and athlete I have been obsessed with learning how the human body functions and how to maximize the performance of this incredible organic technology. The first 20 years were mostly focused on performance from an athletic standpoint. This gave way to learning about the rehabilitation arts as a way to help heal injuries and recover from intense training sessions. This then opened me up into the world of holistic health therapies and devoting a decade of my life to the studies of organic whole food and super food-based nutrition for optimal performance and the reversal of lifestyle-based diseases. Throughout my deep digging into the fields of healing and longevity, I began to observe what I now understand as the metaphysical influences of our bodily health. I began to become incredibly fascinated with what is known as the placebo or nocebo effect of healing. This is essentially the psycho-somatic aspect of physical health, which over time I began to recognize that this may have the single greatest influence over all other aspects of the body.

The psycho-somatic connection is the interplay between the mind and body. It is not exactly accurate to individuate the mind and body as two separate components however, because they are more accurately one in the same. The body is a direct feedback reflection of the state of our mind at any given moment. The state of our mental landscape is also a direct reflection of the state of our body. Are you confused yet? Well, think about it this way. When we have a nagging injury or digestive inflammation it is incredibly difficult to override that experience by focusing on the tasks at hand in our lives. All of our mental energy redirects itself to the inflammation because the pain signaling from the body is taking priority. When the body is out of balance, the mind becomes disorientated and scattered, thus the mind slips out of balance. This is also the case when we are holding too much mental stress and our body begins to reflect this in the form of muscle contractions, cramps, sore tendons, liver stagnation, kidney/adrenal weakness, and lower levels of bodily energy. The pairing of the physical body and the mental body correspond to one another and in this sense, they are one in the same as a whole feedback system.

This brings us to the most significant dimensional understanding in terms of addiction and recovery, which is trauma. To be specific it is the understanding of the trauma-based pain body, which is the energetic sensitivity layer within the physical body. When the pain body is triggered, our nervous system reacts in a defensive state and we become extremely protective of ourselves because the experience of held trauma is being surfaced. This can manifest itself in any forms such as panic attacks, nerve twitches, emotional overwhelm or outburst, highly reactive thought patterns, shortened respiratory breathing, and even extremes such as fibromyalgia or some kind of allergic reaction such as a rash. The traumatic flare ups are far more common than we would likely think, and they arise in different forms and flavors. Some people have less overt trauma in their lives thus smaller reactions and some people have experienced a lot of trauma in their lives, which tends to mean more overt reactions and longer sustained durations.

We have discussed trauma in many instances throughout the book up to this point but now we are going to take it a bit deeper. You see, our issues in our life live in our tissues. We cannot escape this reality and that is the exact issue when it comes to addiction. Our addictions or vices tend to reflect our need to escape our own reality and detach from the issues that are swelling up from underneath the surface. In this case it's underneath the epidermal surface of our skin and deep into our cells and DNA. When a trauma is being triggered up to the surface what we see manifest itself is the old conditioning that was set in place to protect against the traumatic event itself. The conditioned response sets into motion a division between the person experiencing the trigger/trauma and their own connection to the somatic(body) sensations they are experiencing. Addictions solidify themselves into the body when we experience too much of a disconnection between our bodies and our minds. When the body and mind go into a state of disorientation and disarray, the system becomes overwhelmed, and the immediate signal is to find something to sooth the experience of pain or discomfort.

The simple remedy for almost all forms of pain body triggering is to quickly go into the experience itself and rest into the sensations arising in the body. Easier said than done, I know! This is why learning how to use your breathing as a tool for self-regulation and relaxation is so important. This is also why practicing shaking the nervous system, just as wild animals do when they experience the peak point of a traumatic survival event. When the pain body is triggered, it can easily feel like our entire system is going into an intense survival mode and that we need to protect ourselves in order to defend against the immediate threats around us. Often times these threats are not around us though, they are living within us and that which has been buried beneath the surface is revealing itself in order to be purged. If we understand what is actually happening in these peak moments of being triggered, then we can use it as an opportunity to heal and grow beyond the moment of discomfort. If we do not realize what is happening, then we risk the probability of repeating this pattern of self-protection and ego preservation every time the same incidence arises.

When unresolved trauma that is stored in our nervous system is triggered, it can lead to a variety of issues. The addiction component is the attempt to self sooth the hyper-arousal that is being activated in the body, which often times leads to the compulsion to repeat the behavior as a way to medicate the sensations. Trauma does not only occur in the more overt ways we may think of, such as an intense experience as a child or a life altering experience as an adult. Trauma can exist from the accumulation of stress patterns from our daily lives that are unchecked and are not released from the body. We can easily take for granted the real effects of the micro-stresses we experience in the hustle and bustle of daily life. It is becoming more well known that PTSD (post-traumatic stress disorder) is not an isolated issue with war veterans and those who have been through very extreme circumstances. Most people in modern society are likely carrying some form of micro-PTSD from the amount of accumulated stress that has built its way into the nervous system and resides below the surface of the conscious mind.

In the medical field of orthopedics there is a term used to describe micro injuries to the bone, ligaments, and tendons of the body called stress fractures. This is very common amongst athletes and recreational sports, where someone overtrains or trains incorrectly thus creating too much impact force to the bone, which can result in a hairline fracture and eventually a total fracturing of the bone itself. This is well regarding the physical framework of the body itself but what about the psycho-emotional body? The physical body, again, is a reflective feedback system of our proverbial bodies and the pain body is the alarm mechanism that the rest of the system is out of synch. I am using the term stress fracture in terms of the wear and tear that occurs to our psyche over the course of our lives, which manifests itself in the symptoms of our pain body. We can develop stress fracturing of the psyche when we are overburdened by all forms of stress. When the psyche(mind) is incapable of handling the amplified electrical activity that occurs due to mental/psychic overwhelm, it divides itself and compartmentalizes it's point of focus. This is a survival adaptation mechanism in order to prioritize an immediate threat in the environment. Once the threat is dealt with the utility of this function is to reintegrate the divided information and consolidate it back into the whole view of an individual's experience.

The great challenge with this is that very few of us were ever taught how to reincorporate stressful experiences back into our lives effectively and safely. This is not a commonly held perspective on trauma and stress, but it is an accurate one based on cognitive and developmental psychology. This is also the reason we may find ourselves avoiding certain tasks, responsibilities, challenging situations, or uncomfortable conversations in our lives. We may just put it off as not important, that we do not have time for it, or whatever other stories we may tell ourselves. The truth of the matter is when we are in a pattern of avoidance, it is likely because the thought of the thing we are avoiding arouses the surface of a wound or trauma and we feel the sensations of stress upon thinking about it. We may assume that the stress of the situation (even if it is only in our mind) simply comes and goes but the reality is that the energy sticks onto us and the micro-stress sensation that arises becomes stored in our physiology. Over enough time (and repetition of stress avoidance) our pain body begins to kick on and if it is not dealt with accordingly the symptoms become more overt and more strenuous.

So, in understanding the holistic point of view in trauma therapies it's important to note that it always has an emotional effect, a psychological effect but all trauma is primarily a physiological process. This is why we have an entire population of people walking around carrying boatloads of unresolved stress and traumatic patterning, despite the best efforts to solve it through psychiatric and psychological interventions. The book, **The Body Keeps the Score** by Bessel van der Kolk, M.D. does a fantastic job at explaining the intersection between the mind and body, relating to the body becoming the store house for unresolved trauma and stress patterns. The book, **It Didn't Start with You** by Mark Wolynn offers a further explanation into the metaphysical dimension of bodily trauma helping us understand that our bodies inherit the encoded information of the unresolved traumatic experiences of our genetic lineage. Although these inherited trauma patterns are 'meta'-physical (beyond physical) in nature they are experienced through the physicality of bodily sensation and that is exactly where they must be dealt with in order to clear out the faulty corrupted software programs that we have unknowingly inherited through birth.

If we return to the orthopedic example of bone stress fractures, then we can simplify this process easily. Once we become aware that there is a problem i.e., stress fracture and we understand how it was caused (overtraining or incorrect training) then the next step is to alter our behavior in order to allow the body to heal itself. Remember, the body is an infinitely intelligent biotechnology that is designed to heal itself. We do not heal our body. Our body heals itself and all we do is support it in this process, which often times really just means getting out of its way so it can perform it's innate healing functions. Dr. Peter Levine, author of the book, **Walking the Tiger: Healing Trauma** beautifully articulates the cause of trauma and equally important, how to discharge the energetic signature of trauma from the body and resolve the reactionary patterning the trauma signature activates. The key to this is to unstick the trauma from the nervous system and allow the body to go into an automatic(autonomic) self-soothing process. Instead of using substances or external recreations to sooth a trigger for a few moments, we want to release the tension point between relaxation and contraction, which is where catharsis can occur.

The word catharsis has two basic meanings. The medical definition is purgation meaning purging. Another is "the process of releasing, and thereby providing relief from, strong or repressed emotions." You see, our emotions alert us to the state of affairs going on within us. For example, if someone feels stressed or overworked, they may begin to harbor all kinds of feelings inside and the emotions that arise could be that of frustration, resentment, and anything else that resembles tension in the system. Emotions are every bit as physical as our extremities and could be describes as the physicalized expressions of our feeling sensations. This is why the emotional catharsis is absolutely necessary in order to help move out stored trauma in the body. It is never enough to simply talk about our issues and analytically piece together the story board of our past. This is not an intellectual or logic process. It is entirely a physical process and as the purgation of emotional trauma begins to release, the psyche also begins to reorganize itself because it now has the safety to do so.

Just like healing a physical stress fracture there is a rehabilitation process to recovering from trauma-based addiction patterning. One aspect is obviously to begin removing ourselves from the addictive tendencies that only mask our symptoms and provide temporary relief. The other aspect is to disengage with our usual patterns that we have habituated too in order to keep things running as normal. This can be a tricky process because once we remove the coping mechanisms that shield us from our emotional sensitivity, we are forced to experience the discomfort of each and every present moment of the healing process. If we continue on as we always have, we will only further injure ourselves due to the weakening of our stress fracturing. Therefore, we must begin to create a self-rehab program that allows us to slow down, rest and relax, and allow the body to enter into those sensitive spaces within ourselves. This is where modalities such as conscious breath work, meditation, neurogenic tremors (shaking), safely administered plant medicines, sensory deprivation tanks (saltwater float tanks), ice baths/cold therapy, frequent napping, journaling and reflection exercises become of paramount importance.

In Dr. Peter Levine's somatic trauma healing work, he discusses the process that animals undergo as a response to bodily trauma that is brought on by a predatory threat. We have discussed this in more detail earlier on in the book discussing the neurogenic tremor phenomena that is innate to all mammalian animals. Well, as Dr. Levine reminds us this is also an innate function built into human beings as well and is the pressure release valve to exercising stored trauma and stress patterns that get stuck in the body. Dr. Levine shares that one of the functions an animal will enact is to immobilize themselves in the presence of a threat, which means that they play dead as to be undesirable to a predator or to counterattack a predator. Once the threat is gone, the animal goes back to normal unhindered by the stress it temporarily experienced. The challenge with humans is that we may get stuck in the immobilization phase of stress and hold ourselves in a semi-immobilized state for fear of experiencing the intense sensations that are being held at bay. After enough repetitions of this pattern, we develop the habit of getting "stuck" between first gear and second, which does not allow us to fully process out the stored energetics of stress and trauma.

The answer to all of this is actually very simple and straight forward. It is to engage fully with our bodily sensations and create a space of safety for ourselves so that we can successfully unhook the pressure valve of stress. This can be done in a variety of ways such as physiotherapy methods involving deep tissue body massage, neuromuscular release therapies, foam rollers and pressure point release methods, and even laying sprawled out on a floor while doing deep diaphragmatic breathing from the solar plexus(belly) region. Other effective methods for maintenance of the nervous system response include hot and cold therapies such as infrared sauna combined with ice baths. The sweating out increases the detoxification effect, while the cold plunge of ice water increases electrical voltage of the body system and helps to process out stagnant energy. It can also be extremely helpful to run a warm bath with essential oils for emotional releasing. We will discuss this aspect in more detail in the following chapter **Healing the Heart.**

It is well worth exploring the work of Dr. Peter Levine as well as Mark Wolynn for more detailed information on this subject and effective measures for releasing stored trauma. It is also worth noting that trauma release is a form of psycho-emotional detoxification and like all versions of a good detox protocol, it can sometimes feel worse before it feels better. It is very common for old memories to resurface and take residence in one's conscious mind that had previously been put on the back burner. This is a process of our own consciousness piecing back together aspects that had been repressed in the past. It is important not to get too caught up in this process but to simply observe what comes up and allow it to move safely through the system. In this process one may experience sensations of anxiety or even temporary bouts of what could be described as desperation. This sensation is a sign that the pain body is being stimulated and the more we can simply breath into this experience, the easier it will be to move through it and beyond it. The past and the future are illusory in nature. The mind can get sidetracked going down memory lane or get lost in future projections as a way to disassociate from the experience itself. The focused breath brings us into the moment and the more we breath into our experience the more we will fully feel our experience and the quicker it will pass through.

The Metaphysical Anatomy of the Body

One of the most profound discoveries in all areas of health sciences and alternative natural healing therapies is the realization that our body is its own inner physician. This is a concept we have expanded upon in multiple ways throughout the book and one I want to drive a bit further in this section. The entire chemistry set of our biology is a self-facilitating homeopathic laboratory that is perfectly designed to produce the chemical measurements of exactly what we need, when we need it, in the dosage required for that moment. This has been discovered and repeatedly proven to be factual based on the scientific experiments done in the fields of metaphysics involving transcendental meditation practices, self-hypnosis, guided breath work, and even measuring the physiological recovery effects of getting consistent quality sleep. This shows that our body is designed to repair and recovery itself as an autonomic response pattern to the wear and tear we accumulate through the course of our lives.

You may be asking what is your point, Ronnie? You have already drilled this point in multiple ways so far. Well, the point is an ever expanding one and, in this context, it is all to set up one of the most incredibly discoveries of the body. Which by the way has a deeply rooted link to all forms of addiction and trauma stress patterns that exists within the physical body itself. Upon a deep research investigation into the nuanced nature of healing I came across an incredible book called **Metaphysical Anatomy** by author, Evette Rose. I had never seen a book like this one before and was instantly enamored by its contents. The book is a literal encyclopedia of the human anatomy and every known metaphysical connection from the psyche to the emotional states of each aspect of the body and the various physical conditions that we accept as common place or simply do not have a deep understanding about outside of the medical approach of cut, burn, poison interventions, as is the case in cancer therapies, for example. For the first time I had access to something that beautifully laid out the mapping of the human body and all known conditions to their appropriate psycho-emotional causes and explaining in depth the childhood associations that could be at play as well.

When we begin to track the tension patterns in our body to their root psycho-emotional causes, we begin to unravel the tension all together. For example, if we have had frequent episodes with our back going out or simply experiencing onsets of stress and contraction, we may find ourselves doing absolutely everything to treat it. Everything except the one thing that potentially caused the problem in the first place. According to the metaphysical anatomy perspective lower back pain specifically is directly rooted to feeling of lack of support in our lives. This could be said with all forms of back issues, including shoulder and neck pain. The sense of carrying the problems of the world on our shoulders can easily manifest itself as shoulder and neck tension. We may get frequent body work to relax the muscles, but it spontaneously arises again shortly after. The back problems continue to emerge despite all of the therapeutic modalities and ointments we employ.

The body as a whole operates as a unified system and one thing effects another and ultimately effects the entire system. As we begin to expand our minds and awareness of how this physical body functions from a mind to body perspective, we discover that all physical inhibitions have a mental and emotional cause. Nothing happens in the body without the mind involved because the body is the physical reflection of our mind, after all. When we clear out the body of residual toxins and clogging foods, our minds begin to open up and newfound clarity emerges. When we practice meditation and breath work to unwind the mind, our bodies unwind long held stress patterns as a natural consequence. They both work hand in hand and in fact are not necessary two separate instruments but two sides of the same coin, so to speak.

There is an ancient metaphysical therapeutic modality that has become modernized in the form we call reflexology. It is said to have derived from a combination of Egypt, India, and eventually China but was introduced to the modern health community through Eunice Ingham who wrote the book **Stories the Feet Can Tell**. Reflexology focuses on pinpointing the trigger points located in our hands and feet that directly correlate to the organ and glandular systems of the body. Just as we now know that all of our teeth are connected to meridian points (energetic vortexes of the body) we also now know that these trigger points in our feet, for example, are connected to our organs and glands which can be profound in addressing deep seeded energetic blockages. For example, the K1 & K2 points in the feet connect to our two kidneys at the lower back underneath our tiny adrenal glands. Using a small ball and placing pressure underneath the soft tissue of the feet can help alleviate pressure in the kidneys, which I have personally experienced many times.

There are more and more organic methods and technologies that help address the multi-faceted nature of the body, but the point is to first expand our minds to the reality that our body is synched up to the happenings of our mind and emotional patterns. In Chinese medicine it is well established how each one of our organs houses specific emotional content depending on the health of both the organs themselves and how much we have processed our emotional experiences in life. For example, the liver is associated with the emotions of anger and the spectrum of heating or yang type of energies. The liver is responsible for filtering toxins and rendering them less toxic in order to metabolize useful nutrients in the body and discard harmful compounds out of the body. When the liver becomes overburdened and does not function at optimal capacity it can become stagnant and sluggish. This can result in a syndrome called fatty liver which can create a heating effect in the body and slows down the body's metabolism. Conversely to the physical effects of environmental toxins, contaminated water, sugary drinks, and processed foods have on the liver, the stored unresolved emotions of frustration, anger, and disappointment can also place a burden which can result in similar physical conditions.

Once we learn how to effectively process our emotional content and trace the feeling sensation to its origin point, the organs begin to work more effectively. The deeper meaning of liver stagnation, from an emotional perspective, is rooted in issues with our father. This could be issues we have with our paternal father or perhaps an even more profound meaning is an abandonment wound we have to our cosmic father i.e., our relationship with God. I would say both are likely the case and it is worth anyone's personal investigation to sense if that rings true for them. When we look at the heart the most common positive emotion associated with it is joy and anything that diminishes our joy can be considered a burden on the heart. Heart disease is the number one cause of mortality worldwide which can be linked to multiple causes, both physical and metaphysical. The heart is also connected to our mother and when we have issues with our mother, we will likely have issues with our heart. It is also worth considering that the worldwide epidemic of heart disease is somehow related to the disconnection from our mother earth and the nurturing archetype we may or may not have received as a young child that organically emerges from the divine mother archetype.

The most important take away in this segment is the deeper inner standing that our mind, our dominant emotional state, and our physiology are inextricably interconnected and rely upon each other for harmonious equanimity. In the fields of health sciences, it is no longer enough to simply preach nutrition, fitness, and alternative healing therapies that only target the physicality of the body. That is basically just scratching the surface. Most physical issues are a combination of bodily imbalances, psychological imbalances, emotional blocks, and spiritual confusion. This is why I was so delighted to stumble upon the metaphysical anatomy by Evette Rose and other works similar in scope to it. The academic textbooks on anatomy, biology, and physiology will have to be rewritten, remixed, and readapted to a much more comprehensive world view of what the human body is, how it heals itself from all dimensions, and what it is truly capable of from we remove the physical and non-physical obstructions.

Nutrition & Biological Optimization

> *"A culture is what it eats, and a human's personality is often largely a reflection of their diet."*
>
> *Terence McKenna*

For the greater part of the last decade, I have devoted my research career and life to the pursuit of natural health, with the specific focus on organic foods, super foods, herbalism, and natural supplementation. Over all these years I have toured around the country and even in multiple other countries giving lectures on a wide range of health-based topics, as well as meeting thousands of people from all different backgrounds, cultures, and belief paradigms around health. Where the rubber meets the road is back to solid nutritional practices and what we choose to put into our body on a consistent basis. Our food should be something of a sacred ritual where we nourish our bodies with organic nutrition that serves as the primary fuel supply to our cells, our tissues, our minds, and our spirit.

I have likely explored virtually every nutritional philosophy and eating paradigm i.e., diets under the sun. I have been a massive proponent of the raw food lifestyle for well over a decade and even wrote multiple books on the subject itself. Since then, I have expanded my personal dietary approach to also include high quality, ethically sourced animal foods after a decade of raw foods, veganism, and vegetarianism. I am sharing this with you because it's important that we avoid the dangers of dietary dogma and rigid concepts when it comes to our nutritional approach. What I have found in all these years is that the bodies biological requirements will always override the minds belief systems of what we think we should do vs what our body really needs to nourish itself. Especially when it comes to the topic of addiction and health recovery, it becomes even more important that we are not trading out one addiction for another i.e., an addiction to food, even healthier foods. Nutrition should be a dogma free zone and each individual needs to find what works best for them to thrive, moment by moment, season by season.

With that said there are a range of solid and universal principles that would assist everyone in adopting healthier nutritional habits and cause them to experience more bodily energy. The first principle is called the acid alkaline PH balance. This is the balance between acidic and alkaline states in our blood chemistry. This is one of the determining factors in overall health, disease reversal, and maintaining optimal energy levels throughout the day. There have been many fad diets stating that we need to be entirely alkaline or adopt a 100% alkaline diet in order to be healthy. This is only a partial truth but there is a condition called alkalosis, which is when the blood PH becomes far too alkaline, and we actually need to establish an acid alkaline balance. This is why high alkaline water systems can produce incredibly healing results in the short term if someone is too acidic from improper eating habits. Eventually though, they will need to strike a balance point between alkaline foods/liquids and acidic based foods. We are not designed to be entirely alkaline or acidic but to reach the balance point which is estimated to be around 7.43 alkaline on the PH blood scale, which is slightly alkaline and above the acidic range.

Keep in mind that our digestive acids are supposed to be at an acidic scale of 2.0 in order to produce what is called hydrochloric acid or gastric acids that digest our food. This is why salt/sodium chloride is important in our diet because it helps to stimulate gastric acids for digestion, among other metabolic functions. The biggest culprit behind many health issues and bodily energy declines is improper food combining (mis combining fats, carbs, proteins) and the lack of digestive acids to properly metabolize the food we eat. These are also the two chief agents behind what is known as candida growth, which can be caused by the small intestine being too "wet" and "damp", meaning there is little to no "digestive fire" to burn up the food, which can lead to parasitic pathogens causing infections due to the fermentation of undigested food. If this is the case for someone then their mental cognition and emotional stability will be adversely affected because there is a direct link between the gut and the brain. In fact, within our gut/stomach is a second brain that feedbacks directly with our primary brain and vice versa.

Eating an organic, whole foods, high fresh living foods diet is a solid foundation for most people which includes an assortment of vegetables, water rich fruits, sprouted nuts, seeds, fermented foods, sea vegetables (high mineral content), and nutritionally concentrated super foods in the form of low-sugar smoothies. This nutritional template will easily upgrade most people's health and steadily increase energy levels. If you want to learn more about the nuts and bolts of this kind of lifestyle along with tons of recipes you read my books **The Holistic Health Mastery Program** & **The Inner Alchemy Youthening Program**. You can also enroll in my online holistic nutrition course **The Holistic Health Mastery Program** to go deeper.

The other principle I will share with you is about reaching the bodies metabolic and hormonal balance through what is called the catabolic and anabolic phases of metabolism. This concept can help simplify your nutritional approach based on which season your body is in and what your body is needing in this moment. For example, sometimes our bodies require more cleaning and elimination of toxins, therefore we would adhere to more of a catabolic approach such as raw vegan or vegetarian diet rich in fruits and vegetables, excluding heavier animals' foods and cooked foods. Sometimes our body needs to rebuild and trigger growth hormones, so we would want to adhere to more of an anabolic approach. This can still include a foundation of living foods or even a predominantly vegetarian approach, but for most people's metabolic needs some animal foods are advised. If you want to go deeper into the nuances here my **Holistic Health Mastery Program** is a great place to start.

Anabolism is where our body goes into a growth and repair phase, such as the recovery phase from working out with heavy weights. The act of lifting weights is technically catabolic in nature due to the breakdown of muscle fibers and only when we sleep, do those muscle fibers repair due to anabolic recovery. Whether we need to be in an anabolic or catabolic phase is entirely due to the state of our body in the moment. If our body is more acidic and coming off a standard conventional diet, then it is likely we need to go into a catabolic phase, which means lowering the animal food (or eliminating them all together) and adopting a primarily plant-based lifestyle. Once we have cleaned out the body sufficiently and are ready to rebuild ourselves, we will want to include more anabolic foods in order to balance out our metabolic needs.

This is also based on the kind of lifestyle activities we engage with every day and our level & type of exercise. If you do more yoga and yin-based movement then you will be better able to sustain yourself on a more alkaline, high plant-based lifestyle. If you lift heavy weights or are putting your body through intense duress, then you will benefit from including higher quality protein and saturated fats to help your body recover and produce longer sustainable energy without taxing your adrenal glands, which is a common issue amongst low-fat high carb plant-based athlete's long term. Ultimately whatever dietary approach you choose for yourself keep in mind that it is all a grand experiment and should be treated just as such. Do not overcomplicate it with preconceptions or other people's ideas or even their personal experiences. Your body is uniquely yours and your metabolic signature i.e., metabolic type is not the same as everyone else's. You must do what works best for you in this moment and make adjustments as needed moving forward.

In addition to this concept on metabolic individuality is the discover that each human being has a unique affinity to different foods that fuel them optimally and sub-optimally. If someone does not know what macro-nutrients i.e., fats, proteins, and carbohydrates work best for them, they could be eating extremely high-quality foods (and high priced) yet getting subpar results. The ultimate point of nutrition is to discover what types of foods and food groups help you produce mitochondrial cellular energy the best. This will require a bit of experimentation and there are tons of different dietary schools of thought to explore. Ultimately it comes down to a simple distinction between high fat - moderate protein - low carb, low fat - low protein - high carb, or moderate fat - moderate carb - moderate protein. Anyone is going to fall somewhere into one of these three basic templates due to their metabolic type, which is classified as either a fast oxidizer (speedy metabolism/higher fat), a slow oxidizer (slower metabolism/higher carb), or a sub-oxidizer (medium metabolism/balanced macros).

The reason this distinction is so important is because food is fuel and certain food types fuel the energy production of cells called our mitochondria better than others. It is estimated that around 70% of the western population are what is known as fast oxidizers, which means they do best on a higher fat-based diet and lesser carbohydrates. This is why the ketogenic trend has become so popular because more people, population wise, will find success vs a high carbohydrate low fat vegan style diet. That is just a statistically probability.

Now, another important distinction to make is that fats and carbohydrates are the only two macronutrients that the body uses as a cellular energy source. Protein is not used effectively as an energy source. Protein is broken down into amino acids, which all have their unique role and function such as repairing neurotransmitters, blood sugar stabilizing, rebuilding muscle fibers, aiding immune function, healing intestinal damage, and support hormone regulation. If someone eats too much protein rich foods but not enough fats or carbohydrates for their metabolic type, they will experience drowsiness, sluggishness, laziness, and general feelings of fatigue or low motivation. This happened to me when I first began including meat into my diet after ten years without it and I had to relearn how to eat high protein with high fat in order to experience stable energy, instead of wanting to fall asleep because of eating too much protein.

All of these concepts I talk about in depth in my **Holistic Health Mastery Program** and **The Inner Alchemy Youthening Program** books. There are great resources online you can easily find as well to guide your investigation. These principles will help you discover what works best for you and how to maintain balanced energy through the day and greater levels of health.

Cleansing, Detoxification, Cellular Regeneration

Over the prior decade of my work in the holistic health and natural foods industry, I would say the hallmark of my focus has always been on cleansing and detoxification strategies for optimal wellbeing. In our industrialized civilization we have been and continue to be bombarded with known and unknown chemical compounds, all throughout the contamination of our conventional pesticide sprayed food supply, artificial ingredients from processed foods, chemical solvents in our atmosphere from trains, planes, boats, automobiles, and fall out from the toxicity that is spewing into the air from buildings and manufacturing facilities. In the last 100 years we have become the very first set of generations in human history to be exposed to this kind of chemical toxicity by way of our day-to-day lifestyles and the way global societies have been designed to operate.

The single most important aspect of overall bodily health and wellbeing in the 21st century is not just about optimal nutrition but even more so about optimal detoxification. It has been shown in varies scientific studies and clinical data that detoxification is even more important than nutrition for overall health and, especially for increasing longevity. This may appear to be a startling statement at first, but once you begin to consider the amount of 'chemical pressure' we have all been under, and for how long these environmental chemicals have accumulated in the bodily tissues of our organ systems, it should not be hard to understand why detoxification is so important in this day and age. Proper nutrition is a foundational principle for overall health, as well as overcoming chemical addiction loops, and rebuilding the neurotransmitters that are associated with addiction. Detoxification helps to purge out the obstructions that are blocking off the bodies innate ability to heal itself and to make best use of the nutrients in our food and supplements so that we can receive the full effect of what we put into our bodies.

The basic premise of cleansing and detoxification is to assist the bodies built in elimination organs (lungs, colon, kidneys, skin) as well as aiding the largest organ inside the body, which is the liver. The liver has a long laundry list of biological functions it carries out in the body but one of its chief functions is to render compounds that are toxic, into metabolite byproducts that are "less toxic". The body has a built-in intelligence for deactivating foreign toxins and then eliminating them from the body. This is done, starting with the liver and gall bladder, and then into one or multiple of what is known as the '4 organs of elimination'. These organs include our kidneys, our lungs, our skin, and our colon. These organs work in a beautiful symmetry with one another and are perfectly designed to cleanse out toxins from the body, so long as we know how to support them in doing their job optimally, and do not unnecessarily get in their way.

The important thing to note about all of this is that when we have become habituated to strong chemical substances, such as the one's listed in the chapter **Culturally Accepted Drugs,** it places a large toll on the liver over time. We know this absolutely the case with alcohol, which can lead to many forms of liver disease and degeneration. Excessive coffee and caffeine can also have a detrimental effect on the liver, especially if someone does not metabolize caffeine as effectively as another person. When the liver gets blocked up, backed up, and stagnated, all other organ systems slow down as a result. This can lead to a lot of metabolic challenges and can certainly result in various forms of physical degeneration and illness. The liver operates as the buffering system between incoming toxins and the blood supply of the body, which transports compounds and molecules into the rest of the body. Eventually as the liver degenerates, its ability to buffer incoming toxicity lessens, and these toxins make their way into the blood stream, leading to all kinds of health issues.

One of the sure-fire ways to ensure an addiction recovery program is successful is to implement intelligent cleansing and detoxification protocols into the recovery schedule. This is not only a strong suggestion, it is actually an imperative to success, both short terms, and most importantly long term. As we discussed earlier on organic nutrition, alkalizing the body is critically important for purging out the chemical residue of whatever addictive substances someone is working out of their system. The constant acidification of processed foods, sugary drinks, caffeinated beverages, tap water, and poor lifestyle habits, on top of the acidification of the other habits involved, will only reinforce the biological addiction cycle even further. It is near impossible to abstain completely from these substances, especially stimulants such as coffee or similar drug like habits if we do not begin cleaning out the blood stream of acid-based compounds. Once we begin to make a change from an acidic lifestyle, into an alkaline lifestyle, the symptoms of withdrawal begin to release and remove themselves effortlessly. A lot of the symptoms associated with habits like alcohol, tobacco, or coffee such as headaches, migraines, brain fog, low energy are based on acidity in the body, and that is why the symptoms can feel so strong and overwhelming.

There are a lot of cleansing programs to choose from out there. It can be hard to know exactly where to get started or what is right for you. There are some simple suggestions I will make below that can help you navigate the options available and begin picking and choosing what makes sense to you right now. I encourage you to do some research on the list of options provided below and reach out to us at _____ for more support.

- *Colon Hydrotherapy - Colonics and Coffee Enemas*
- *1 Liter of Spring Water in the Morning*
- *Green Vegetable Juices - Celery, Cucumber, Ginger, Turmeric, Beet Root, Cilantro*
- *Green Powdered Super Food Drinks - Green Grass Powders, Spirulina/Chlorella*
- *Liver Gall Bladder Cleanse - Master Cleanse | Dandelion Leaf, Milk Thistle, Apple Cider Vinegar, Activated Charcoal*
- *Niacin Flush Protocol - Dr. George Yu Niacin Flush Protocol Specifically*
- *Purium 30-Day Ultimate Transformation Program - Green Super Food Cleanse Program*

The final word I have on this topic is that cleansing should be built into our daily lifestyle and part of our dietary strategy long term. Many of the foods and liquids we consume each day should have cleansing properties to them which help to alkalize the body and remove harmful toxins. I talk extensively about this in both of my prior books, **The Holistic Health Mastery Program** & **The Inner Alchemy Youthening Program**.

"Cleanliness is next to Godliness."

Unknown

Restoring Natural Sleep Cycles

I have been waiting months to write this section of the book but wanted to get through a lot of the other heavy hitting topics before diving right in. Why have I been so eager to focus on a section about sleep so much? Well, simply because this topic could make the biggest difference in all areas of someone's life, especially their sense of wellbeing, and most certainly their physical health. In fact, sleep quality is so important that it trumps the importance of both fitness and nutrition combined. If we are

307

eating the best quality organic super foods in the world and have a solid exercise routine but completely neglect our sleep, then we are setting ourselves up for a big downturn in our overall health. If you combine the quality nutrition, with the specific exercise patterns that best for you, and also place your sleep as a high priority, now you are stacking the deck in your favor for incredible health, heightened mental and emotional wellbeing, and a better quality of life overall.

The irony to this though, is that people who struggle with substance addictions or whatever kind of addictions, tend to prioritize sleep very little, and that is part of the problem with their recovery process. We can easily see how something as simple as a coffee habit could play a significant role in interrupting our natural sleep cycles. Caffeine is a powerful central nervous system stimulant and if consumed in the afternoon, it can keep someone up until the later hours of the night. This is also why substances such as alcohol or sleep medications are frequently used, as a way to counterbalance the stimulatory effects of too much caffeine and/or a bad sugar addiction. Alcohol of course, can feel like it is a sleep aid tonic, helping one to feel a bit more relaxed, drowsy, and ready to "pass out" at night. Well, it does seem to help people "pass out" but that does not mean that someone is getting great quality sleep. It is exactly the opposite in fact. Alcohol will throw off one's quality of sleep by putting them in a particular brain wave state that does not support the deeper, more restorative brain wave states needed.

When it comes to making the proper lifestyle adjustments to ensure we get the best quality sleep possible, there are a few considerations to focus on. The first thing to think about is how we prepare for sleep as the day begins to transition into the evening. Most of us were not taught to wind down with sundown as we normally think of winding up with sun rise. Due to the excessive artificial lighting of our houses and technological devices, we tend to remain in a moderate sympathetic state throughout the night, where in a natural environment without artificial lighting, we would naturally wind down much sooner than most people do in society. One of the most important principles for priming the body and brain for deep restorative sleep is to create a transition point between the activities of the day and the activities of the evening. Most people simply carry over their daily activities into nighttime and wonder why they either have such a hard time sleeping or end up going to sleep at the middle of the night.

This problem can be easily worked out, but it is going to take a bit of discipline and consistency to retrain the brain to naturally unwinding from the cortisol inducing activities of the afternoon.

What you need to know is that upon waking up in the morning, due to sun or light exposure the brain signals cortisol and serotonin production. This helps to alert the nervous system that it is time to awaken from sleep and "rise and shine" as they say. The body goes into "activity" mode due to the rise in cortisol, which in this case is very healthy and natural. When the sun goes down, the brain begins to calibrate to its wake-sleep cycle and darkness signals melatonin production in the brain. Melatonin is the brains primary tryptamine neurotransmitter, produced by the pineal gland, that induces deep restorative sleep. Melatonin is also anti-inflammatory, anti-cancerous, and a powerful antioxidant that is important for all healing factors of the body. When our melatonin production cycle is interfered with our bodies ability to heal and restore itself from the day's prior is significantly lowered, which is one of the many factors involved in age associated degeneration and illness.

Sleep issues such as sleep apnea and insomnia are extraordinarily common in our society these days. Insomnia is one of the most common reasons for doctors' visits in the US, ranging in the upwards of 30-35% of adult population report having mild to chronic sleep issues. It is estimated that at least 4% of the US adult population uses prescription sleep medications and the majority of these individuals are women it appears. According to the National Survey on Drug Use and Health, more than 500,000 people in the US are currently abusing Ambien, which is the single most prescribed sleep pill on the market. There are plenty of variables involved in this staggering discovery we could point too, and of course we do throughout this book. The main contributor I would draw our attention towards, however is the obsession and addiction we have to our handheld digital devices i.e., our "smart phones" and wireless tablets. There is a clear scientific link between the amount of time we spend on our devices in the evening and a significant drop in our brains melatonin levels, which result in poorer quality sleep, reduced healing, and restoration of the body, and waking up unrested.

There have been many studies to demonstrate the fact that the more 'blue light' exposure we receive through the 'photoreceptors' of our eyes, the less melatonin our brains produce. Harvard researchers have discovered that, for every hour we are exposed to the blue light emitting from our computer or phone screens, suppresses melatonin for at least 30 minutes. This means for every additional hour we spend on our screens in the evening there is a 30-minute biological debt that is incurred due to blue light exposure. Blue light is part of the visible light spectrum, which has the shortest wavelength and highest concentration of energy. It typically is there to boost energy, raise alertness, increase cognitive function, and for all intents and purposes, helps to keep us awake. The blue light that we receive from our digital devices is an artificial form that we would receive from the sun, for example. It is also a fractionated form of short-wave, high-energy light on the overall spectrum and this can cause many problems if we are overly exposed to it over time, including eye problems and cognitive challenges.

Let's also consider another element of this situation as it relates to the principles and philosophy of the dopamine reset method. When we are plugged into our digital devices at night, most likely scrolling back and forth on social media undoubtably, we are also triggering the dopaminergic feedback system as well. So, we are interacting with the dopamine system at the same time we are increasing cortisol levels and reducing our melatonin production. This is not a great recipe for biological success, especially if we are trying to recover from addiction at the same time! Think about this for a moment. You can be focusing on something very important to you in the evening time, maybe writing an article, a book, or moving towards your goals. Out of nowhere you get the urge to check social media or maybe that dating site you signed up for. Before you know it you just spent 15 minutes, no more like 30 minutes. Maybe even an hour or more on that side diversion and completely forgot about the thing you were focused on.

Now what? Instead of completing your task and feeling really good about the progress you intended to make, you just spent that extra time in distraction land, and are getting to sleep, yet again at a much later time than you would have hoped for. This is the common cycle of self-sabotage in our day and age, which unknowingly by most people is causing a huge bulk of health and life challenges that go undiagnosed and unresolved. This is partially why the rates of sleeping pill medications, herbal supplements for sleep, and all the other industries that relate to sleep are booming like crazy but the people themselves are struggling. This is where we need to get a sober outlook on the effects poor sleep has on our lives because unless we can remedy this single issue, then all the other work around addiction recovery is going to be very challenging, at best!

First of all, poor sleep can often lead to specific types of food and stimulant cravings during the day. We have all had the experience of staying up too late partying or maybe just scrolling on our phones until the wee hours of the night. When we wake up the next morning, feeling unrested and a bit anxious, we tend to lean on certain foods and/or substances to help us get through the challenging day ahead. Coffee and caffeine are obvious culprits here and that should come as no surprise. Common food cravings that emerge tend to be sugar and starchy carbohydrates, for many people things like pastries, cookies, donuts, muffins, and whatever else people are into these days. This is all due to the fact that when we get poor sleep it effects our blood sugar regulation and throws our metabolism out of balance. This is also due to the fact that one night of sleep deprivation can significantly increase cortisol production (fight or flight hormone) leading to increased muscle wasting/atrophy/soreness due to the catabolic nature of both excessive cortisol in the body, combined with the effects of sleep deprivation itself.

There are many other detrimental consequences of not getting enough sleep over days, to weeks, to months, and over into years of our lives. I know for me, there was a period of time where it had felt like I had not gotten a really good night's sleep in a matter of years. This was due to prolonged stretches of life stress and not prioritizing my sleep as I knew I needed to do. I was engaged in my own dopamine feedback addiction cycle and when we are caught in this cycle, we tend to not make the wisest decisions for our future. That is possible the biggest problem with prolonging quality sleep is that it causes us to live in a very short term, reactive minded state, where we are always on the defensive, and living out of reaction, instead of being proactive, and taking the initiative to change ourselves for the better. This is largely due to the effects on the brain itself that are caused through sleep deprivation, which leads to reduced critical thinking, memory loss, brain fog, irritability, and cognitive challenges.

Now, let's discuss some of the amazing things your body does when you are actually getting the deep restorative sleep you need. One of the main functions your brain does while in deep sleep is 'memory-spatial-processing" which is a combination of 'synaptic-pruning', meaning auto-deleting old neurons or old circuits that no longer have any relevancy (like old tabs on a desktop browser), and processing "information" i.e., organizing miscellaneous "files" of the mind that do not happen in the waking state of consciousness. This is what happens when we wake up feeling clear headed, enthusiastic or motivated, and simply overall feeling good about ourselves, and the day ahead. When we wake up feeling anxious, irritated, uncertain, or confused that is a sign that spatial processing was not successful, and we are carrying over the unprocessed data files from the day or days prior. Have you ever heard the phrase "Just Sleep on It"? Well, this phenomenon is where that phrase comes from.

During sleep your body goes into what is known as an 'anabolic' rest, recovery, and repair state. There is a cascade of hormones that flood the body assisting with the repair and regeneration process. This is how men build back the testosterone they used up from the day prior. As we discussed, melatonin is released from the pineal gland. The pituitary gland releases human growth hormone, which is one of the most powerful anabolic substances the body has for muscle cell growth, cellular recovery, and neuromuscular and skeletal repair. Another interesting fact is that we have a biological clock where certain organs go into their own repair process at specific hours of the night. The liver for example goes through a cleansing cycle between the hours of 1-3 am. So, staying up consistently beyond these hours can slow down the function of the liver. The dark circles around the eyes associated with fatigue can often times be related to the kidney-adrenals but often times are more specific to the liver.

With all of this information you may now be wondering when exactly you should plan to get to sleep. This is an interesting area of research because there are many different opinions and perspectives to choose from. It is important to understand that our bodies have a biological clock called a 'circadian rhythm'. This is the bodies built in wake-sleep cyclical system and is affected by environmental influences of light and dark. There is a field of study that explores the scientific research on our circadian rhythm called 'chronobiology', which is the study of our bodies internal biological clock. There is a unique systematic schedule our internal clock goes through based on the rising of the sun, the afternoon, and the downing of the sun into nighttime. The basic premise to this research is that everyone has their own "peak state" at any given day. Some people peak in energy in the morning, which apparently constitutes 80% of the population, and then has a lull sometime in the afternoon. Some people even peak in the nighttime, which would associate these people as "night owls".

The study of chronobiology can be a very interesting field to research, because it helps to illuminate a lot about why we do what we do, and how we can adjust our routines based on our biological clock time. There is also something called 'chronotypes', which Dr. Michael Breus, PhD bases his entire book **The Power of When** around. This is the idea that there are 4 distinct chronotypes that exist and based on what your chronotype is determines when you tend to go to sleep, wake up in the morning, how much sleep you require each night, and how to gage your gradual energy levels through the day. I won't spend any time going into these types as you can research this concept deeper for yourself. It is a very interesting perspective and worth deeper investigation to see how it applies to each individual. One thing I will add to this is that when we begin removing the stimulants like caffeine/coffee, tobacco, energy drinks, junk food, and other substances such as alcohol, cannabis, and late-night internet scrolling, our natural biological clock comes into its natural rhythm. If you think you are a night owl but simply stay up late because of addictions and dopamine triggers, it is likely you are designed to sleep earlier and for longer than you typically do but are artificially inducing a late-night sleep routine. Keep that in mind when studying the chronotype and chronobiology information.

From a physiological level, when structuring your sleep schedule, it is important to note that between the hours of 10 PM - 2 AM is the window our brain secrets melatonin as a way to prepare for deep sleep. This is the 'anabolic' window of recovery where the body is more prone to produce human growth hormone, which helps to signal healing factors that result in feeling well rested and recovered the next day. According to Shawn Stevenson, the author of the book **Sleep Smarter,** when people are better rested at night, they can burn up to 50% more excess body fat than they can when they are sleep deprived. This is due to the hormonal regulation that takes place in this anabolic window of recovery and when we consistently miss this window it becomes much harder to maintain base metabolic health and hormonal balance.

There is a lot more that can be elaborated on the benefits of prioritizing sleep. I highly recommend Shawn Stevenson's book on the subject as it goes deep into the research and provides a lot of practical tools for how to maximize sleep quality. The important take away from this section is simply to acknowledge how important our sleep routine is, for overall health and wellbeing, as well as overcoming any form of addictions, especially those that we lean on like a crutch to get through the day because we are operating from a biological deficit due to poor sleep and lifestyle habits. Making simple changes in our sleep routine can make the biggest difference in our experience of life and how we feel in our own bodies. This requires sound lifestyle changes we mention in this chapter in addition to structuring our morning and nighttime routines.

Healing the Heart | Emotional Trauma

"The empathic wave form of the actualized human heart
will traverse universes."

Dan Winters

Our journey together has been a long and deep one. We have explored the topic of addiction from all different angles and touched on aspects of it that may have never been discussed together before. Now our exploration takes us right into the heart of the matter itself. Underneath all problems with addiction and recovery can be traced back to the health of the human heart. I mean this both literally and also metaphorically. The number one reason for death worldwide is due to heart disease. It outranks diabetes, all cancers combined, suicide, automobile accidents, drug overdose, and all other known fatalities. The subject of heart disease itself is very interesting to unpack and we will do that a bit in this chapter as we move forward.

The underlining causal mechanisms in addiction are rooted in some form of trauma, which leads to emotional instabilities. The inability to effectively cope with our emotions and ultimately integrate run away emotional states, leads one to medicate themselves as a strategy to suppress the imbalance within. This is due to the trauma that one carries with them, as part of their nervous system complex and the belief patterns that are programmed into the body itself. The body cannot heal itself independent of both the mind and heart. In this way I am both speaking of the physical heart and to a greater degree what can be called 'the sacred heart'. This is a term coined by my close friend Steve Adler who is an ordained essence minister and has devoted his life to unpacking the physics of love. That is a bit of a topic in of itself which is beyond the scope of this discussion, but it is worth saying that there are quantum physics/mechanics that govern our healing process, which can be found inside of what we are calling the sacred heart.

This is explained as a kind of portal that exists within us and is the source point for the particle physics of love. What I am talking about is known as 'adamantine particles' which are crystalline molecules that are intrinsic to all sentient biological life forms and are said to hold the energetics of pure love. Now whether you believe this or think it's some strange 'new age' concept is entirely up to you. What I will tell you is that this concept bears enormous weight because it produces immediate results in real time. The literal power of love is the thing (the only thing) that actually heals anything, or anyone. It's not the food, supplements, exercise routine, or workshop seminar that causes a healing to happen for someone. Those are complimentary additions, but it is actually the manifestation of love within someone's heart that causes healing to occur. Without this generation of love inside the heart all the diet plans, super foods, and supplements make very little difference, unless of course the food is grown with love, and the soil of that food is rich in minerals, which actually hold loving frequencies. Yes, minerals are actually points of light frequency that hold a vibratory charge that our bodies respond too and are powered on by.

So then, this begins to beg the question. If all of our health and addiction challenges are due to a literal lack of love in our heart, then what in our lives is blocking out to the love from emerging? Well, this is a fantastic question to ask, and the exact question that leads to the answers our heart is seeking. It had become abundantly obvious to me in the beginning of my journey into the natural health world that people are not only suffering from malnutrition, but also from a severe disconnect to their hearts. I had studied heart disease inside and out. There are clear physical reasons for heart disease, that point is very obvious. It also become clear that the reason heart disease is the number one killer in society is partly due to the fact that most people have closed their hearts to love. In fact, their hearts have developed a type of plaque-based calcification within the arterial walls, which constricts blood oxygen flow, and also scars the inner lining of the arteries themselves.

So, in essence, what we are dealing with is a situation where the physical heart is degenerating, which leads to ventricle atrophy. And also, we are dealing with a situation where the sacred heart has become calcified and, in some cases, turned into a hard stony rock. You have probably met people who are very abrasive, defensive, paranoid, and seem to have a very hard way about them. These are the kinds of people who tend to get heart conditions over time, and I can assure you this is not

316

by accident or coincidence. It is simply due to the fact that all of our organs represent a metaphysical connection to something going on within the human being themselves. For example, long suppressed grief and sadness tends to manifest itself as lung/respiratory problems i.e., lung cancer. Specific behavioral patterns such as smoking become adopted as a coping mechanism to deal with the unprocessed grief and sadness that rests underneath the stress one experiences, which leads to the smoking habit. Eating fast food, processed junk food, soda drinks, and even sugar habits can be traced to unprocessed emotions relating to one's own heart.

Unless we deal with what is going on at the emotional level of our lives, we will find ways to medicate ourselves as a way to avoid feeling what is there. In order to do this, we have to get past the stories we have about the varies dynamics in our lives, and especially in our relationships. There is no bigger area of most people's lives that have the biggest emotional impact than our intimate relationships. When someone is experiencing major ups and downs in their general lives it can likely be traced to a disturbance in their relational life. Our relationships set the foundation for every other area of our life, and that is why we devote an entire section in this chapter to discussing relationships as an essential element of recovery and emotional healing. Healing after all tends to happen through the reflection of relationship and what is known as 'co-regulation', which is the empathic connection between two or more human hearts in resonance with one another.

There is a lot more to cover in this discussion and so much more we can elaborate on the fundamentals of the heart, and its role in healing trauma in our lives. One of the major coping strategies to deal with emotional trauma is to live in our heads and to over analyze our life experience, opposed to simply feeling the experience itself within our bodies. There is a lot of discussion about living in the heart as opposed to living in our heads but what exactly does that mean? Well, in simple terms it means to live in our bodies because our heart is part of our physical body. When we do not feel entirely safe in our body we tend to disassociate from the sensations of the body and pop up into the mind because it feels safer and easier to control. This is a compensation strategy to deal with the sensations of anxiety, overwhelm, stress, frustration, and all the like. These are perfectly normal sensations we all experience at different times in our lives and the only way to overcome them is to learn how to engage with them.

The key to accessing the stored trauma imprints in the body is learning to tap into our 'autonomic nervous system', which is what governs the holistic functionality of the overall nervous system itself. The autonomic nervous system (ANS) controls all of the involuntary functions of the body that do not require any conscious participation in order to function. We discussed many of the concepts related to the nervous system in the prior chapter **Healing the Brain.** I am bringing awareness to this aspect of the conversation as it relates to emotional dynamics of the heart and more specifically as it relates to the healing of stored trauma in the body. We have all heard of the difference between the parasympathetic nervous system (PNS) and the sympathetic nervous system (SNS). The PNS is geared towards rest, relaxation, and recovery whereas the SNS is geared towards activity, alertness, and heightened focus. This is all true in essence and also an oversimplification because it is actually the ANS that controls the scales of balance between the PNS and the SNS and to what degree we are in an imbalanced state or a balanced state.

When trauma is triggered and activated in the body, we tend to go into a heightened SNS state, which promotes sensations of stress, anxiety, fear, or defensiveness depending on the individual's conscious awareness and their ability to remain stable as they are experiencing a trauma activation. This is a major challenge for most people in society, one of which I have had years of issues trying to overcome, and even make sense of while being catapulted into experiences of surfacing trauma that I did not entirely recognize that I had stored in my system from many years prior. There are a lot of very useful tools we can utilize to help regulate these extreme states when they onset and many of them are identical to the dopamine reset protocols in this book. Ultimately what the experience of trauma onset is showing us is the degree that we do not feel safe and secure in our own bodies, especially when we feel threatened or triggered. With this broad view awareness, we are able to take more ownership of our experience and implement effective tools for navigating the onset of trauma without it overtaking us in the moment.

There is a very interesting perspective on this subject that is articulated in the concept of the 'polyvagal theory', which is a term coined in 1994 by Stephen Porges, who is the director of the Brain-Body Center at the University of Illinois at Chicago. The introduction of the polyvagal concept is extremely important because it points to another aspect of the human nervous system that has only more recently made its way into the wider lexicon of neuroscience and holistic health. This is the understanding that our 'Vagus nerve', otherwise known as the pneumogastric nerve, is one of the master regulators between the head and the body, which means that is greatly influences the autonomic nervous system and all of the downstream effects that has on our parasympathetic and sympathetic functions. The Vagus nerve is the tenth cranial nerve that interfaces with the control system of the heart, lungs, and digestive tract. When the Vagus nerve is in a state of imbalance, we can develop cardiovascular, respiratory, and/or digestive issues simply due to this one issue, which ultimately creates more stress on the system.

There are a lot of well discussed methods for down regulating and soothing the Vagus nerve such as cold exposure (cold showers/ice baths), deep slow diaphragmatic breathing, chanting and singing, breath work and meditation, appropriate exercise, hands on touch and massage, as well as something called 'co-regulation'. Co-regulation is a very important concept as it relates to this chapter on the heart and healing trauma because this may be the single most important aspect of healing traumatic imprints that result in emotional instability, particularly within our intimate relationships. Co-regulation is basically the heart-to-heart empathic connection between two or more human beings, in real time. This is where we feel 'connected' too another person and 'felt' by that same person. When we feel safe and secure around another person it allows for a nervous system regulation to occur inside someone's body and through connection, stored emotions can safely arise to the surface and be felt when there is a space of compassion available to do so. This helps one to drop out of the analytics of the mind and sink into the felt experience of their heart.

"To switch effectively from defense to social engagement strategies, the nervous system must do two things; (1)

319

So now we are going to connect all of this together in order to move forward into the rest of the contents of this chapter. When we are in an 'autonomic' state we are now in our involuntary reactions of whatever default program that our unique nervous system is set for. For some people, this will result in the 'fight' response, which means defense or attack. For others this will result in the 'flight' response, which means run away or protect. For some others, this will result in a 'freeze' response, which means they get locked into place, frozen by indecision, and resemble a deer stuck in the headlights of an incoming car. Now, what if I told you that depending on how your nervous system is entrained through childhood trauma and accumulation of life experience, you are likely to display one of these three typical states as the primary response pattern to situations or circumstances that your autonomic nervous system interprets as a threat of some sort.

This autonomic sensory interpretation system becomes the filter for how most people's brains experience the world around them, and to some degree the world within them as well. This helps to explain why someone can experience a trigger activation based on seemingly benign things such as a taste, a smell, a tone of voice, or even an unconscious similarity in a total a stranger they have never met before but elicits a response in the threat detection software of their nervous system. This entire process of neural circuits in the brain that distinguish whether a situation or a person feels 'safe' is called 'neuroception'. This is the built-in safety valve or measurement system within our brain that helps regulate our autonomic response patterns. The challenge is when someone has stored trauma in their body and experience repeated triggering events due to a circumstance, experience, or a person that feels similar enough to the event that caused the trauma to occur in the past.

I began this chapter by doing a deep dive into the nuances and unearthed science on the autonomic nervous system as a way to bridge these discoveries with the subject of trauma and living a heart centered life. It is very easy to simply talk about the intellectual concept of living from the heart, but it is a much different thing to actually do this. The reason is because most of us have experience some form of trauma and accumulated stress patterns that cause us to eject from our hearts and occupy far too much time in our heads. If we try to live a heart centered life but have stored emotional problems due to traumatic experiences that have not be resolved, then all we will be left with is an intellectual awareness of living from the heart but wonder why we cannot seem to experience it consistently. This is the source point for most substance abuse issues, repeated toxic relationship patterns, binging on 'comfort foods', as well as getting addicted to 'altered state experiences' such as plant medicines and psychoactive compounds that could otherwise be very healing and beneficial.

Now that we have a solid foundation to stand on in this chapter, we will move forward by exploring some unique and lesser-known concepts in order to awaken our hearts. The first thing to awaken in this process is the mind itself. Once the constraints of the ego-identity begin to lift, then the higher mind can slip into our conscious awareness and provide enlightened insights to help move our internal energies towards healing. Following this is the awakening of the human heart itself and allowing for the emotional purge of unsupportive energetic states such as anger, resentment, pride, jealousy, depression, sorrow, and sadness to move about. These energetic deposits of emotional states can be called 'molecules of emotion' and that is exactly what we are going to discuss now.

Take a sacred pause right here, close your eyes, place your hand on your heart, take a deep breath, or two, or three, and let's proceed.

Molecules of Emotion

"Most psychologists treat the mind as disembodied, a phenomenon with little or no connection to the physical body. Conversely, physicians treat the body with no regard to the mind or the emotions. But the body and mind are not separate, and we can't treat one without the other."

Candace Pert, Author of Molecules of Emotion

The concept that our emotions are not simply points of invisible "energy" but contain within themselves a molecular basis in the physicality of our body is becoming much more common place. Most of us have been taught to assume that our emotions are simply passing waves of feeling states that generates in our bodies due to what we are thinking and/or as a response to circumstances we experience. This is true in part but also a gross simplification of what emotions are and how emotions influence the physical state of our overall health and wellbeing. Emotions are not simply substance-less feeling states, but more so experiences that carry a certain type of 'weight' in our lives, particularly within the physical body itself, leaving a residue in the cells of our body when these emotions are unexpressed or unprocessed.

The traditional model of how our conventional theories of science and western medicine began could be summed up in this simple way. Let the churches and religions deal with the spirit and other "non-physical" matter (such as thoughts and emotions) and designate the hospitals, along with pharmaceutical drugs to deal with the physical body itself. These elements of the whole human being had been entirely compartmentalized and assumed to have little, to no direct interaction or connection to each other. As insane and unbelievably misinformed this perspective may seem, this was the general ideology and paradigm of the last century of western medicine and materialistic science. In the last few decades, we have been making our way out of this wrong turn in science and discovering that our physical body is directly affected by the interplay between our thoughts and emotional states, maybe more so than anything else for that matter.

Candace Pert, PHD is the author of a classic book called **Molecules of Emotion** which makes the convincing case that our emotions have a molecular reality within our cellular bodies. The sub-title of the book is "the science behind mind-body medicine" and that is exactly what this section of this chapter is pointing too. We are going far beyond the allopathic drug-based model of medicine, and even beyond the organic supplement and food-based model of medicine in order to tap into the connection between the mind and the complex workings of the body. Candace Pert was a neuroscientist who is claimed to be responsible for discovering the opiate receptor in the brain which is the binding mechanism for endorphins. One of her quotes to describe her body of work is *"since emotions run every system in the body, don't underestimate their power to treat and heal."*

She also said, *"we've all heard about psychosomatic illness, but have you heard about psychosomatic wellness?"* which means that just as the body can become overrun by negative thoughts and emotions, it can also be healed and brought back to vitality through loving thoughts and emotions. Candace also has said in one of her audio recordings that *"Your body is your subconscious mind"* which is a statement I have said many times with all of my clients and in my lectures over the years. The body and the mind are not separate entities onto themselves, they are actually one in the same. Whatever is going on in the conscious and more so the unconscious mind, the physical body will pick it up and seek to express it in some form or variation. They are a direct feedback of each other but again, not of two separate "things" but of one unified "thing" called the body mind or mind body. What determines the quality of our physical bodily experience is largely connected to the molecular quality of our emotional experience.

"Music, like our bodies, is structured vibrations."

Candace Pert

One of the most profound discoveries Candace Pert made in her work was that our brains contain neuroreceptors, such as opioid receptors that can plug into what she calls the molecules of our emotions. Dr. Darren Weissman, who is a proponent of her work, has said that drugs such as heroin bind onto the same receptor sites as emotions do. What this means is that our physical brains can become addicted to sub conscious emotional states the same way as they can to the chemical molecules of external drugs or substances. There is an information exchange that occurs through the chemistry set in our brains, based on the molecular deposits of the emotions we experience and revisit repeatedly. We have discussed this idea multiple times throughout this book as the addicted brain phenomena that happens when the brain wires itself to dopamine response patterns. It turns out this is just as real when it comes to the emotional stimulation we experience, which tends to come from the traumatic imprints of our childhood and/or intensified life events that have not been fully processed and resolved.

Many years ago, I became very interested in the scientific discovery of the psychosomatic(mind-body) effects on health, which is an entire body of research called psychoneuroimmunology (psycho-neuro-immunology). This is an emerging field of science that looks at the interactions between the central nervous system (CNS) and the immune system. These two systems of the body, being the brain-nervous system & immune cells and organs, communicate with each other by producing protein molecules to defend against opportunistic organisms that cause infections. The immune system is always looking to protect against any biological threats to the human body, as well as neutralize any current threats that may already exist such as a viral or bacterial infection.

When the central nervous system is put into a prolonged stress state (fight/flight/freeze) it sends the message to the immune system that there is a detected threat in the system. Because there is no detected infectious organism present in this situation the immune system can go into a 'red alert' response due to heightened signals of stress, and result into what is often experienced as an autoimmune response. This can cripple the immune system over time and be detrimental to our physical wellbeing. We may find ourselves chasing our tail trying to find the right supplements, eating strategies, alternative healing modalities, and all the rest, when in fact the source of the problem was not due to any of these things, but entirely due to the psychological conditioning that had manifested because of an unconscious pattern in the mind itself. The emotional deposits that are created as a result of this create their own chemistry, which the body now has to processes as if there was a foreign organism or toxin that needs to be expelled from the body.

One of the primary examples of this phenomenon I commonly share is that of a mid-life checkup or simply when someone receives an unexpected "diagnosis" from their doctor upon a routine checkup to the doctor's office. They are in relatively good health and do not exhibit any known symptoms they are aware of. Everything appears to be just fine according to their personal experience. When they do a routine scan, the doctor comes back shortly after, and tells them they discovered some kind of abnormality such as a tumor, for example. All of a sudden, the individual becomes consciously aware that there is a tumor in their body and depending on the attitude and cadence of the doctor delivering the information, the patient will receive the new information a particular way. If the doctor presents the information with fear, urgency to act, and pressures them to get some kind of operation to deal with the new discovery, the probabilities of the patient starting to exhibit immediate symptoms increases dramatically.

Now, remember, this patient came in without any detectable symptoms to begin with. According to them they were just fine and feeling well. Upon receiving the information and the energy behind the information, they may now begin to feel increasingly unwell, even sick as a result of that exchange of energy between their doctor and them. The more dramatic example of this is when a doctor tells their patient, in no uncertain terms, that they have an exact amount of time to live. Let's say they tell their patient they have 3 months left to live and that they should get their accounts in order to prepare for their death. Well, statistics reveal that in these cases that a patient tends to listen to their doctor and believe what they tell them as concrete fact. So, what we find is these individuals often times really do die in the approximate, if not exact time they were told they had to live.

What exactly just happened in this situation? What happened is the negative consequences of the psychoneuroimmunology effect. What they believe as absolutely true in their mind created the emotions relative to that person's perception, and those emotions directly affected the functions of their immune system, which prior to this diagnosis was working just fine without their interference whatsoever. We also call this the placebo effect which is the irrefutable scientific understanding that if someone believes a sugar pill (they do not know it's a sugar pill) is a medication that it tends to work just as well as the medication or in some cases even better. These experiments have also been conducted with surgeries, which are called 'sham-surgeries' where a patient will be told that they had a certain type of surgical procedure and upon coming out of the anesthesia they have the effects of someone that had gone through an actual surgery.

Now I am not saying the placebo works 100% of the time. There are variables involved but both of these examples, and many more are all well documented, and prove that the power of the mind-body connection is far too real to ignore. The placebo works both ways, positive and negative. What we believe about ourselves illicit emotions that correspond perfectly to our self-perception. If we believe that we are truly healed and recovered then the molecules of our emotions will issue themselves in our body the sensations of someone who is healed, integrated, and recovered. If we believe we are hurt, wounded, and disadvantaged the molecules of emotions will produce the sensations of someone who is hurt, wounded, and always feeling like a victim. Remember, the body keeps the score because it is recording the emotional deposits of how we really feel about ourselves, not just what we would prefer to feel through an intellectual pursuit of positive thinking or self-help tactics.

> *"It seems to me that everyone on this planet whom I know or have worked with is suffering from self-hatred or guilt to one degree or another. The more self-hatred and guilt we have, the less our lives work. The less self-hatred and guilt we have, the better our lives work, on all levels."*
>
> *Louise Hay*

In closing in this powerful section, I want to direct our attention to a pioneering figure in the transformational industry who is Louise Hay. In 1984 she released her classic book **You Can Heal Your Life**, which set a standard and foundation for which much of the personal growth industry has been built from. She is also the founder of the now Hay House publishing company, which has supported countless legendary teachers over many decades. Louise Hay's work was centered in and around the understanding that not only do we have the innate power to heal all aspects of our lives, including our physical bodies, but that the quality of our overall life is reflected in the quality of our bodies. It would be impossible to give a full discourse on her entire body of work in this section, but her work is an important insight into the nature of healing and overcoming one's personal circumstances through transforming the emotional deposits in the body by simply observing the feedback our body is giving us.

There is a brilliant lecture online by Louise called **Conversations on Living by Louise L Hay** that anyone can easily look up. In this presentation she provides an in-depth road map of how each part of the body carries it's only unique mental and emotional blueprint. She takes the audience through a description of many common physical ailments and discusses the metaphysical cause behind these conditions. For example, she discusses that when children experience ear aches it tends to be because they are constantly being told something they do not want to hear, such as the word no. It is common knowledge that the single word a child hears more than any other is the word no and this also reinforces a negative association as they development into adolescence and into adulthood.

Another example she makes is that when people have persistent lung issues it is a sign that they are cutting themselves off from life itself, therefore reducing the amount of oxygen in the respiratory system as a result. She makes the point that most of us take for granted the single most important element we all need to live, which is our breath or oxygen. She explains that most people have been conditioned to believe that they do not have a lot of value and do not deserve to take up "too much" space in this world, thus limiting the amount of oxygen they take in since that is the essential molecule for life. What is interesting about this idea is that most people actually do reduce their oxygen intake through shallow breathing patterns. It is also true that most people have a negative self-image of themselves and tend to not have a lot of self-esteem or self-worth as a result. Louise simply is revealing the connection between the perceptions we have of ourselves and the physical symptoms that manifest as a result of this.

I discussed this concept in more detail in the chapter **Mastering the Body** in the section **Metaphysical Anatomy of the Body,** so I do not want to belabor the point too much. What is critical to inner stand, however, is that the molecules of our emotions are generated from the perceptions and consistently repeated behaviors we entertain every day and into every year of our lives. One more example Louise shares is when someone has chronic headaches it tends to be related to the habit of invalidating oneself, meaning self-criticism and self judgement. I have known many people who would be otherwise extremely healthy and upbeat but seem to have chronic headache or migraine issues where they are constantly taking some medication to sooth the problem. I could also see those same individuals having these kinds of self-criticisms and that being the primary cause of the physical symptom of a migraine or headache, aside from any environmental toxicity issues that may be involved also.

So, here we have it my friend. This section in of itself is a bit of an emotional journey into the deeper inner standing that our emotional states are not simply an ephemeral phenomenon that passes through us from time to time. There is a very real molecular physicality to our emotions based on the crystallization of molecules formed from the energetic vibrations we entertain and maintain over time. I hope that you can use this knowledge to help shift any negative or heavy emotional processes you may find yourself in, simply by knowing that the body always keeps the score, and the longer we linger in these states of emoting the more we will have to move them out through the tissues of the body itself.

To go deeper into this, I highly suggest the work of both Candace Pert and Louise Hay, who both are now passed on but their immortal impact in this field of discovery will always live on, which is partly why I found it so important to make mention of both their names and their invaluable works.

Life is Based on Relationships (Core Wounds)

"The wound is the place where light enters you."

Rumi

Out of all areas of life that has the biggest impact for most of us is undoubtable the arena of relationships. This is both true in our intimate romantic relationships as much as it is true in our familial and friendships. Relationships are the corner stone to the human experience because they provide a mirror for us that nothing else really does. It could be said that if one wants to see themselves better, they should seek to see themselves through the eyes of the people they are in relationship with. I know this has been the truth for me, albeit a very uncomfortable and confronting truth at times, and yet a truth all the way around. It can be much easier to go through life by isolating ourselves from getting too close to others and staying within the narrow bandwidth of our preferred habits, patterns, personal beliefs, and chosen addictions in order to remain comfortable. The problem here is that being too comfortable with the version of ourselves we are accustomed to leads to stagnation, which does not provide the necessary feedback we need to learn and grow from.

Relationships have a unique way of revealing the aspects of ourselves that we would prefer not to see, acknowledge, and certainly rather not experience altogether. The more a relationship bond has been created, and the deeper it is between two people, the more potency it may have to trigger the exact thoughts, emotions, and bodily sensations that already exist underneath the surface of our conscious awareness. This is most pronounced in our intimate romantic relationships for sure, which is also why these relationships tend to be so difficult, full of potential complications, and 'triggering' for most of us who choose to get involved emotionally and sexually with another. It certainly does not have to be this way but because of the depth of wounding and trauma most people have experienced that has gone unhealed and unresolved, these patterns repeat themselves in future relationships, that is until the pattern is interrupted and resolved.

Now I am not going to go into a full-blown discourse on relationships and certainly not going to go into giving relationship advice. That is for the hundreds of other teachers who have made that topic their focus and life's work. I want to provide a different perspective on the topic, as it directly relates to addiction, recovery, and healing the core wounds that unavoidably will unearth themselves due to the alchemical process of relationships themselves. What is very important in this context is that each of us has carried some kind of core wound within us over the course of our lives. In my own life there have been a few distinct core wound patterns I have discovered through the course of multiple long-term

329

relationships, as well as friendships and professional partnerships. When we are dealing with core wounds, they act as an archetypal theme, which repeats itself in different relational dynamics, in different situations, but there is always a similar theme or pattern to them.

For me, the primary core wounds I have experienced were/are abandonment, betrayal, and inadequacy. This was not always entirely obvious to me before, in fact, to be honest with you, I only became crystal clear about these three truths while starting to write this chapter on healing the heart. You see, the thing about this is when we are in the thick of an emotional trigger and experiencing the physiological effects of heightened stress, it is next to impossible for most of us to accurately see what is actually happening. Our nervous system goes into an immediate fight or flight state, blood is rushing into our extremities as if there is a dangerous wild animal in front of us, and we are automatically put into a defensive psychological position. I cannot even count anymore how many of these triggering experiences I have had in relation to an intimate partnership problem where I felt like I was losing control of my sanity, liable to break anything around me, and/or simply wanting to run away from the situation all together. I have found myself shouting at the top of my lungs, punching walls, stomping my feet, throwing something across the room, and at the end of all that, finding myself completely breaking down inside and crying due to the exhaustion of it all.

This is an example of a core wound being unearthed inside of someone's nervous system and that person either not having the tools to deal with it or likely not even knowing that it is a core wound that is causing the defensive, seemingly irrational set of behaviors. When I would feel the triggering of my abandonment wound, I would quickly feel defensive, hurt, and even a bit like a victim in any given situation. This is the same basic response when my betrayal wound would surface, which was never far away from the abandonment wound. These two primary wounds would contribute to my feelings of inadequacy, where I never really felt totally "good enough" or that I "was never enough". In fact, I can remember in one such relationship where I would repeat statements such as "I feel like nothing I do is ever enough!" or "I cannot seem to do anything right". These were authentic feelings I felt but they also were based on the fact that I felt wounded and inadequate in the relationship, which in truth was simply a mirror for how I felt in my overall life at that time. It was not until I began to take responsibility for my wound, began to consciously engage with them, rather than suppress them, that the triggers became easier to manage.

Now, it is important to consider that there is a reason for how these core wounds have developed inside of us. They are not simply something we inherited in our lives, although there can be a significant relationship to the epigenetic transference we received from our parents and grandparents. But even still, most of what we receive from our familial blood line is the conditioning and belief patterns they had and gave us during our developmental years. For me, these core wounds were traced back to the earliest years of my childhood, so early that I do not even have a conscious memory of them, but I recognize where they came from and how they imprinted into my consciousness. You see, I was raised in what I would describe as a functionally dysfunctional family situation. There was love and care in my youth, but it was somewhat of a random upbringing due to the fact that my parental caretakers really had little to no clue what they were doing, and it really felt like they were just "winging" the whole thing.

The biggest point of reference I have is the fact that my biological father was never in my life. I grew up without a father and to make matters more confusing I was never told by my mother that I even had a father, until I was 12 years old, and finally pressed the issue when I saw one of my friends getting picked up from school by his father. Prior to that experience I had never even considered that not having a father was somehow abnormal or strange. It was simply the situation I was familiar with and it felt as "normal" to me as it would be for someone else to have two healthy, present parents in the household. Once I became aware that I did have a father my mother asked if I wanted to meet him. Well, of course! You might assume, and strangely enough, it was that easy for her to make a call, arrange a meeting, and so we did weeks later. That was the first and last time I ever met my biological father, when I was 12 years old, and interestingly enough, since I was so used to not having a father in my life, it did not seem to faze me that he would no longer be in my life following that one week we spent together.

I went on with my life after that, thinking little to nothing of the whole thing. It was not until almost two decades later that I would discover how much of a deeper impact this made on my young psyche, and the core wounds of abandonment were instilled in me nervous system. I remember a specific moment, around 5 years ago (30 years old) my mother was encouraging me to reach out to him and try to develop a relationship with him before he died. I was very resistant to doing this, simply because I felt no obligation to do so, and if he wanted to have a relationship with me, he simply could have reached out all this time. My mother pressed on and I finally agreed to give him a call. Now mind you, this is 18 years after the fact of meeting him in person. I had no idea what to say but I decided to make the call. This experience would help to begin the process of revealing just how deep the core wounds I inherited and held inside me really were.

I called him on Father's Day. The phone rang a few times and finally there was an answer, "Hello?" I fumbled over my words, as if I did not expect that he would actually answer. I basically told him I was his son and ten seconds into talking, the phone hung up! I was a bit shocked and confused. I paced around a bit and then decided to call him again. Same thing, "Hello?" this time I tried again, and maybe got 15 seconds into it, and he hung up again. This time I was furious! I called my mom, told her what happened, and said I was done with him, and would not call back. She then explained to me that he was not a very confident or courageous man. He was scared and probably embarrassed or something. I felt more compassion and softness in my heart, so I decided to give it one more go-round. He answered "Hello?" and I told him "Do Not Hang Up", "You do not have to say anything but please listen." I proceeded to tell him I was not angry at him and that I just wanted to let him know that I forgave him for not being in my life and that I loved him. I think I got 45 seconds into it this time before he would hang up again, without ever saying a word.

That moment was the very last time I ever attempted to reach out to him, but it was a defining moment because I chose to overcome my immediate feelings of anger and chose compassion instead. After that I found myself processing the experience, crying a bit, and finding resolution in the fact that I had done my part, and that was all I was meant to do in this situation. That was also a moment where my own core wound healing process would begin because prior to that I had little to no clue that I had been carrying a major burden of abandonment inside of my heart, my psyche, and my body this whole time.

332

I share this all with you to help illustrate that there is a personal story that we all carry inside of us that is directly linked to the core wounds buried inside of our cells. These cells contain the molecules of stored emotions that Candace Pert so brilliantly discussed in her work. These molecules of emotions had also carried themselves out into my most intimate and personal relationships beyond that point in time, and it was not until very recently that I began to really see the patterns that would play on repeat, all due to this singular core wound that happened at the earliest years of inception. I would strongly suggest that for most people there is such a core wound that was imprinted into them at their earliest years and that is very likely the source point for the triggered trauma patterns that result in problems in our intimate relationships.

The surfacing of our core wounds can easily lead into the resurfacing of old or current addiction tendencies we are trying to overcome, or perhaps have had success in abstaining from but the urge is intensified once an emotional trigger surface.

There is one other piece of information I would like to provide which can be very powerful for understanding the unique dynamics of different intimate relationships and what is called our "attachment style" in relationship. During one of my prior relationship challenges I was recommended a book called **Attached** by Amir Levine and Rachel S.F. Heller which sheds light on how each of us has an 'attachment style' that plays out in our relationships, depending on the types of relationships we tend to get involved in. The basic concept is that each human being has what is explained as an 'adult attachment style', which breaks down to the anxious, avoidant, or secure attachment. These are not fixed in place, they can be altered through working on the core wounds i.e., emotional triggers that come up in relationships, but this is the starting point that is used to gain more awareness of how an individual tends to respond in relation to their partners attachment style.

So, if one person has an avoidant attachment and the other has an anxious attachment this will create a push and pull type of dynamic, where one person tends to avoid conflict and the other tends to become anxious when they feel their partner's avoidance. The avoidance tendency is also a pattern that can persist to feeling the anxiousness of their partner. It should be semi-obvious to see how this dynamic can create conflict and trouble in the relationship. I have personally experienced this dynamic in multiple relationships where I felt my partners anxiousness and found myself avoiding confrontation due to the energetic discomfort this dynamic creates. Both of these attachment patterns tend to feel much safer when their partner has a secure style, which simply means they are secure in themselves, and do not feel anxious in the relationship, or try to avoid conflict when it arises.

There is a good passage in the book that explains this really well:

> *"As adults we don't play with toys anymore, but we do have to go out into the world and deal with novel situations, and difficult challenges. We want to be highly functional at work, at ease and inspired in our hobbies, and compassionate enough to care for our children and partners. If we feel secure, like the infant in the strange situation test when her mother is present, the world is at our feet. We can take risks, be creative, and pursue our dreams. And if we lack that sense of security? If we are unsure whether the person closest to us, our romantic partner, truly believes in us and supports us and will be there for us in times of need, we'll find it much harder to maintain focus and engage in life. As in the strange situation test, when our partners are thoroughly dependable and make us feel safe, and especially if they know how to treasure us during the hard times, we can turn our attention to all the other aspects of life that make our existence meaningful."*

So, my take on the attachment style concept is that the ultimate goal is for both individuals to find their own inner security, both in themselves, and within the relationship. This can only really happen when both individuals do the work on themselves to excavate their core wounds, emotional triggers, and fears that are prompting the avoidant or anxious reactions. When one person is secure and the other is anxious or avoidant, the relationship can still "work", and this tends to be the case in most longer-term relationships, more than not. But ultimately the goal of the entire process is for both people to feel security in the relationship by finding security and certainty within themselves, as well as obviously feeling totally secure and safe with their partner.

Long-term loving relationships, and especially marriage can be something of a crucible these days. The common saying that relationships are not easy and take a lot of work is very true. However, relationships can be significantly easier and far more harmonious when both individuals in the relationship choose to adopt total responsibility for their personal core wounds and triggers. When we begin panning off our "issues" onto the other, this is the start of what will turn into a very tumultuous endeavor, if not total collapse of the relationship, resulting in either divorce/break up, or a slow drain of life force in the individuals which will lead into falling back on addictions and dopamine dependencies to compensate for the lack of fulfillment and connection they are not experiencing in their relationship.

"All relationships have one law. Never make the one you love to feel alone, especially when you're there.

Unknown

Final Thoughts on Healing the Heart & Trauma

There have been a lot of books written on both the topics of emotional healing and resolving childhood trauma. This chapter is meant to serve as a detailed introduction into these topics for those sincerely looking to purge the negative influences that have affected their lives and successfully move forward towards greater health and fulfillment. The key inner standing in this chapter is recognizing that our 'core wounds' influence every aspect of our psycho-emotional experience and can trigger defensive reactions in our nervous system when we feel a lack of safety or security. This is why relationships tend to be the container where our core wounds are most triggered and also serve as the primary space for true healing to occur.

The most important relationship in our lives will always be the one we have with ourselves. How we are with ourselves is how we will show up with others. How we show up with others is simply a reflection of our we are showing up with ourselves, whether we are consciously aware of that fact or not. Using our close relationships as a direct mirror can be very empowering, because it then becomes a tool to receive feedback as to how much healing we have done with ourselves or how much healing is still required. When we personalize the triggering, we may experience and attach a story to it we can easily get locked into the fight or flight sympathetic nervous system response. This only keeps us stuck in the trauma or emotional trigger but does not allow for true healing and reconciliation to take place.

Use the information provided in this chapter to help navigate the molecules of emotion that bubble up to the surface so you can better identify what is rising to the surface, where it is coming from in the body, and breathe deeply into it as a way to provide safety instead of defensiveness. Safety is the key to healing our psycho-emotional pain points that get locked and stored in the body. Meditation and breath work become highly effective tools for self-soothing, internal processing, and integrating the lessons that exist right below the surface of the trigger itself.

Section 4

The Integration Phase

We have now reached the single most important phase of our journey together. This is where all of the road work begins to really pay off and produce fruitfulness. We have now stepped fully into the integration phase, which represents the starting point of a completion process from one phase of a journey into a brand new one. This is the moment where all of the conceptual knowledge on addiction becomes embodied wisdom. This is where what you have learned begins to manifest immediate and long-term results in your life that are palpable, experiential, and deeply felt. This is the moment the challenges of the past begin to fade from memory, and the triumphs of the moment begin to really come alive.

The single biggest challenge that most people struggle with is integrating the knowledge they have gained and turning it into brand new habitual patterns that create entirely new results in their lives. We are going to remove the common struggles of this transition out of the equation and move right into the embodiment process. But remember, this process is still entirely dependent on whether you really want it or not. I cannot do it for you. All I can do is provide the blueprint to help you navigate the journey ahead. The rest is entirely up to you, but I know you have what it takes to radically transform your life and who you choose to become in that process.

Once one has taken themselves through a proper initiation, as we have in the last series of chapters, the remaining element is to integrate what has been learned and experienced. This requires a kind of self-reflection and vulnerability that many are simply not willing to feel. This next phase of our journey will require you to feel everything that arises in your body and begin purging the parts of your psyche that no longer serve your future. This is not a complicated or drawn-out process. We have moved through the complexities of the process and now are going to simply face the pure truth that resides at the final destination of the noble journey. Your willingness to confront the truth and look squarely into the mirror

337

of your own reflection will determine how much you are able to integrate all that has been brought forth.

It's time. Let's proceed.

Listening to the Soul

"Wisdom is reading the mind of God."

Wallace Wattles, The Science of Becoming Rich

We have now reached the final stage of this journey together into the nature of addiction and all that has been explored, from start to finish. This has been a journey unlike any other, and if you are anything like myself, then it is safe to assume that much has been brought to the surface, as it certainly has been for me, as well. We began this exploration by discussing the subtle nature of addiction and how the spirit of addiction enacts itself in our lives, as well as the various tools it uses to entrap us in its grip. The key concept here is that the spirit of addiction has its own consciousness and its own motivation, which is why it feels appropriate to describe it as a spirit, instead of simply saying we have an addiction, or we are simply addicted to a certain pattern, substance, or tendency. We are not addicts, in and of ourselves. We, as human beings, are incredibly powerful beyond measure, intelligent beyond comprehension, and full of untapped potential but when we are in our lower states of conscious awareness, we are easier to manipulate by forces that exist outside of our common senses.

The common struggle of addiction tends to be a tug-o-war between the archetypal forces of the victim persona and the hero or victor persona. This is the eternal conflict that all human beings seem to struggle with, and it is also written into the mythology of all spiritual teachings and allegories throughout recorded history. In my own struggles and challenges with the subtle nature of addiction, I have been brought face to face with my own inadequacies, insecurities, limiting beliefs, and cultural programming that aided and abetted the spirit of addiction to maintain its influence over my life, and reinforce the patterning of self-defeating behaviors that kept me in a cycle of struggle. This cyclical pattern of struggle is very nuanced and not entirely obvious at first glance. It can feel like we are making great progress when we overcome a particular habit or refrain from engaging in a habit when the opportunity to engage presents itself. This causes us to feel greater self-esteem and confidence in that moment but if we do not remain focused and centered in the transformational process at hand, we can easily find ourselves slipping hard at another moment, which can lead us back to our old habits, thus causing us to feel disempowered and as if we have made little to no progress at all.

The struggle of addiction and recovery tends to be a hard-fought battle for many of us because we can often find ourselves fighting against ourselves, which can only bring forth further inner conflict within ourselves. The real battle at play is not with or against ourselves at all, but more so a conflict between our lower nature and our higher nature. Our lower nature reveals itself when we sink into the mindset of victimhood and find ourselves placing blame and judgement onto others or even onto ourselves. When we are in this state of victimhood, we become the judge, the jury, and the prosecutor as a compensation for feeling disempowered in our personal situation. This is a psychological maneuver to avoid the pain and discomfort we may feel in the tension of our own struggle. The problem with this is that what we judge and prosecute outside of us eventually becomes redirected back to us and thus reinforces the cyclical nature of inner conflict and struggle. It's like finding ourselves struggling with the tension of having our fingers caught in a Chinese finger trap, only to discover that releasing the tension, and letting go of our need to fight with ourselves that the trap expands and easily releases our fingers.

The greatest discovery I have made in my own explorations of the nature of addiction is that it is entirely a spiritual process that leads to complete healing and total recovery. When I say that the nature of addiction carries a spiritual energetic to it, I mean exactly that. In my own experience with overcoming addiction energies in my life I found myself smacking up against roadblock after roadblock. Hard wall after hard wall. I could not figure out for the life of me why I could be hyper intelligent and still revert back to the same behavioral patterns, time and time again. It became obvious to me that I was not going to be able to transcend my own limitations on my own or by myself. I needed an extraordinary source of support that led me to reviving my inquiry into the timeless teachings of certain biblical principles that I had been exposed too in my younger years. I thought I knew the basic teachings, but I began to suspect that there were deeper layers of meaning imbedded in the principles and passages that could assist me in overcoming the spiritual obstacles of addiction.

Now, without going into a theological discussion on the validity of the Bible or the potential hijacking of certain versions of the bible by the victors of history (and trust me, I can easily go there) I want to share a famous passage from Ephesians 6:12 which perfectly articulates my own process with overcoming the spirit of addiction. "For we wrestle not against flesh and blood, but against principalities, against powers, against the rulers of the darkness of this world, against spiritual wickedness in high places." I have had to read and reread this passage many times in order to allow it to land in my heart and help illuminate my consciousness to the blind spots of my own ignorance that had blocked my inner vision as to what was tethering me to various forms of addictive habits and most importantly the spiritual nature behind it all.

The struggle of addiction is when we are in conflict with ourselves i.e., flesh and blood. When we are at odds with ourselves, with our short comings, with our inherent flaws, and are in judgement of our humanness, we become self-inflicted victims of circumstance. This is the ultimate trick that has been played upon us, which is to convince us that we are to blame for our inferiorities and that we must engage in some form of inner civil war with ourselves as the path towards salvation or liberation. This is the same enslavement program the social engineers of organized society implement to create social unrest and cause division amongst a growing population. Virtually every social justice movement that was rooted in division, separation, and conflict was manufactured with the purpose of driving a wedge between the people of a community or nation. We fight amongst ourselves and others because we think it will produce some form of positive change, but this has never been the case; history is riddled with example upon example that this only furthers the cycle of struggle.

So, what we must understand is that in order to override prior psychological programming and overcome our addiction patterns, we must put our faith in something greater than just ourselves. Otherwise, as the passage in Ephesians 6:12 teaches us, we are only wrestling with flesh and blood but distracted from the source of our struggle all together. I have found for myself that it is very difficult to fully excavate myself from a hole I dug myself into, especially if that hole was created through years

341

of unconscious digging. This is why we need to surrender our will to a higher power that can help carry up back into a place of inner balance that only comes from living in alignment with our soul. When we choose to ignore the whispers of our soul calling, the transmission of the mind gets backlogged with static and noise. We attempt to figure out how to solve problems using our mind, without realizing most of the problems we have created for ourselves came from listening exclusively to the programs of the mind. It's like trying to dig deeper into that hole we got ourselves into as a desperate attempt to dig ourselves out of the hole. The reactive mind on its own will tell us to keep digging and dig faster yet logically we can see how that approach would only drive us deeper into our problem.

When I say we must surrender our will to a "higher power," what I am saying is that the addiction frequency resides at the level of the reactive mind, whereas the triumphant frequency of grace resides at the level of our soul. The higher power I am suggesting is really all about tuning into and attuning too the still point that exists inside of us when we allow for the inner space/silence to receive what our soul is guiding us towards. In my own personal relationship with the heavenly father i.e., God, I relate it to a divine intelligence that is both everywhere and nowhere at the same time. It is omnipresent and omni supportive in its nature and it is giving off blessings at all times but much like a radio station, we have to tune into the right frequency channel in order to receive what is being put out. The way I do this is to still my breathing cycles, close my eyes, place my hand on my heart, and silence the noise of my mind. One thing I know for certain is that the divine intelligence that is my/your soul will not raise its voice in order for me/you to hear it. We have to turn down the volume of our mental chatter in order to hear its whispers. And make no mistake, it communicates in whispers, sensations, hunches, intuitions, and subtle visions.

There is a simple way to distinct between the communication of our soul and that of other forces that we will simply call the spirits of addiction. The whispers of our soul/higher divine intelligence are subtle, inviting, detached, calm, and expansive, if received and felt into long enough. What is good for us tends to have a softer, smoother, and uniquely inspiring energetic tone to it. What is good for us does not tend to trigger the addiction frequency, in fact it may bring our addictions to the surface because what is good for us is often times simply doing the opposite of what we have an addictive relationship with. The spirit of addiction tends to be subtly manipulative, casting all kinds of promises, alluring, and carries the energy of temptation. It also tends to get louder and more overt in its sensations if we create enough space between ourselves and it. In other words, the spirit of addiction is that of possessiveness and control. Our soul never needs to possess or control for the simple fact that it is the authentic core essence of who and what we actually are. The spirit of addiction is the inauthentic core essence of who and what we are not but tirelessly tries to convince us otherwise, and in this confusion is where we run into problems, such as a spiritual identity crisis.

Think about something for a moment with me. If we are truly the core essence of what we are told in spiritual, religious, and mystical texts, alchemical and hermetic teachings, as well as the countless reporting of near-death experience survivors, that our soul is immortal and timeless, then how could we possibly succumb to any form of identity confusion. We would have had to have had our memory of who we really are erased or perhaps we just went through a dream spell of temporary forgetfulness. That would explain why so many aspects of the material world we experience every day can feel painful, and why it can feel very heavy, hard, and frustrating. This also explains why we allow ourselves to compensate by medicating ourselves through all forms of substance abuse or activity overload. Because of the overload to our senses via all forms of cultural and digital distractions, we have simply forgotten who we are. The good news is that we are almost one step away from remembering the truth of our soul and this begins from simply turning down the noisiness of the world, putting down our compulsions, and simply practicing the sacred art of listening.

Moving forward in this chapter we are going to go through the art of listening and also the art of receptivity, which is an important part of the equation. Many of us where taught to listen but did not necessary receive good instructions on 'how to listen' and what listening really entails. For most people, in the busyness of their lives and the world around them, can only partially listen, at best. For many people, listening tends to look like one person speaking, the other appearing to listen and at the same time thinking about what they are going to say in response to what is being said to them. This is not truly listening to another person. Imagine if we are doing this in our daily interactions with other people, then how much true listening and receiving are we practicing with the divine intelligence of our soul?

The Power of Prayer

Throughout all of the Biblical scriptures and spiritual development teachings in the world, there is one consistent theme that shows up and that is the power of prayer. The interpretation of what prayer is and how to pray has become confused, misunderstood, watered down, and convoluted over the modern techno-centric era of the last 100 years. The materialistic Newtonian based scientific movement has been positioned as a replacement for spirituality, prayer, and faith by making the claim that science and technology allows us to know based on material evidence, instead of relying upon what is commonly called 'superstition' and 'blind faith'. This is one of the great tragedies to the developmental process of children into adults and adults into role models of the following generations. The more spiritual principles and practices have been weeded out of our daily life, the more problems we seem to have accumulated in our world. This is where a remodeling of our understanding about the power of prayer is needed, more than ever before.

Most people's form of prayer seems to be in response to a situation or set of circumstances that they do not want. People pray for better times but how many of these people take the time to sincerely pray during good and prosperous times. The act of prayer has been demoted from its original importance in our lives and used as an attempt to bargain or negotiate with God when we fall upon tough times. Ironically, for these same individuals it tends to be tough times they got themselves into and once it gets painful enough, the last desperate act is to plead with God to change their favor. For example, one time in high school I had drank too much at a party and became so intoxicated that my head was spinning, I felt nauseous, and it felt like it was never going to end. I remember going into a fetal position and begging God to bring me out of this drunken spiral. I even began to bargain that I would never drink again if only I could get out of this situation. Of course, eventually I sobered up, slept it off, and went about my life as if it never happened. I doubt God had anything to do with that incident, but I know that if I had made it a point to intently pray prior to that event, then I likely would not have drunk that night (or ever!) and I would not have had to experience that situation at all.

In the case of dealing with our addictions or even avoiding unnecessarily difficult situations of our own creation, prayer can be the difference maker in our lives. Prayer is not about getting something from kneeling down and making a wish to the universe. This is how most people go about it and that is also why most prayers seem to go "unanswered". If we are attempting to use the concept of prayer as a wishing well or a transactional exchange, as if God was our vending machine, then we have some serious growing up to do. Prayer is serious business, and we have to be serious in order to receive the benefits of this sacred practice. The thing about true prayer is that it requires us to leave our ego at the doorstep and drop into a sincere and authentic communication between our soul and whatever exists beyond our physical senses. Prayer absolutely works and when done effectively, it can work wonders in our lives.

As this chapter opened up, I began to discuss about the spirit of addiction and that addiction energy carries its own form of consciousness. When it is said that what we wrestle with in our lives is principalities and powers it is referring to the principalities of man-made institutions i.e., our cultural indoctrination system and powers referring to the unseen spiritual forces that act as the invisible hand, orchestrating chess pieces on the physical chess board of life. We have discussed the principalities elements in prior chapters and as for the spiritual forces behind all addiction phenomenon, that is where prayer becomes an essential tool. We cannot fight what we cannot see with our 5 physical senses and we certainly cannot defend ourselves with only the utility of our mind alone. Prayer is the armor that we raise up to deflect the temptations of addiction and ward off the parasitic spirits that probe for our weaknesses, whisper false promises of immediate pleasure, and tell us it's ok to compromise today because you can always start back up tomorrow.

There are three distinct aspects of prayer from my own perspective I think would be useful in this discussion. One is the act of praying for protection, one is the act of praying for strength, and the other is the act of praying for grace to pave the way forward. Praying for protection simply means to ask for assistance, support, and guidance. The spiritual armor analogy merely means that we ask our soul to stand guard at the gateway of our mind and defend against negative thoughts or victim-based stories to take hold. This results in a strong mental attitude and clear focus on what needs to be done. The protection prayer simply provides us assistance in any and all forms that we may require support in the journey ahead. Knowing ahead of time that we will encounter our insecurities, weaknesses, and temptations provides us the wisdom to ask for help and guidance to avoid the booby traps ahead. It also provides any extra help from unseen forces that very well may be angels following our steps and guarding against accidents in our life, that we may have never known were moments from happening. It would be a good idea to simply pray and express gratitude for that, just on the off-shoot chance it is true.

The act of praying for strength is to tap into an inner fortitude and conviction that already exists within you to move through any temptation or distraction that meets your path. This is not about physical strength, although working out the body and physical training are recommended practices for holistic empowerment. There is a reason that serious body builders consider the gym to be their church! The strength I am referring to is the strength of mind, strength of heart, and strength of purpose needed to reach your next level. We all face trip wires along the way and life can sideline us pretty hard sometimes. When we have made great progress and all of sudden our life gets turned upside down, this is when the spirit of addiction comes back to us because we are at our most vulnerable. Life is going to happen. So, preparing ahead of time by instituting an intentional prayer practice for the strength, discipline, and commitment to follow through when the going gets tough, because it will, and you already know this.

Finally, the act of praying for grace is what activates the trifecta of this entire prayer circuit. We discussed some of the brilliant work of Richard Rudd in his Gene Key's book in the chapter The Dopamine Dilemma relating to addiction and the epigenetic concept. When I began to dive deeper into the Gene Keys material, I began to see a common theme arise in all of the teachings. The common thread is a return back into a state and frequency of grace. You have probably heard the concept of the fall from grace which describes a fall or departure from our highest virtues as human beings and falling into the darkness of ignorance. This of course is depicted in the biblical story of Adam and Eve being evicted from the garden for disobeying God and partaken in the forbidden fruit. Whether you believe that story or simply interpret it as a metaphor, as I do, the theme itself has been playing out through human history and is best represented within each of our lives, through our struggle with addiction. The fall from grace is not something that happens to us but something that happens through us as we consciously choose to lower our vibration by participating in behaviors that lower our energy, limit our mental capacities, and hold us back from excelling in our lives.

Because the fall from grace is a result of our own choices, the return back to grace is also a result of our choices. We are always standing, front row and center, at the choice point of our own destiny. This is why prayer becomes so instrumental in overcoming and recovering from the addiction frequency that has been implanted into our psychology, as modernized people's living in organized society, that thrives from turning creators into consumers. Grace is what happens within us when we move closer to our divinity, which is a feeling of wholeness, integrity, and inner peace. The act of prayer invokes an energetic activation within our hearts that opens us up for receptivity. Receptivity is the state of being required in order to receive the grace of life that is always available to us but must be chosen by us. Many times, we block off our abundance, resources, and support simply because we do not know how to receive it or understand that it is always with us in the first place.

This is where the power of prayer comes in to turn on the switches within our mind and hearts to allow for the physical (and non-physical) support to assist our path. Even the simple act of praying, with a sincere intent, can radically alter our state of mind to a point that solutions to our problems emerge and our perception of a situation changes in a few moments. This is what I call a powerful moment of grace. These moments of grace have a way of reorganizing our priories, helping to reveal what is truly important to us, and letting go of the weight that comes from overthinking about the things that really do not matter in the big picture of things.

We are now going to discuss how to turn on the power of prayer as a practical tool that you can make use of at any moment you wish. There is both an art and science to this process and unfortunately it is one that has been misunderstood and a bit convoluted through the indoctrination of "Churchianity", which is very different from the pure teachings of Christian mysticism. Jesus was a true mystic, if there ever was one, and a master of the prayer process. His teachings were tried and true but have been misinterpreted over the course of organized religion, which we are going to completely bypass here and go straight into the pure truth of how to enact prayer, sustain its potency, and allow prayer to empower our lives.

How to Turn on the Power of Prayer

"When we know beyond any doubt that we already speak the feeling language of prayer, we awaken that part of us that can never be stolen, lost, or taken away. This is the secret mode of prayer."

Greg Braden

Now that you better understand the power and potency of prayer, let's discuss the mechanics of how this art form can truly work wonders in our lives and reshape our faith in life itself. Most of us were trained to use prayer as some sort of repentance token to get ourselves out of a situation that we got ourselves into or maybe we did not see coming but are struggling to overcome none the less. The concept of repentance is an important one because it basically means to offer up our mistakes (often referred to as "sins") to a higher power (God) in order to cleanse our minds and return us back into a state of inner peace (Grace). This is true enough and can help us recalibrate ourselves when we have missed the mark of a higher direction in our lives. The problem for many people is that they do not autocorrect their behavior because they somehow assume that they can just 'repent" for any indiscretion they create, and all will be forgiven as long as they simply pray for forgiveness.

The act of praying for forgiveness, in my perspective, is not about something outside of us forgiving us but more so, us forgiving ourselves, and then making the changes necessary to balance our lives. There is still a major victim archetype/attitude playing itself out in the religious circles and it tends to be more of a passive form of prayer, instead of a sincere, heartfelt form of prayer. In the bible it even says not to be 'lukewarm' in your prayer but to be hot or cold because lukewarm (comfortable/passive) does not create the results we want. When I speak about the power of prayer, I am not speaking about acting like a victim and being a passive passenger in the process. What I am saying is that in order for prayer to work, it must be done with genuine energy and with direction. What are you praying for exactly? Why are you praying? And what are you willing to let go of in this prayer? These questions must be known in order for it to work.

The real "secret" to the magic behind prayer is contained within the energy that the individual brings to it. Expecting that prayer work is going to magically change our circumstances in of itself is still part of the passive spectator attitude and that has to change. It is very much the same analogy of going to the gym, working out on the weights, and reaping the rewards of the effort and energy you put into the practice, on an ongoing and consistent basis. True prayer is an act of full embodiment between mind, body, and spirit. You have to know what you are entering into when you begin the process and what exactly you are wanting to get out of it. Prayer is an amplifier and multiplier to what is already inside of you. The beauty of this is that what is held deep inside of you can be brought out of you through the sincerity, directness, and conviction of your prayer.

This is best explained from a story I heard the author and metaphysical teacher; Greg Braden describes in one of his lectures. He spoke about how he was on a drive one evening with a close friend who happened to be a Native American steeped in the traditional wisdom teachings and was encountering a rain drought in his community. This was a serious drought that struck a large portion of the population in the state they were in and according to the weather "experts", there was no sign of rain in view. His friend said he was going to pray for rain in hopes it would cause a spontaneous rain shower to occur. So, he began to close his eyes, go into a trance like state of meditation, and connect with his higher "guides" on the matter. Not long after this process clouds began to form over the men and water droplets started to land on the car windshield. Before they knew it had begun to rain in the presence of what was a drought.

Now, I admit I likely am getting a few details off about this story, only because it has been a few years since I had listened to it but what happened next in their conversation is crystal clear in my memory. Greg was astonished and asking his friend what exactly he did for this miracle to happen. His friend responded by telling him that he went into a meditation where he began to experience the palpable sensations of being in the midst of a rainstorm. He could smell the rain, he could feel the rain on his head, he could taste it, and he could take himself to such as place where it was a full-blown experiential reality for him. He explained that this was a traditional understanding of prayer taught throughout the mystic teachings of his culture and all you had to do was allow yourself to fully embody the experience you are praying for. He jokingly said after that the only thing he had not figured out was how to make the rain stop after it had begun!

So, whether you believe this story or think it's a bit far-fetched (Greg tells it much better than I!) the principle should be self-explanatory. The true teachings of prayer work is to allow for a direct connection between yourself and the experience you are wanting to have. A full embodiment of sensation, just as if it was a physicalized experience happening right now. The wishy-washy passive approach to prayer taught to us by organized religion, although with good intentions, simply does not work and only positions us in the victim role, but never in the creator role. When we understand that we are the creators of our own experience and we can create a brand-new experience at any given moment than the power of prayer turns on for us like a cosmic light switch. We have to feel it in order to reveal it. We have to attune our energy fields to match the energy of what we wish to experience and often times that means refraining from doing things that lowers our energy levels, otherwise we will never be a match for the higher rates of energy we are trying to call forth in our lives.

So, again, the idea is that we want to get into a meditative state of stillness, where the mental chatter and emotional worries remove themselves. This happens through focusing on our deep inhalation and exhalation of our breathing cycle. This helps to move the current of energy through our body. This is called somatic processing. Now we must begin to exercise our imaginative powers to envision what we want and allow the sensations of our body to feel it as if it is happening. One of the ways I do this is by focusing my intent on what would it feel like to fully feel total abundance in every cell of my body, right now! What would it feel like to feel the healthiest I have ever felt in my life, right now! How would it feel in my body to know all of my needs are covered, all of my concerns are gone, and I have overcome all addiction frequencies in my life, right now! Those simple inner statements combined with my breathing cycles and making sure I have a big smile on my face completely change any energetic stagnation I may experience and redirect my mind towards what is possible, instead of drowning in despair.

There is another key to this practice you need to inner stand in order for it to work for you. You have to completely detach from any outcome that this prayer may or may not produce for you. Sound counter intuitive? Well, here's the deal. Most people pray for what they don't have in hopes of getting what they need. They assume that God or the universe is a vending machine and them once in a while, reactionary prayer is some sort of get out of jail card. This does not work if someone is in a state of desperation, fear, doubt, or scarcity. This only works if the person is willing to sacrifice their doubts, fears, shortcomings, and insecurities on the altar of truth and the altar is the space we show up to in order to conduct our sacred prayer ritual. We must know that our prayers are always answered but due to the laws of electromagnetism and quantum physics, we can only experience that which we are an energetic match too. This is why many sincere people feel abandoned or unfairly delt bad hand after bad hand, yet they are good people and pray regularly.

I really hope what I am sharing makes sense to you and lands somewhere in your heart. This is the truth behind why passive prayer falls short and only leads to someone fantasizing about their life but never truly experiencing what is possible for them. We have to do the inner work and release the addictive obstructions that are keeping us in emotional states of fear and insecurity in order to experience life at a higher and higher level. If you practice this regularly and with an intensified conviction, it is impossible that you will not experience moments of absolute grace. These moments will spontaneously occur within you as you do this, and productive ideas will flow freely into your mind as a result. As you take steps on those ideas, circumstances, and situations will connect themselves for you, bridges in the form of people or opportunities will emerge, and your only work is to maintain and sustained a heightened prayer field where the highs only get higher, and the lows begin to only get higher as a natural consequence of living from your faithful heart.

Richard Rudd, founder of the Gene Keys and the man who wrote the forward for this book contributed his own personal prayer mantra to help the reader establish their own prayer practice. Richard is a seasoned mystic and spiritual practitioner who has explored the far ranges of metaphysical practices. Below is his personal guided prayer mantra he uses each day. Also, if you want to explore his material further you can go to this website for instructional videos to help you. https://genekeys.com/videos/the-holy-incantation-of-solace/

Richard calls this Holy Incantation of Solace. It is a prayer for the new humanity. You can think of all beings, and especially all human beings when you use the word 'we', it's protection, strength, and grace all in one according to Richard's wisdom.

May loves to pour through our soul - *binding us together as One*

May light flower in our heart - *lending us the Grace to transform all fear*

May warmth radiate our belly - *bringing prosperity to all*

May purity shimmer in our bones - *filling us with the essence of the stars*

May kindness resound in our voice - *softening the path that lies ahead*

May clarity shine through our mind - *as we rest in the arms of the infinite*

May solace abound in our life, *touching all who we meet*

May solace abound in the world, *bringing all beings into perfect union.*

The next and final topic for us to unpack in this chapter is the power of faith in your journey. Faith is absolutely everything and creates miracles out of anything it comes into contact with. Faith is just as misunderstood as prayer for many and that is why we are going to unpack it, especially as it pertains to the whole subject matter of this book and the unique exploration we have been on together. The kind of faith I am talking about is the result of living from that prayer field we just discussed and beginning to see from the inner vision instead of waiting for things outside of us to change.

Let's go deeper now!

"Faith is taking the first step, even when you don't see the whole staircase."

Martin Luther King Jr

The power of faith can never be underestimated, nor could it ever be overstated. Faith is the foundation for which all things are built, just as it is the wellspring from which miracles and all forms of healing emerge from. When it comes to overcoming any kind of addictive pattern in our lives, we must exercise our faith muscle when times get tough, our mind get tired, and our heart feels weak. Faith is not simply an idea that we leverage when we feel low or out of steam. Faith is a superpower that we access within ourselves by digging deep into our soul and facing our challenges head on. Faith is the corner stone of all spiritual traditions and mystical practices worldwide. Without faith, all the action steps in the world can only take us so far. With faith and calculated action combined, anything is possible, and an entirely new world begins to reveal itself to us.

In my own life I have had to rely upon faith when nothing else seemed to work for me. In my hardest moments where I felt backed up against a wall, I had to fall back on my faith in myself, and in a higher power to navigate through what felt like a no way-out situation. For me, faith is the inner sight that comes from practices such as meditation, breath work, and prayer. When one is going through a challenging withdrawal period in their addiction recovery process, it can feel like the world is caving in around them, and things are feeling heavy or disorientating. I know this feeling very well; it is something I have experienced on many occasions in my life. I have had to let go of old habits and strategies I used to simply cope with my discomfort in order to overcome these habitual patterns that did not serve me. The only way I had found to successfully overcome these challenging moments was to humble myself, ask for help in the form of prayer, and sit quietly in silence until I felt my faith begin to emerge once again.

Faith is not something that we have to wait for when times get tough, and we have no other option. Granted, this tends to be the tendency for most people, which is to wait until things get so bad that they humble themselves enough to ask for help, from others or from a higher power. Faith is something that can be practiced each and every day, in all moments of our lives. Again, faith is like a muscle, and the more we exercise this muscle, the more accessible it is to us at any given moment. Faith can be likened to a positive optimistic attitude one develops as a normal way of being in their daily lives. Faith can be generated, simply by the dominant perspective one holds for their lives. Everything in our life is shaped by our perspective, therefore if we maintain an attitude of gratitude then we are better able to see things we can be grateful for. If we fail to maintain a grateful and optimistic attitude towards life, then we will default into negative thought patterns, and as a result we will lose our faith in the process.

Faith is the inner standing that something better exists beyond the surface of our temporary circumstances. It is the innate ability to see beyond our circumstances by using our heart to touch the possibilities that exist in front of us, and beyond us. In order to cultivate this heightened state of awareness, we need to set up rituals in our daily lives for meditation and stillness. In our fast-paced world we tend to get caught in the mad scramble of busyness and constant doing. We are in great need of a counterbalance to constant movement, which is reflection and presence. It is only in the awareness of the present moment that we can see through our doubts, worries, fears, phobias, and concerns. Fear and doubt is what diminishes faith in our lives and when faith begins to go away, so does happiness, joy, inspiration, creativity, and gratitude. Therefore, we are required to create more balance and equanimity in our daily lives, where cultivating faith becomes central on our priority list, because without faith, everything else falls apart, and with faith, everything comes together.

One of the main ways I cultivate greater faith in my life is to focus on who I am becoming instead of obsessing over who I have been in the past. Every day I place special attention on my daily, weekly, monthly, and yearly goals for my life. I remind myself that life is all about flow of motion and that my top priority for my day is to keep my energy in motion, moving towards the direction I have set forth for myself. If you remember in our chapter on **Purpose | Goals | Vision,** there are two distinct types of goals we discussed: Outcome Goals & Process Goals. I place a small percentage of energy on the outcome I want to achieve, and the rest of my focus is on the process in order to get there (or beyond!). The process is the most important because that is the way in which I am creating the next level version of myself, leading towards achieving whatever goals I set out for myself. By focusing on the process, I am developing a greater sense of faith, not simply in my goals or direction in life, but in myself, and my ability to stay disciplined, committed, and steadfast in my pursuit of becoming the best version of me I can be.

The biggest dream killer of all is self-doubt and self-criticism. These negative forces in the human psyche are byproducts of stagnation, which is to say when we stop focusing on who we are becoming, and marinate too long on our faults, our failures, and the judgements we have about ourselves. These are the psychological roots of all external addictions, which is why the process of cultivating faith in oneself is the antidote to absolving addictions from one's life experience. If we have allowed ourselves to get stuck in the weeds of negativity and doubt for too long, then it will take an extraordinary effort to break free from these bondages, but it is not simply a Herculean effort of action that is required. It is a deeper kind of effort that needs to take effect. It's a spiritual commitment to one's own purpose and destiny that must emerge within one's heart to unlock the chains that bind them to their addiction patterns. For only faith in oneself and faith in life as a whole can break the bonds of self-doubt and judgement that holds them back from their God given birthright to something far better than they have ever known before.

There is a practical application to this discussion on faith that I would like to share now. Something we should all consider is how we structure our days, from start to finish. When we awaken in the morning it is crucial to transition from the astral realm of sleep state into the waking state, slowly and gracefully. The common tendency for most people is to wake up with an alarm clock, put on a pot of coffee, and rush into their morning. This is a big mistake and one that does not allow for the human nervous system to acclimate properly into the day ahead. What I suggest is when you wake up in the morning, take ten deep breaths while lying flat on your back before getting out of bed. This will help to prime your body and brain to easily move forward into the morning. Following that begin to take a few intentional moments to feel the sensations in your body and gage your emotional readiness for the day ahead.

What this does is sets up what I call a 'transition point' for the start of the day. Throughout our day all kinds of 'random' situations can manifest themselves in our experience. If we are not properly primed up, then we can easily get knocked off balance and resort to our default coping habits out of stress. In any given day there should be at least 3 main transitional points from morning, to mid-day, to evening prior to going to sleep. A mid-day transition point may be following the workday. When someone comes home from work (if they work outside the home) they can easily bring the stress of their day home with them. I tell my clients to set up a transition point prior to going home or prior to entering the home to release any energies of the day. This can be something as simple as doing another ten deep breaths in the car in the driveway or even taking up a yoga class or work out after work. Whatever works for you is fine but make sure you install a transition point before completing the workday.

The final transition point is before going to bed. One of the biggest epidemics in our world is sleep problems and without deep restorative sleep, our entire nervous system begins to shut down. I recommend creating a ritual for going to sleep such as taking an Epsom salt bath, doing a meditation session, reflecting on the day that is past, and doing a simple prayer before going to sleep. People would be surprised to discover how much better they sleep when they prepare for it like a ritual instead of just rushing into bed in order to wake up and do the same thing, they did the day before. Transition points are a way of resetting the mind and body between stages in our day. If we never reset the system, then we are going to carry the day with us and eventually all that stuck energy just becomes heaviness in our body. This is why I believe most people do not get the deep sleep their bodies really need.

So, there you have it. These are some of my thoughts on the power of faith and some practical tools you can utilize for optimizing your bodies nervous system, which is an essential element of maintaining faith as a resource to empower your life. Also consider that when you develop more discipline and consistency in your actions you will automatically develop more faith and confidence in yourself. The two-work hand in hand together. One does not work without the other. Action without faith is simply just busyness. Faith without action is simply delusion. Faith with action creates miracles and moves mountains.

> *"My faith helps me understand that circumstances don't dictate my happiness, my inner peace."*
>
> *Denzel Washington*

Integration & Recovery

"The meaning of life is to first give life meaning."

Bruce Lee

We have finally made our way to the conclusion point of our journey together, on the road to recovery and holistic transformation. It is worth taking a moment to become present with the grand adventure we have undertaken and to slow down our attention before rushing to complete the journey. This journey is not to be taken lightly and all that you have unpacked within yourself up to this point deserves the space needed to fully integrate it into your life moving forward. I hope you have figured out by now that this book is not any ordinary book on addiction or even health for that matter. It was designed to be an interpersonal journey, as much as it was designed to be highly educational and practical. The journey from addiction to total recovery is one of the most honorable and courageous paths anyone can undergo. For this, you deserve a major "pat" on your back and a huge sigh of relief, knowing you have done something that very few in our society ever accomplish.

No transformational process is ever complete unless there is a final integration phase built into it. Without integrating what has been uncovered and learned in this book it will only remain conceptual knowledge, but concepts do not change lives. Consistency, discipline, commitment, and practicing what we learn every day does. We are going to complete the "recovery" phase imbedded into the addiction free lifestyle roadmap and cross the final bridge towards ultimate success. We have explored so many nuanced ideas, many of which have never been connected to the general discussions of addiction before. You will likely need to reread and continue reviewing these ideas over time in order for them to come totally alive in your mind. Once we cross over this final bridge that is really the new starting point in your upcoming life journey. The road does not stop here, it merely begins a new trajectory for all that is possible by releasing the strangle hold of outdated identity software programs, belief systems, and habits that do not belong in your future.

This next idea that we discuss may prove to be the most important and if you interpret it the way I do then you may find that it has a way of revolutionizing the way you perceive addiction, all together. I arrived at this perceptive through my own process of shedding away outdated belief systems and addiction patterns I had struggled with, some, for many years ongoing. I had to go deeper and deeper into myself in order to figure out what was pulling my chains every time I felt like I was starting to make solid progress. Every time I felt I was closer to my own inner freedom, something kept pulling me back into it and I become terminally frustrated by this because I had no answers to identify the cause to my effect. This soon began to change as I explored new concepts around spirituality, metaphysics, psychology, and exploring mystic traditions that spoke about these things in a way I had never heard of from western medicine or conventional psychiatry.

A number of years ago I came upon the work of a man named Michael Tsarion, who has now been a frequent guest on my podcast and become a close colleague and trusted advisor. Michael is a developmental psychology expert who merges the worlds of spirituality, mysticism, and real-world practical teachings in a way that is incredibly unique. He explained the interplay between what he calls the inauthentic man and the authentic man. Of course, we have all heard the ideas of being authentic and what it means to be inauthentic, but Michael brought a brand-new understanding of what that actually means. He related it to the eastern teachings of karma and dharma. Karma representing the expressions of the inauthentic person playing out their lower-level drives and motivations. Dharma representing the authentic person embodying their highest virtues and living in a way that is truly authentic to their core nature.

As I began to do the inner work within myself while taking in these unique perspectives, I began to see another parallel to this connection, which was the root cause of all addiction. The single thread that connects the cycle of addiction itself, and what determines whether someone breaks free of their addictions or remains entrapped to their addictive patterns. Karma represents the repetitive behavior patterns of the inauthentic self or should we say, the socially conditioned self. There is a significant reason why addiction carries with it an energy field, all of its own. Anyone who struggles with any manner of addiction knows that it can feel, as though they are possessed by their addictions. As if their addictions have a hold onto their better judgement and can even influence one's consciousness to convince or persuade them to use faulty logic to repeat the cycle. This is the karmic pattern playing itself out within the individual who is still living out an inauthentic identity and the only way to freedom is to break down the manufactured identity altogether and choose the Siddhartha path. (We will discuss what that means.)

So, in our finale point here we are going to explore two profound concepts and teachings to tie this entire journey together, in a way that has never been done before. We have a bit more spiritual lifting to do before we conclude this journey, but you are well equipped by now and have everything needed to cross the finish line.

The Karmic & Dharmic Journey

"People's dogma tends to get run over by their karma(carma)"

David Avocado Wolfe

The word karma may mean different things to different people but according to the Hindu and Buddhist interpretation, it simply means the sum total of persons actions, in this life or in previous lives have an effect on their daily lives, now and into the future. Karma is considered the result of someone's actions as well as the intent behind their actions. Whether you believe in past lives or not is not totally relevant because we live multiple lives wrapped up in this one physical incarnation itself. We take on different roles and identities at different developmental stages and the actions of each stage set the framework for our actions and patterns at the next stage of life. If we had not completed the developmental stages of our childhood and adolescence, then we would likely carry some of those undeveloped patterns into our adulthood.

Some people misunderstand karma as some kind of punishment or reward system by the universe. This is a very childish perspective to have because the universe is not some sort of vending machine or proverbial Santa Claus picking through the little boys and girls who have been naughty or nice. Karma is not personal, and it does not play favorites based on good or bad behavior. Karma is not dependent on human morals or social ethics. Karma is neutral and exacting in its distribution in each of our own lives. Karma is the positive or negative result of our prior habits, actions, thought forms, relationship dynamics, and the unresolved trauma that we carry within us. Karma is not our punishment in life. It is our greatest lesson in life and shows us exactly where we need to learn and grow.

The concept of karma alone is a big subject and carries a lot of baggage that should be unpacked for a more comprehensive understanding. There is a great book called **Healing Ancestral Karma** by the author Dr. Steven D. Farmer that does a remarkable job at helping the reader to discover how their personal challenges in life can be influenced by the epigenetic and psychic transference from our familial blood line. We discussed this idea in depth in the chapter **Mastering the Body** in relation to unresolved familial trauma, that is stored in our genetics (and psyche) from birth. In his book Dr. Farmer states *"as you heal yourself in any manner whatsoever, your ancestors and your descendants are healed in turn."* Here we find that what we call karma in our own lives could be, in part a result of the unresolved karmic patterns that had persisted through our genetic lineage and had been passed down to us. It is hard to know if that is exactly the case but what we can be sure of is if a pattern repeats itself in our own life, it is ours entirely to heal and work out of our lives.

So, let's take this conversation a bit deeper and more to the point of this book, which is about living an addiction free lifestyle. In my own interpretation and conceptual understanding, karma is simply the patterns and habits we consciously (or unconsciously) choose to repeat, day in and day out. The results of our "karmic patterns" are simply the direct byproduct of the patterns themselves and a feedback mechanism to show us the effect these habits have on our lives. It is easy to get caught in the effects themselves and simply label those effects as "our karma", but that is not really the truth. The bigger truth is that our unique karmic patterns are played out within our addictive habits and until we make the connection that our addictions are really manifestations of our soul karma, then we may never discover the lessons wrapped up within our struggle towards personal salvation. Salvation really meaning inner freedom and self-mastery.

In the spirit of my friend and colleague Michael Tsarion, it would be appropriate to bring in some of his esteem wisdom into this explanation on karma and dharma. The easiest way to inner stand this karmic dynamic is through the distinction of authenticity and inauthenticity. Authenticity, meaning the embodiment of our values and virtues and inauthenticity, meaning the misalignment between who we are being and who we really are. The inner tension and inner conflict that exists within all struggles with addiction is really just us living out of alignment with our core values. The inner conflict tends to dissolve itself once we make the consistent effort to correct inauthentic behavior and live our lives congruently with the values, we know that we 'should' but for some reason avoid doing.

The inauthentic person who is caught in the spiral of their own addiction cycle is placing greater emphasis on their shortcomings than on their untapped potential. The struggle of addiction is a karmic knot that continues to get tighter and tighter the more it is allowed to take priority in one's life. In essence, what is happening is this individual is submitting to the mediocrity they feel within themselves and arresting their higher nature from liberating them from the shackles of addiction. It is a form of subservience and submission. Subservience towards lower human drives that lead to addiction. Submission to the dictates of social consensus that go against the dictates of the authentic expression of one's own soul. Remember, organized society is construed in a way to create consumers, which tends to go against the authentic man or woman's true spirited essence.

When we consciously choose to play into our shortcomings and reinforce our addictions, what we are actually doing is creating more karma for ourselves. If one has a pornography addiction and they keep feeding that addiction, they are reinforcing the strength of it, and in so doing, will create a bigger karmic feedback mechanism to snap them out of the looping cycle. This is also the same with any addictive feedback cycle you can think of. The increasingly detrimental effects they have on our lives, the more karma is created for us to overcome. The releasing of karma in our lives is the release of the habitual patterns themselves and the energetic cord that is tethered to the compulsion we feel prior to acting the habit out. The habit is just a habit, it is virtually neutral, other than the physical effects it has on our health, our mind, or our overall life. That is basic cause and effect. The karmic imprint itself is sealed within the energetic cord that binds our consciousness to the habit and compels our mind to fixate on it in order to cause enough psycho-emotional friction so that we cave in and submit ourselves to the behavioral pattern.

This is why addiction recovery work must incorporate the psychological and emotional development aspect, as well as the physiological and biochemical (dopamine reset) methodologies for total success. When we begin to grasp the concept of karma in our lives and apply a depth of spiritual wisdom to each challenge we face, both internally and externally, we discover that our struggle with addiction is actually a struggle for inner freedom. To the degree we are beholden to any addictive tendency, is the degree we do not feel free within our own skin and that lack of autonomy is a very uncomfortable thing to sit with. It can feel like we are at odds with ourselves, in a bind of sorts, playing out some kind of wrestling match between our higher virtues and our lower basal desires. Well, this eternal conflict between the higher and lower nature is the perennial conflict built into the human condition. This eternal conflict is the tension we humans find ourselves in is not really between flesh and blood but between our karmic and dharmic nature.

This brings us to the next concept we should inner stand, which is the nature of dharma and its role in salvaging what was lost in the karmic cycle of chaos and bringing us into our ultimate redemption moment. This redemption moment was beautifully illustrated through the mythological wisdom teaching that Joseph Campbell brought forth in his classic book, **The Hero with A Thousand Faces.** The distillation of his work is in the telling of the 'hero's journey' template, which is the secret script behind all major Hollywood movies and successful stories. It is built into every iconic tale we have ever heard and more interestingly, it is built into the fabric of the human story, which includes each and every one of our lives. The alchemical transformation from transmuting the density of our karma into what is known as our dharma, is the great mythology of the human condition, which is also the same story of addiction to recovery.

When I talk about dharma, I am speaking about the unified thread between our true purpose/mission in this life and the authentic version of us, that had laid hidden beneath the layers of karmic patterns. When I trace back through the memory banks of my own life, I can see a common thread that has existed throughout all of the ups and downs. It has been this search for meaning and an internal quest to strive for truth amongst of world so heavily invested in falsehoods and uncontested theories. I had always had a sense that things where not as they appeared. This sensation I could not shake, despite how much I may have tried through trying to fit in with my peers, medicate it with substances, or avoid it through adolescent rebelliousness. No amount of trying to fit myself into the social order provided for me (and for us all) ever compensated for this feeling of hollowness I felt every time I went away from my authentic path. It was only a matter of time before the karmic patterns(addictions) would fall off and something much stronger, much more powerful began to emerge from within.

This really is the essence of what it means to recover from addiction. Have you ever considered what the word recovery really means or implies? This term addiction recovery is so easily thrown around, but it seems to me that not a lot of people have taken in its real meaning. The word recovery means to recover and when we think of someone who is recovering from something, we tend to think of a disease or debilitation of some sort. That is layer number one to its overall meaning. The realization is that an addiction is a form of disease, but not in the conventional allopathic meaning of a physiological/biological disease such as cancer, diabetes, heart disease, etc. Those conditions themselves are the result of the real disease itself. The disease of addiction is really a pathological infection that is rooted in the psyche/mind and the poison goes downstream into the sacred heart, which ultimately manifests itself in the physical body as a final outcome. This understanding changes our entire conception of disease management (allopathic medicine) and opens us up to what true healing is all about.

The karmic imprints that have been encoded and encrypted within our genetic coding throughout all of our familial lineages are rooted underneath our addiction patterns. Until we learn to authentically address the root of our issues, we will simply be spending all of our time rearranging the furniture in our lives, wondering why we feel so unproductive and exhausted. It is exhausting to keep moving the furniture, over and over, yet nothing really seems to be changing. This is the trap of the logical mind attempting to solve a problem that it cannot see or accurately detect. This is where the sacred heart comes into play.

The sacred heart (not to be confused with the organ) is where our dharma resides and also where our recovery blueprint exists. We have likely spent so much of our lives chasing things outside of ourselves that we may have lost or had misplaced aspects of ourselves along the way. The path to true healing is built into the quest for recovery and recovery is simply the process of recovering the innocence that was lost through the trauma of our life experiences.

Our karmic addiction patterns are the access point to our dharmic destiny. Without knowing our karma, we could never know our dharma. When people spend all their time 'searching for their purpose', they continue to find it alluding them. This is because there is no bypass or shortcut hack to discovering who you really are. There are no short cuts to life. There is only a straight and narrow path towards the truth. It is always right there in front of us, inviting us into it, but we may have become so numb or guarded against it that we miss it every time. This is why we cannot avoid our pain, push away our discomfort, or pretend that we do not have emotional triggers that come up from time to time. These are the dimensional gateway points within our own DNA that allows us to go from a life of karmic cycles into dharmic purpose. This is the access point from "disease" to healing, from addiction to recovery.

One of the unique nuances of this transitional process is in becoming aware of your own guilt complex. Most people, if not all people (aside from psychopaths & sociopaths) feel various dimensions of guilt. There are two specific versions of guilt that are important to become aware of because the distinction between the two reveals the karmic and dharmic influences in our lives. There is primary guilt and secondary guilt, which I call the guilt complex. Primary guilt is more aligned with what I would term the authentic nudging from our soul when we have gone off course and are living out of alignment. This is the persistent discomfort that subtly arises in our belly, sometimes in our chest when we know something is not right in our lives. This is the nagging feeling that we need to make a course correction but sometimes do not do, out of fear and avoidance. This is the sensation of guilt that we suppress, sedate, and numb out when we are in the throes of our own addictions. This is the shaking of the boat that is coming from our soul.

There is a secondary guilt complex that everyone (with an honest heart) has experienced, and it is a manufactured guilt from society, politicians, authoritarian "leaders", fundamentalist religion, and most often from our own parental figures. This is the guilt that has been put onto us as children through conditioning, trauma, and giving away our own sovereignty to the control system of society itself. This guilt is simply a complex of programs, belief systems, social consensus, ideologies, and abstractions of the human mind. Another way of describing this phenomenon is living inside of our head. It is a function of a control mechanism conditioned into the impressionable psyche of innocent children (all of us!) as well as the psyche of well-intentioned adults doing what they 'think' is best for their children. It is the socialized guilt complex that actually holds our addictions together, because the root of the control in our society is dependent on ensuring addicts remain addicted and never break free from the programmed response pattern.

It is critical to discern between these two sensations of guilt because one keeps us in bondage to inauthentic patterns and the other liberates us from it all together. Primary guilt can feel like an existential crisis, such as an identity crisis that arises after a divorce, a bad breakup, a career plunder, encountering a loss of a loved one, and anything that turns our sense of reality upside down. These are always the moments where the opportunity for transformation is at its highest. These are also the moments where we are most fragile and susceptible to reinforcing addictions as a way to cope with what is happening inside of us. The false secondary guilt can easily creep in due to social conditioning, which can lead to us blocking out the authenticity of what is trying to emerge within us, in moments of personal doubt or life change.

The primary guilt is really a form of existential guilt from living an inauthentic life or holding onto elements of inauthenticity. The false guilt is from cultural programming, based on what we believe is right and wrong. There is in fact a clear distinct right and wrong, correct and incorrect but often times these lines are blurred due to societal guidelines, which does not allow very much room for the authentic nature of one's own soul to emerge. The existential guilt I am referring to is not to be confused with ego-based judgements, labels, belief systems, or even shame, for that matter. Those are all byproducts of cultural conditioning and are not part of the dharmic path. If we find ourselves in bouts of judgement, towards others or towards ourselves, we can be sure that we are operating out of the secondary guilt complex.

Primary guilt is pure in its nature and only serves to bring us back towards the light of truth, but never to distort or confuse the truth. Social programs distort and contort truth and produce what we know as 'little white lies' that so many have become accustomed to living in. A so called little white lie is a blend of partial truth and partial falsehood. This can seem tricky to navigate in our 'moral realistic' world, but we all know when we are telling a partial truth, because the guilt of the lie is always tied to it. It's the same dynamic when we are negotiating with ourselves, while still entertaining our addiction patterns but with the wholehearted intention of quitting tomorrow or another day, other than the one we are living now. Addiction recovery requires a move from partial integrity to whole embodied integrity. The split between the two is what creates internal tension and causes the struggle between our karma and our dharma, our inauthentic patterns and our authentic nature.

This is the fundamental and perennial struggle of the human condition in modern times. The struggle to overcome our lower desires and make the continual commitment towards our higher nature. This does not happen in a single day and the results of our labor are not produced in an instant. It takes time, a lot of time, and a dedication towards patience. Without patience we fall into patterns of frustration, scarcity, not feeling enough, and due to the weight of our own inner judgements, we simply give up, again and again. This is where we step off the wheel of samsara (wheel of suffering) and end the conditioned cycle of suffering, once and for all. One day at a time. One moment at a time. One breath at a time. One workout routine at a time. One green juice or super food smoothie at a time. One loving act of kindness at a time. One thing leads to another and one success builds upon the last.

Now that we have covered one of the most unique (and important) concepts relating to the transformational process of healing and recovery, we are ready to take the final step into total integration. This is a journey that has played itself out throughout history and one that is timeless in the history books of humanity. It is the life story of the enlightened being that we all simply know as Buddha, and how he went from riches to rags, and then rags to riches again. This has been one of the most enduring philosophical studies of any human being, next to only Jesus, in my mind. It is basically the same iconic mythological story as Jesus, but the archetype is played out a bit differently and relates specifically to the theme of this chapter perfectly.

You will have a brand-new understanding of the story of the Buddha, as well as its direct reflection of the road to recovery, and inner freedom from the addictions of our seductive world. This is the hero's or heroin's journey that each of us must embrace, as it is written into our genetic code, and unique life incarnation.

The Siddhartha Path (The Story of the Buddha)

Our entire journey throughout this book has led us to the final lesson, and what a profound lesson this is. The hero's journey that each of us is on in our lives carries immense wisdom and insights born out from our own direct experience. These insights that we arrive at through the trials and tribulations of life are, in one part unique to our own experience, and in another part, are central to the human mythology itself. The paradox of life is that our own journey is wrapped up in a greater collective mythos that has played itself out from the beginnings of time. The road from addiction to recovery is the central story that each of us share, with no exceptions to this fact. No one, regardless of how successful or "enlightened" as one may seem, has made it through the journey without passing through the initiation of addiction. The road to recovery, integration, and embodiment is the hero's journey, and once we realize that each of us shares this journey, it becomes much easier to cross the bridge towards health and wholeness.

One of the most enduring mythoi in our world culture is that of the story of Siddhartha Gautama, otherwise known as the Buddha. One of the most well-known "religions", if you want to call it that, is Buddhism, which has countless devotees and followers worldwide. Many people know Buddha as an enlightened master spiritual teacher who is more of an iconic mythological figure in history than a real, flesh and blood man, in most people's minds that is. Buddha represents an archetypal embodiment of human potential and what is possible when one devotes their entire focus on a single idea that transforms their entire being. Buddha was not always the end product of who we believe him to be

368

however, he was a very real flesh and blood man, who walked a very intense path towards his own enlightenment. He was born as Siddhartha Gautama

The story of Siddhartha is the consummate story of everyone who is seeking out their own potential in life, and especially those of us who have had to confront varies forms of addictions and limitations, whether self-imposed or otherwise. The Siddhartha path is the path of self-discovery towards personal truth, which tends to mean that the path forward is going through all of the limitations that exist within us, confronting them one by one, and persisting through each challenge until victorious. Although his story is set in a different time period and different cultural traditions, it does not take away from the universal patterns that play out in each and every one of our own lives. This is why the Buddha story has remained so universally relevant and has been a source of incredible inspiration and hope for many on the path of self-development and healing.

The word Buddha is said to mean "awakened one", someone who has awakened from the dream spell of the world around them, and the false pretenses they have had about life, based on belief systems, religious indoctrination, and other forms of conditioning. The central theme of this story is around dealing with the suffering of life and embracing suffering as an unavoidable fact of living. Shortly after Siddhartha was born, 7 days to be exact, his mother Maya died due to complications in childbirth. 10 months before his birth, his mother had a visionary dream where a rare white elephant offered her a lotus flower and then entered the right side of her body. This is meant to mean that she had conceived an especially gifted child. When her and her husband, who just so happened to be a king, consulted with a sage on her dream, they were informed that this child would either grow up to be a greater leader or he would grow up to be a spiritual teacher. He would either conquer the world or become an enlightened being.

As the story goes, being the son of a king, he was raised within the confines of the palace walls and did not see anything of the outside world until his later adult years. He had access to every imaginable luxury and was encouraged to keep inside the palace as a way to block from his view the suffering and poverty of the commons outside of the palace. He was raised in such a way to keep protected from any perceivable threats or simple discomforts. The reason for this is because Siddhartha's father, upon hearing of the sage's prophecy, wanted his son to become a king, therefore wanting to shield him from any sense that there was anything wrong with the world outside of the lifestyle they were accustomed too. He was afraid his son would discover the poverty and plight of the world outside the palace walls, which would spark his son to follow the path of the monastic spiritual holy man archetype, which was cause him to leave his home, and seek to help heal the suffering of the world.

Siddhartha spent 29 years of his life secluded inside the amenities of royalty and privilege. He was arranged a marriage with his cousin, which was not uncommon in that time, and they both fell deeply in love with each other. It seems like Siddhartha's path of following in his father's footsteps is clear, cut, and dry. There is no possibility of him diverting from this path, simply because he is now an adult who has been entirely accustomed to a particular lifestyle and had been buffered from the outside world his entire life. Well, one day Siddhartha became increasingly curious about what existed beyond the palace corridors. Who knows where this sudden spark of curiosity arose from but arose it certainly did? He finally made his way outside the palace and as the story goes, he encountered 4 milestone moments that would radically change his life forever and cause him to question everything he had ever known up to this point.

The first encounter was with an old man. He asks his attendant he is with what that was. His attendant responds, "Oh, that's change", as he explained that eventually our bodies will change and grow older as time goes on. The next encounter is him stumbling upon a sick man, of which he had never seen in such an impoverished condition before. His attendant tells him "that happens to all of us", as he explains that everyone will experience some kind of sickness in their life, even if you're a prince or a king. On his third encounter he comes up upon a necrotic human corpse. This encounter shocked Siddhartha, as the realization of impermeability and mortality often does for us all at first. The combination of these encounters began to stir inside of him as he realizes that this is also his fate as well. He is not somehow immune to getting old, getting sick, and ultimately dying. He begins to recognize the fact of impermanence and the wisdom of uncertainty.

The fourth encounter would seal his fate moving forward and set him off on a path entirely contrary to the one he had been on his for his first 29 hears of life. He came across what was described as a "spiritual seeker", someone who has devoted to seeking enlightenment and contentment outside of the worldly affairs that Siddhartha was all too well accustomed too. Through this entire journey Siddhartha begins to have a traumatic encounter with the pain and suffering of life. His father, out of love and care, tried to protect his son from the dark side of life by keeping him insulated in the palace walls. But unfortunately, for all parents and children alike, we cannot protect our loved one's from experiencing the suffering of life, simply because it is a hard fact of life, and to try to dispense with that aspect of life is to live in a one seasonal reality. This was Siddhartha's reality, one of opulent pleasure, indulgence, privilege, and relative happiness. Even for a prince, intentionally protected from the atrocities of the outside world, his father, a king, could not stop the fates from confronting his son with his true purpose and destiny.

Siddhartha was placed into the moment of destiny, where he would either remain as he had been raised to be, which was a prince who would eventually become king, or to sacrifice everything he has ever known in order to pursue the inner calling that emerged due to the loss of his own innocence. The loss of innocence is a classical theme in the hero's journey, which is the initiation point between adolescence into adulthood, naiveté into maturity, boy into man. It is impossible to say what the "right" decision was for him to make, because he had left behind a beloved wife, a newborn child, and his father all in the same moment. Of course, he chose to silently slip away from his home, and embark on his inner journey without ever saying a word to those he had now left behind. All we can say about this moment in time, is that he chose to do what he did, and as painful as it must have been for both him, and his loved ones, it is clear that there would have been no Buddha Gautama if he had stayed back in the palace walls.

For the first time in his life, Siddhartha was now alone in the world, in the wilderness of an unforgiving nature environment, and all he had was his own newly awakening instincts to guide him in the journey. He had gone from prosperity to poverty, from having a home into homelessness, from total security and certainty into insecurity and total uncertainty, on a primal survival level at least. There was definitely a significant degree of certainty he had within himself or perhaps, maybe just in the calling that propelled him to make such a life altering decision. Perhaps this is all any of us have in the moments of destiny, where we are confronted with an impossible decision, and somehow, despite the lack of certainty, we still make that decision, and somehow put one foot in front of the other on our way into the unknown. It is said that Siddhartha made mention that he had been wounded by the enjoyment of the world and now he longed to obtain true inner peace.

Well into his solo journey, Siddhartha came across many seekers, who had all forfeited their prior lives in search of some semblance of truth, likely spawning from some similar calling that Siddhartha experienced back beyond the palace walls. These individuals are what are called 'renunciates', which means to renounce the material social world and pursue a life of poverty and celibacy, living entirely on the edge of life and death. It is important to mention that the said purpose for why so many people in Indian tradition became renunciates is because they believed that by abstaining from worldly "pleasures" and material comforts, they could escape the wheel of suffering, which was associated with the reincarnation cycle of life and death. The central problem that Buddha had faced was that "suffering" did not begin at birth, but it was a cyclical existential problem that carried over from lifetime to lifetime. So, the idea was that, by abstaining from the world itself, one could become "enlightened", and escape the reincarnation cycle all together, which would allow them to become free of the wheel of suffering.

What I find interesting about this stage in the journey is that there is both truth and abstraction of truth laid out in this belief paradigm. On one level it is absolutely true that suffering or trauma can pass over from generation to generation through the epigenetic transference of grandparent, to parent, to child, and that is detailed in the earlier chapter on **The Dopamine Dilemma**. As we discussed in the previous section of this chapter karma, which is a heavy focus in the Hindu culture, is associated with personal suffering. As we discussed, karma is the addictions in our lives playing out on a looping cycle up until the point we become conscious of them, and then break the cycle of addiction, which also means to break the cycle of suffering. The abstraction in all of this is the notion that we need to escape the "trappings" of life itself in order to liberate ourselves from the karma of life. There is a fine nuanced distinction in our story that separates Siddhartha, who later becomes Buddha Gautama, from the thousands of other "truth" seekers who seem to become nothing more than vagabonds who wonder aimlessly from place to place, with no clear direction as to where they are going, or any real care as to where they may end up.

There is a saying that states "not all who wonder are lost," which I feel fits perfectly with Siddhartha. He was not what we would call a 'lost soul' wandering around planet earth like a vagabond, shipwrecked at sea, and tossing with the tides. He made a conscious decision to separate himself from luxury and prosperity of his former life to explore a life of ascetic monastic discipline. This of course did not spare him of the intense experiences that would befall him as he embarked on the journey, but I believe it is this distinction that allowed him to summon the power that existed deep inside of him, and pulled him through those challenges, to ensure he would become exactly who he was destined to be. We will explore some of the pivotal trials and obstacles he faced as we progress into our story.

Let's keep going now.

Along Siddhartha's journey in the wilderness, he came across what is sometimes labeled as a "guru", which simply means a spiritual teacher. This was his first real encounter with a teacher who could help guide him towards the development of the path he intuitively struck out towards. What Siddhartha was beginning to learn is that he could use practices such as yoga and meditation as a way to tame the reactivity of the mind. That the self-reflective nature of our minds could be put to productive use for self-development and the pursuit of "enlightenment". This concept of taming the mind through mastering physical practices is central to the yogic philosophy, where of which was just as prevalent in Siddhartha's time as it is now a days. Siddhartha was said to be an extremely fast learner to all of the yogic and meditation practices he was provided. He was already something of a master, but make no mistake, he was completely devoted to practicing them every day. These did not just come without effort or merit. He had to earn it, just as we all do in whatever our endeavors are, even the ones that come naturally to us.

As time goes on, Siddhartha continued to bump up against the same pain and toil that he originally set out to liberate himself from. No matter how many practices he did, he kept finding himself unable to transcend the pain body and the existential concerns around suffering. It is said that he ascends to very 'rarified' states of consciousness, literally transplanting his mind into new dimensions of reality, similar to how plant medicines can do that through altering the pharmacology of the brain chemistry. The problem he kept finding is that none of these experiences were permanent, they were all transitory in nature, and the higher in consciousness one goes, the lower one can also go as a necessary balancing phenomenon. He found that none of these experiences brought forth a penetrating truth into the nature of reality. They simply become, more or less, a temporary escape from the physical shackles of the body and all of the emotional sensations experienced in the body and in the mind.

So now Siddhartha leaves the guru's he studied with and seeks out another route to find the answers to the problem of suffering. He had already experienced extreme luxury and prosperity in the first 29 years of his life. He now goes into the opposite extreme, which is to experience deprivation. He remembered amongst the renunciants he encountered that asceticism was a way to find enlightenment, through "punishing" the body, and depriving it of food and material comforts. This was thought of by many people to be an effective way to obtain states of serenity and wisdom, by forgoing the needs of the body all together. In this belief paradigm, as crazy as it might sound to the reader, was centered around the idea that the body itself poses a big problem, which is that the body weakens, gets older, succumbs to disease and degeneration, and is unavoidably intertwined with the experience of suffering. The idea behind pushing, and sometimes punishing the body, in a variety of rituals, was to transcend the mortal flesh, and liberate the mind from the constraints of the body.

This pursuit of emaciating the body lasted for 6 years or so. Constantly doing whatever he could to put an end to the sensations of suffering and quill this nagging problem once and for all. He, like so many people in ascetic spiritual pursuits, were trying to destroy anything inside of himself that he perceives as "bad", "detrimental", or what we would call in this book "an addiction". The more he fought against his urges and cravings, the more pain and suffering he would in turn experience. This was the most perplexing of problems to contend with, where no answers could be found, and only more pain and suffering would arise. The spiritual traditions of that time preached that one could liberate themselves from pain and suffering if they could eliminate all comforts, pleasures, and attachments to the physical realm. Essentially one would have to do away with everything that makes them uniquely human. Siddhartha tried all of that, maybe more intently than anyone before him, and yet the problem of pain and suffering had only persisted.

After enduring this long-drawn-out bodily deprivation experience and having his question of human suffering unanswered, he had a spontaneous vision arise in his consciousness. He had taken himself almost to the edge of death, extreme fasting, and physical punishment. At this edge point he remembered a memory of him as a child with his father sharing with him the perfection of the world exactly as it was. The life and death cycle of all things came over him and he was stricken with a bout of sadness in a moment of his childhood memory. He could see how every living being and organism on this planet is interconnected together. He then found himself sitting into a yoga meditation pose, almost entirely based on instinct, and all of a sudden, he began to experience a feeling he had not in so long. He began to experience the sensation of pure joy.

The joy and peace that came to him was due to him accepting the pain and suffering that exists in the world. Accepting the "brokenness" of the world helped to allow true healing to emerge at the same time. He was no longer fighting himself or parts of himself that he felt were intolerable and negative. His great insight was that underneath the suffering and pain of the world existed peace and joy. He also made the discovery that he would not be able to sustain this newfound joy if he did not eat anything, so he began to consume food again. Out of nowhere a woman appears carrying some kind of rice porridge and offers it to Siddhartha. This is a very meaningful moment in the story because the decision for Siddhartha to accept the gift of food being offered to him was not just a choice to survive, it was a choice towards life itself. It was a moment of pure grace.

There is a profound teaching in this part of our story because in most spiritual traditions the 'grace' moment is looked at as something that can only come from the 'divine' i.e., our interpretation of God. In Siddhartha's case the grace moment came from a simple offering of generosity from an ordinary girl upon a chance encounter where he was at his edge. The moral of this moment is that none of us can go through our journey in life entirely alone by ourselves. We all need help from others and others need help from us. Siddhartha had exhausted all possible approaches to self-enlightened and inner peace through aloneness and solitude. It was not until he encountered this young woman who offered him love and compassion in the form of food that his heart cracked open, and he was met with the inner peace he had so persistently sought out through traditional methods. In that moment he had memories of his wife, his child, and his family whom he had left behind. A flood of powerful emotions came through him and it is safe to say it likely soaked his entire being in that moment of being touched by divine grace.

Following this encounter with grace, which had literally saved his life, he was still confronted with the insight that life is full of suffering and pain, therefore the problem still had not gone away. Now that he was eating food to nourish his body, the extreme ascetics around he disbanded from him, claiming that he had forsaken his devotion in exchange for the comforts of the body. Siddhartha was set into a new direction in his journey after all he had been through. He entrusted his life to two spiritual gurus', punishing his body, and starving the cravings of the mind only to almost die in the process. Now he was beginning to discover that the path to enlightenment could not be found in external teachers, traditions, or depriving the body of what it needs to thrive. He realized, as most of us do after a while, that one can eat, drink, and be a "normal" human being, all while pursuing a life of moral virtue and spiritual growth. His next realization was that the answers he was seeking would not be found in external sources. They could only be found by going within and trust himself.

Following this phase of Siddhartha's journey awaited his ultimate initiation into the embodiment of what we all know him as, the Buddha. After all the experiences he had endured since leaving his familiar palace home, he was beset upon a path of voluntary struggle, hardship, loneliness, and spiritual endurance. He finally found himself ready to make the final commitment to his own evolution. For Siddhartha, this meant that he would sit beneath a classic bodhi tree and he said that he would not leave this spot until he had finally solved the problem of pain and suffering, that no other practices could offer him. He accepted that his body may begin to wither and dry up in this spot, but he was resolved in his decision. This is indeed the spot in which the Buddha was born but it would not happen just because he decided it would. He would have to pay a price for his transformation to manifest, just as each of us do in our own individual lives.

"It is better to conquer yourself than to win a thousand
battles. The victory is yours. It cannot be taken from you,
not by angels or by demons, heaven or hell."

Buddha

There are multiple interpretations on how this part of the story actually goes. Some a bit more fantastical than others but the archetypical relevance of this initiation is what is most important. This is the single moment that defines Siddhartha's entire life journey and the moment the weight of all his experiences would carry him through what would scare and intimate most anyone else. As he began to untether himself from all of his worldly desires, he was quickly confronted by the demon king 'Mara', who is said to be the demon of desire, lust, and temptation. It is not exactly clear if Mara appears in physical form or more likely as an apparition within Siddhartha's consciousness as he sat closed eyed underneath the bodhi tree, as is told in the legend. Mara is said to have approached Siddhartha accompanied with a band of demon minions in an attempt of intimidation. Siddhartha remained poised, still, and unwavering in his seated position, as if to barely notice the perceived threat in front of him.

Mara orders his minions to thrust bladed arrows at Siddhartha and as the arrows approached him, they all began to turn into soft flowers before landing on the ground in front of him. It was as if there was an energetic force field surround Siddhartha which transformed the deadly arrows into harmless flowers upon contact. Following this Mara sent out his three daughters which each represented a principle of addiction and deception. His daughter Tanha represents thirst and hunger, Arati represents aversion and discontentment, and Raga represents attachment, desire, greed, and passion. These are known as the three temptations, which can be simplified as thirst, desire, and delight, which were used to seduce

Siddhartha, but they proved completely ineffective as Gautama paid them no mind, thus disabling their powers of seduction and diversion. It then became apparent that Siddhartha was not going to alter his unalterable attention and move from his sitting position.

As the story goes, Mara tells Siddhartha that he is sitting on his seat and that it belongs to him. All of his minions yell out in agreement and say they are Mara's witness, that it is in fact his seat. Mara asks Siddhartha, "where is your witness that this is your seat?" In that exact moment, without hesitation, Siddhartha places his fingers onto the earth to gesture that the earth and all of nature is his witness. All of a sudden from there, the earth began to tremble, and a huge thunderous noise emerged. This completely shocked Mara and all of his minions because it became clear that Siddhartha was in fact witnessed by the entirety of nature herself and was chosen as the enlightened Buddha from that moment forward. The demons vanished from sight and Siddhartha had undergone his complete transformation from the young prince into the legendary Buddha, who would go on to become one of the greatest spiritual teachers in all of recorded history.

At the age of 35, Buddha would go on to devote the rest of his life to spreading the teachings of what would eventually become Buddhism and overcoming the wheel of karma. Through his entire life he had explored and experienced the two polar extremes of asceticism and of opulent abundance. He discovered that the path to inner peace, healing, and enlightenment was not found in completely abstaining from the pleasures of life, nor was it found in pleasure sensory overload. His ultimate discovery was that the answers to the problem he spent years trying to answer were found in what he would call 'the middle way'. As he discovered and as he would teach his disciples, the answers to life's challenges are always found in-between the extremes but never found entirely on either side of an extreme itself. Everything is balance and by walking the straight and narrow path, as the master Jesus also taught, our perceptions of the world will remain in balance, thus helping us stay out of the zone of human suffering.

This is the first 35 years of the life of Buddha and the legends that accompany his remarkable story. There are some deeply penetrating lessons for us all and it would be worth your time to either reread this section or explore more resources on the life of Buddha to see how his journey is simply a mirror for our own. In the final section of this chapter, we are going to discuss some of the seminal lessons relating to the trials and recovery process of addiction from Siddhartha's transformation. That is of course why I chose to complete the book with this mythos in mind, because it is very much the same story, we all have experienced, and can provide incredible practical wisdom for us all.

"We are what we think. All that we are arises with our thoughts. With our thoughts, we make the world."

Buddha

Lessons on Addiction from the Siddhartha Story

"Any idea that is developed and put into action is more important than an idea that exists only as an idea."

Buddha

When we do a comprehensive analysis on the life of Gautama Buddha and explore what we are calling the 'Siddhartha path', it should become somewhat obvious that the overarching theme of the story is about overcoming addiction. This may not have been entirely obvious to all historians and those who chronicled the mythology of famous spiritual figures in history. I would assume that this insight was not lost on the countless followers of Buddhism itself and those who sincerely study the life of the man behind the legend. The intensities of Siddhartha's life path after his departure from his palace home is not very much different than the internal journey, we all make from addiction to recovery, and from recovery to wholeness still. The external landscape may look very different than it did for Siddhartha, including all of the obscure practices he put himself through in a Hindu cultural setting, but the path itself is very much the same, and requires a similar level of conviction in oneself, and in something bigger than themselves in order to pull through onto the other side.

379

There is so much we have to learn from this story, which is exactly why I chose to use Buddha as the role model for overcoming the most persistent of all addictions we know of. You may ask yourself; what addiction did Siddhartha have exactly? It is not mentioned that he had a drinking problem, gambling problem, or even a sex addiction. In fact, from all best accounts it seems like he was a very happy, well-adjusted young man who had fathered a child with the woman he loved and was surrounded by loving parents. This appears to all be true and it may not be easy to spot out what he affliction he was suffering from by just looking at his life prior to the affliction becoming more pronounced in the years following his departure. The addiction or affliction I am alluding too, is more so one of the minds than it is a biological addiction such as the common dopamine feedback loops, we are all too familiar with now a day. Siddhartha's biggest problem up until the age of 29 was that he was all too complacent and comfortable in his sheltered bubble that he had become a bit numb to the world that existed outside of his point of reference.

This is clearly depicted once he makes his way outside the palace walls and encounters the harsh reality of life that he was not properly introduced too by his parents. Due to the lack of a proper initiation as a man, he was still very much a boy i.e., a prince archetype, and underdeveloped psychologically, which is why it was such a rude awakening for him once he encountered poverty, sickness, and degeneration. This lack of awareness kept him a child in many respects and as a result caused him to be far too comfortable with being comfortable, which is a major issue for so many countless souls in the world today.

Siddhartha was not only confronted by the harsh realities of life upon contact with the outside world. What he was actually confronted by was a deep seeded trauma that had existed within his own being that he was completely unaware of prior to these encounters. This trauma is very much the same trauma or core wound that exists within each of us as we make our way through the rigors of life. As we have learned in prior chapters, trauma can be inherited through our familial bloodline and trapped inside of our genetic template, waiting for the perfect catalyst to bring it to the surface of our conscious awareness. Well, there is also another perspective on this same phenomenon, which is that the core wounds of humanity also exist within each of us, independent of our direct genetic familial bloodlines. What Siddhartha was confronted by was the core trauma of humanity, which was the wounding of poverty, disease, degeneration, isolation, abandonment, and ultimately the pattern of suffering.

All addictions are merely coping strategies to "deal" with the pressure and pain that arises in the psyche, as a downstream result of the core wound of suffrage. Everyone that has experienced the trials of addiction has also experienced the pain of suffering. The life path that Siddhartha was led into was to discover the way out of human suffering and that is exactly how you know that his pursuit was actually to find the way out of human addiction. Addiction is not something that suddenly manifested itself in the twentieth century, due to overindulgence in substances, social dynamics, pornography, and more recently with the advent of technology. Addiction is one of the most basic universal themes that has existed from the very dawn of human history, tracing back to the biblical accounts of Adam and Eve, descending down into their offspring with the parable of Cane and Abel. The central wound pattern of the human heart, which translates into each and every human heart, is that of addiction and the cycle of struggle and suffering that accompanies it.

As we follow Siddhartha through his experiences with asceticism and into self-punishment as a way to disavow the carnal desires of the body, we find a man who is seeking to escape his own felt sensations of pain and suffering. He is instructed to punish the body as a way to ascend spiritually but this becomes a futile endeavor, and only amplifies the very sensation he is trying so hard to become free of. This kind of pursuit can become an addiction all of itself, one that I have witnessed throughout the varies spiritual and health orientated communities worldwide. People go on long extended water fasts as a way to abstain from the desires of the body in hopes that they will break free from desire all together. Fasting is a powerful practice for growth and healing but taken into its extreme, it becomes detrimental to the body, and detrimental to the human being who is trying to escape their body. Anything that is done in the extreme for extended periods of time becomes an addiction, and that addiction is one that can only be remedied by coming back into the natural balance of life.

One of the main messages that Buddha taught following his transformation was about desire and how we need to balance our desires, as opposed to disown and reject them all together. We are never going to get rid of our desires, they are here to stay. So, the objective is to manage our desires with discipline, intelligence, and acceptance. The core principle here is accepting our desires, instead of rejecting them, because if we reject our desires, what we are doing is rejecting a part of ourselves, and this only leads to an overcompensation of an unmet desire. When we sense a strong desire for something that we associate as "bad" or "unproductive", the appropriate response is simply to feel where that desire is coming from in our body. The idea is to remain balanced in our emotions and simply allow the sensations of the body to be fully felt, acknowledged, and met with loving awareness. It is only when we begin disowning our desires and rejecting them, that we experience a strong amplification of bodily sensations that lead us into reaching out for coping mechanisms to numb, sooth, medicate, or override our own temporary discomfort.

"Addiction is not your problem. Addiction is your attempt to solve your problem."

Dr. Gabor Mate

In Buddhism there is a concept called 'the hungry ghosts', which describes the sensation of craving, thirst, and hunger we may feel when in the experience of addiction. The famous lecturer and physician Dr. Gabor Mate, who is one of the world leading experts on addiction, speaks a lot about this concept. He wrote an incredible book on addiction called **In the Realm of Hungry Ghosts**. The hungry ghost concept is explained from the Buddhist perspective that there are multiple realms in which the human experience exists. The two primary polarizing realms of extremes are the hell realm and the god realm. The hell realm is where the deepest states of suffering and bondage exist, which is what we may likely associate as the general states experienced in serious addictions. The god realm is the transcendence from the issues of survival, sensual desires, and material worldly concerns. We as human beings tend to exist somewhere in-between these two extremes, some more to one than the other at different seasons in life.

In Dr. Gabor Mate's book, he articulates the realm of the hungry ghosts; *"The inhabitants of the hungry ghost realm are depicted as creatures with scrawny necks, small mouths, emaciated limbs, and large, bloated, empty bellies. This is the domain of addiction, where we constantly seek something outside of ourselves to curb an insatiable yearning for relief or fulfillment. The aching emptiness is perpetual because the substances, objects, or pursuits we hope will soothe it are not what we really need. We don't know what we need, and so long as we stay in the hungry ghost mode, we'll never know. We haunt our lives without being fully present."*

This is a brilliant description of the concept at hand, because it explains the fundamental theme that plays itself out within all of our lives while we are caught in the hook of addiction, which produces increased sensations of anxiety, self-doubt, and suffrage. The realm of hungry ghosts is oftentimes a place that people seek out as a possible escape from dwelling to much in the lower "hell realm" they may have found themselves in. As Gabor says, "addiction is not your problem. Addiction is your attempt to solve your problem" and once we become aware that our addictive tendencies are a strategy for relief, then we can begin to work ourselves out of this no man's land called the realm of hungry ghosts. As the name suggests this is an experiential realm where we are feeding our cravings that have a bottomless pit but cannot effectively digest what it is consuming. We may think we are feeding a substance or object of our insatiable desire, but what we are actually feeding is our vital life force energy, and the only possible result of this kind of dynamic is loss of life.

This circles back to the central teaching of Buddha around managing and discipling our desires. Where exactly are our impulsive desires coming from? What is the craving behind our desires? What is the payoff from feeding our desires? These are all important questions to ask ourselves as the desire emerges and to choose whether we are going to feed a hungry ghost or we are going to empower a genuine impulse to grow and evolve as a human being. As the Buddha learned, everything comes down to personal choice. Everything we do is a choice, even if we slip into autopilot or simply pretend to be a victim of our addictions, it is all still a choice we make in the moment. When we are feeding our hungry ghosts, it is usually as a form of pain relief or to ease the pressure we feel inside. When we feel these heightened states of internal imbalance it can become very difficult to make rational and logic decisions. All we want to do is escape from the temporary moment of discomfort and the allure of the hungry ghost suggests that if we just feed it, all of our problems will go away, for a moment that is.

This was likely the same temptation Siddhartha faced while being confronted by Mara and his three daughters of deception, lust, and trickery. The allure was to make him fall off his center, out of his balance, and tempt him to give in to these lower states of addiction. He had effectively purged himself of any temptation or addiction to escaping his own humanity by this point, which is how he was able to so easily remain still, poised, and balanced, while perceived chaos was breaking out all around him, even if it was only in his own mind. He was able to fully accept all of the spectrum of human emotion and integrate it as an embodied state of being. This is the same test we all face in our daily lives, in the battles we experience with our addictions, with our inner discomfort, and it all begins to soften the moment we choose to accept that discomfort and pain is simply a part of life, just as joy and happiness is a part of life as well.

The greatest lesson I take away from the Siddhartha legend is the power of persistence and the pursuit of achieving a noble ideal for one's own existence. Addiction is simply the initiation points we all face in our road towards greatness and recovery. It is the necessary process of integrating the lessons we learn along the way. It is a long road to recovery, because recovery is a life path in of itself, but it is not the ultimate conclusion of the path, it is simply the bridge between the addicted version of ourselves into the liberated and empowered version of ourselves. The moment Siddhartha became the Buddha was in a moment of absolute wholeness, where he touched the earth as his ultimate witness, requiring no approval from anyone or anything around him, and in that moment he truly became enlightened.

This journey we are all on is a transformational process and one that must be walked one foot in front of the other, one breath after another, and one day followed by the next. You, nor I, nor anyone on this recovery path requires the approval of our family members, our peer group, our clients or customers, or anyone else for that matter. The only approval we truly require is between us and God, or between us and life itself if you prefer to use that phrase. It is all the same at the end of the day. In order to truly heal our addictions, we must learn to heal the inner divide that has caused a trauma inside our beating hearts, because that wound is what has caused the addiction to manifest in the first place. Just as Siddhartha was able to heal the core wound of humanity within his heart, we too can do the same. And that process my friend, is incredible personal and incredible sacred. In fact, it is the single most sacred act of self-empowerment anyone can ever make in their lives.

Section 5

The Return Back to Wholeness

We have finally made it to the final frontier of this incredible journey into the exploration, unpacking, and recovery phase of our addiction free lifestyle adventure. This is truly a moment of triumph, grace, and achievement for anyone who has endured the rigors of addiction, self-sabotage patterning, and has continually chosen to rise from the ashes of their prior setbacks, only to remerge as a human being who is far more capable of greatness, disciplined in their actions, confident in themselves, and focused on their life direction. There are no words to properly articulate how proud of you I am but suffice to say, that you are standing on the shoulders of all the giants who have come before you, come before us all, and have paved the way for us to do incredibly remarkable things in the world.

Just as we have passed through the sections regarding karma and dharma, we too have moved through our own karmic holding patterns to addiction, only to realize a greater power of healing that has existed inside of us all this time. This moment is the moment of all moments. This is the moment of decision, where we choose who we will be from here on out, and what our lives will be for all of time. We have explored the spiritual roots of addiction and how it takes a spiritual commitment, not just an intellectual one, to truly overcome the addiction frequency that is ravaging the planet right now. Addiction is a spiritual affliction more than it just is a psychological or chemical one. The story of Siddhartha was the testament to this fact, and you can include yourself in the halls of great beings who have conquered their innermost addictions, and transmuted their weaknesses into immense strength, courage, and spiritual fortitude.

The final segment of this book will dive into the practical application of the 21 Day Dopamine Reset - Reboot - Recovery Methodology, which provides a holistic blueprint for resetting the dopamine addicted brain, rebooted the brain and nervous system complex, and stepping into the recovery phase of whole healing and integration. This is where the next journey of life begins but certainly not where it ends.

The 21 Day Dopamine Reset Protocol

The dopamine reset protocol is the most important element of this entire book because it provides the clear-cut road map for optimal health, internal motivation, and overall success. Dopamine is the biological trigger point for impulsive tendencies that are associated with addiction and reactive habits. In order to overcome any form of addiction we have to overcome our biological dependency on dopamine triggering habits and balance out the neurotransmitter system of the brain. The dopamine dependency phenomenon not only creates addictive habits, but it is also creates an addicted brain due to the rehearsed patterns influencing the neuropathways that guide our thoughts and behaviors. There really is no alternative or bypass to this process other than doing a full dopamine reset which involves abstaining (detoxing) from all of the dopaminergic triggers in our day-to-day lifestyle.

As you begin implementing this protocol it is important to utilize the principles and holistic strategies laid out in the book to support yourself while you undergo the bio-chemical rebooting process. Remember, healing is a holistic process and requires us to address the whole human, not just the body alone. As the body goes through its own alchemical process of transformation the mind will also begin to undergo its own process. In fact, the mind begins this process far before the body itself and once someone has made a decisive commitment to follow through on a particular path, the body begins to respond in like fashion. The discomfort, tension, and doubt that kicks on in the beginning is the indication that this process has begun and that it's time to push through that doubt in order to take the next steps forward. The doubt is a signal that there is change on the way and what lies on the other side of this change is something completely different than what the conditioned mind has become all too familiar with.

There are stages to this protocol, and it does not have to be done all at once. It certainly can be done at the same time and that would be the fastest way to go. Not everyone is ready to begin untethering themselves from each and every dopamine triggering habit right out the get go. The important thing to remember is this process is all about making consistent progress, not about perfection. The most critical place for everyone to begin is unhooking their own biology from the foods, substances, and overt influences that have the biggest impact on their neurochemistry and nervous system response. This would be the processed foods, the sugary drinks, the synthetic supplements, the coffee and caffeinated teas, the blood oxygen reducing tobacco, brain stunting alcohol, and escapism through cannabis, and anything else that has a significant effect on altering one's brain state which includes pornography, excessive social media exposure, and aimless online scrolling.

When these things have been conquered all the other little distractions are easy to manage and eliminate. Life becomes far more enjoyable, manageable, and free of unnecessary stress because the chemistry set of the brain is operating as it was designed to do. In the beginning everyone feels a bout of withdrawal and all of the emotions that arise due to resetting the system. This is normal and should be expected for the first few days to a week. This protocol is designed to help you cruise through the withdrawal process as easily and effortlessly as possible but that does not mean it will always be easy or effortless. You are going to have to work to redirect your attention towards the things you have been avoiding due to the distractions of what you are now letting go off.

You will likely notice a need to sleep longer the first few days and some energetic lows through the day. Again, this is normal, and you will need to remind yourself that nothing is wrong with you if you experience a heightened negative self-talk arising to the surface. You may even experience a bit of what is considered depression and how you deal with those temporary states will determine how incredibly good you feel on the other side. Give yourself a few days to be unproductive, unfocused, unsettled, and to sleep as much as your body needs. This is not the time to begin stacking your schedule. You will not feel like a superhuman right away but give it some time and I can assure you that you will feel a greater depth of motivation, energy, and mental focus than you had ever felt while under the influence of mind-altering stimulants and dopamine triggering behaviors.

This is an overall lifestyle upgrade, so treat it as a whole lifestyle makeover and you will find that success is not only achievable, but you will feel far better than you could even begin to imagine before. Health is about a lifestyle that supports the functions of the body, the mind, the heart, and the soul. When we think of recovery from this perspective then we become less inclined to do anything that would infringe upon any of these considerations. It always allows us to easily discern between what is supporting us and what is slowing us down. When we create a lifestyle map for ourselves, we begin to create greater momentum in our life and all of the pieces tend to fall into synchrony together from there. Then all we need to do is remain consistent with the momentum and keep it going. It's really that simple!

The Three Phases of Progression: Reset - Reboot – Recovery

The three phases of progression is a concept I developed almost a decade ago in my original book, **The Holistic Health Mastery Program**, which takes people through the three phases of healing the body goes through from a disease or degenerative condition into balanced health. This starts with detoxification as phase one. This leads into experimentation as phase two. This then goes into integration as phase three. The simple concept is that we have to cleanse and detox the body of all prior indiscretions of poor food choices, chemical toxins, and destructive habits that led someone to their state of poor health. Following the detoxification phase is experimentation, which is where someone begins to explore the wider array of organic fruits, vegetables, super foods, tonic herbs, and other whole food options as a way to discover what works best for them moving forward. The integration phase is where someone finds what works best for them at this point and solidifies their new lifestyle habits as a consistent approach to life.

I readapted this concept to match the dopamine reset, because it is very much the same identical process, but the framework is a bit different in this regard. I am going to take you through the three phases of dopamine resetting and brain-based recovery so that you have a working model for how to get started, what to consider as you make your way into phase 1 and two, and how to remain consistent as you enter through phase 3 of the process.

Phase 1: Reset

The reset phase is likened to what we would call the "withdrawal" phase of any addiction or persistent habit that has a neuro-chemical response in our brain. The withdrawal phase is the hardest part of the journey for most people who seek recovery and freedom from addictions. This is where the brain is in most resistance to getting started and/or making that full departure from its accustomed dopamine feedback stimuli that it has become all too comfortable with. Remember, the brain itself can become addicted to the dopamine-serotonin feedback loops, and when we are resetting our neuro-chemical receptor pathways, we will likely experience various forms of discomfort during this period of time.

Withdrawing from a habit means to abstain from the habit itself in order to create enough space between the cognitive association of the habit and the desired effect it causes in our brain. For example, if you use coffee or caffeine as a way to stimulate your brain to get into gear and start out the day, you will likely experience resistance when you choose to remove it from your morning routine. Trying to do this in moderation could be beneficial in the very beginning as to not disrupt your daily flow too much, especially if you cannot simply take a week off from work, but do not fall into the trap of living in the moderation mode, because the point is to completely remove this pattern in order to help the brain reset itself. The brain will not be able to go through a full reset until we remove the substance for long enough period of time, which tends to look like multiple months at minimum.

The reset phase can last anywhere from a few weeks to a little over a month, perhaps 6 weeks depending on how insulated the habits have been. What will shorten this reset phase is when you replace old stimulatory habits with healthier habits that help to repair the brains neurotransmitter set, specifically dopamine and serotonin as the chief brain hormones being exhausted from addictive substances or excessive habits such as social media or pornography. The reset is phase one i.e., the withdrawal phase, and this leads us into the second phase, which is where we begin to experience the emerging benefits that come on the other end of a good cognitive reset.

Phase 2: Reboot

The reboot phase is where our brain and nervous system has properly withdrawn from the chemical feedback loops, they had been addicted too, and running on autopilot with. In this phase we are no longer running on autopilot, we are fully conscious, and entirely anchored in the cock put of our bodily operating system. Like a computer processor, it has to sometimes go through a rebooting phase in order to delete old files, programs, and malware viruses in order to run more efficiently. Well, this is exactly the same with our brains that process incalculable amounts of information, life experiences, belief programs, and absorbed data of the world around us. When we have too many tabs open in a web browser, the processing speed slows down, becomes less efficient, and it takes much more time to move from one window browser to another. Our brains happen to be far more advanced than a simple CPU processor, but they function very much the same.

The reboot phase is where upgraded information in the form of brand-new lifestyle habits, dietary practices, exercise routines, self-care rituals, and new life skill sets are uploaded into the operating system. The brain has an auto-delete process called 'synaptic-pruning', where it will delete old neuronal circuits associated with prior habit patterns that are no longer useful or relevant to the new brain that is being formed. Yes, I said NEW BRAIN that is being formed! That is exactly what is happening in this process, which is why it is so important to maintain consistency to your chosen upgraded habits, because this is a very sensitive and fertile period where the operating system of the body is deciding what it will let go of and what it will include, based on the information it is being provided.

Most people get completely stuck in the reset phase, which is why they rarely ever experience the benefits of removing destructive habits, and simply maintain a dysfunctional relationship with their addictions. This is the phase where we begin to experience more bodily energy, better recovery from sleep, increased mental clarity and emotional stability. This is where we begin to get enough positive reinforcement from our efforts and are shown a glimpse of what is really possible by living an addiction free lifestyle.

Phase 3: Recovery

This phase is where all the effort and persistence count the most. This is the phase of total integration of one's intentions, goals, commitment, and hard work. This is where we recover from the afflictions of addiction and transition into wholeness of self. This is where true confidence emerges as a byproduct of staying steadfast on the path, making it through the reset and reboot phase of the dopamine recovery process. The brain itself goes through a complete recovery, because as I mentioned, it is not only us that goes through addiction, but the physical brain that has its own addiction loops as well. The result of the brain recovering from addiction is increased processing power, which looks like greater memory recall, both short term and long-term memory. When we are unable to remember things easily, that is a sure-fire sign that our neurotransmitter system is greatly out of balance. This is not something that has to happen with age, it is something that happens when our brain ages due to poor health choices, chemical influences, and neurotransmitter short circuiting.

As I always explain to my audiences, clients, and podcast interviewers, the recovery phase is not simply recovering the physical addictions. It is more so the process of recovering the lost pieces of ourselves that had gone missing earlier on in our childhood due to traumatic events that we were unable to process or simply did not realize had an effect on us. It is the recovery of our innocence that was assaulted in childhood, sometimes due to familial trauma, and sometimes due to the fact that we had to grew up far too fast, in order to get through the world, and become an adult the way society told us we had too. So, in a sense, the recovery process is a form of self-parenting ourselves into a fully integrated state of healthy adulthood, where our traumas have been healed, our wounds have been cleared, and the addiction patterns we used to medicate our pain have completely been released as a result of the healing that has occurred.

This is where we truly discover who we are, without our dopamine crutches, without our dependence on false stimulation, without our limiting stories and excuses for why we do not feel like we are good enough. This is the moment of integration and the word integration really just means to be in integrity with ourselves, our core values, our authentic beliefs, and the daily actions we carry out for our lives.

The Dopamine Reset Guide

The Ultimate Dopamine Reset - Reboot - Recovery Method is a 21-day process that I adapted from all of the research and practical tools I have garnered over the years of being a professional nutritionist and transformation coach. This is a very simple yet sophisticated approach to repairing the dopamine receptor sites in the brain and rebooting the entire operating system of the body itself. This process can be done in conjunction with other approaches such as specific cleanses, modified diets, and other holistic health-based strategies. The important part about this is adhering to the foundational principles which act as a guiding light for success. There is a lot of flexibility built into this protocol and the most important principle is consistency over all others.

The first place we begin is the preparation phase which is to set up the framework for the next 21 days and get clear on the principles that need to be followed in order to ensure success.

Prep work:
- *Creating a Winning Environment*
- *Have a Dopamine Detox Buddy*
- *Have a Journal Ready*
- *Clarify Your Goals / Intentions*
- *Hydrate & Nourish Yourself*
- *Identify Stress Patterns*

What to Avoid:
- *Stimulants (Caffeine, Nicotine, etc.)*
- *Unnecessary Stressful Situations*
- *Being Overly Logical / Heady*
- *Judging Yourself & Others*
- *Comfort Foods / Sugary Drinks*
- *Staying Up Too Late (After 10 PM)*
- *Too Much Social Media*

Nutritional Protocols:

- *1 Liter of Spring Water + 1/4 tsp Sea Salt*
- *Purium Core 4 Products (More info provided below)*
- *High Quality Magnesium (More info provided below)*
- *Full Spectrum CBD*
- *Green Vegetable Juices (Celery, Cucumber, Green Apple, Ginger, etc.)*
- *Green Powdered Super Foods*
- *Balance of Fats, Protein, Carbohydrates in the Diet*
- *Calming Evening Tea + Apothacherry (More info provided below)*

Tech Protocols:

- *Delete Social Media Apps on Phone*
- *Clarify Your Purpose for Using Social Media*
- *Get the Flux App on your Computer (blue light dimming app)*
- *Get a Pair of Blue Light Block Glasses for Evening Tech Use*
- *Leave Your Phone Alone Prior to Sleep (On airplane mode)*
- *Only Check Emails & Social Media Twice a Day*

Integration Practices:

- *Breath work*
- *Meditation*
- *Cold Shower / Ice Plunge*
- *Emotional Processing / Somatic Work*
- *Journaling / Reflection Time*
- *Tapping / EFT (Emotional Freedom Technique)*
- *Daily Naps / Deep Restorative Sleep*
- *Movement Practices / Preferred Exercise Routines*
- *Yoga / Stretching*
- *Sweating / Infrared Sauna / Sun to Skin Contact*
- *Float Tank - Sensory Deprivation*
- *Nature Time - 1 Measured Hour in Nature Each Day*

The Dopamine Reset Daily Flow Chart

The dopamine reset flow chart is a simple daily mode of operations for structuring the rhythm of each day by following a simple action-based framework. There is flexibility and fluidity to how this works and as mentioned before, there are basic principles to help keep you anchored to the overall goals and outcomes you desire. The main outcome is to reset the dopamine receptor pathways of the brain and begin what I call the "rebooting" process for the bodily operating system. This flow chart lays out a morning, afternoon, and evening structure. I kept this very simple because each person's lifestyle, diet, supplement needs, and overall situation is unique, but the core principles remain the same.

Morning
- *Wake Up Without an Alarm*
- *Take Ten Deep Breaths*
- *Drink 1 Liter Spring Water + 1/4 tsp sea salt*
- *Take Supplements*
- *Journal / Map Out the Goals for the Day*
- *Postpone Tech for 1-2 Hours if possible*
- *Movement / Exercise Routine*
- *Pray / Meditation / Energy Work (Somatic Work)*

Mid-Day - Afternoon
- *Super Food Smoothie and/or Healthy Meal*
- *Engage Top Priorities for the Day*
- *Mid-Day Nap / Rest & Reset (Nap if needed otherwise take 30 minutes to simply rest)*
- *Access Energy Levels*
- *Do What is Nourishing, Fulfilling, & Important to Close Out the Day*

Evening
- *Transition from Technology*
- *Read / Movement / Write / Art*
- *Eat a Nourishing Healthy Meal*
- *Take Evening Supplements*

- *Prepare for a Deep Night's Sleep*

Down Time Activities

The biggest challenge in this process can be feelings of boredom and loss of interest in "normal" activities. Because the dopamine receptors become blunted due to pleasure sensory overload or due to excess stress, we can find ourselves losing interest in what may feel like mundane or trivial daily functions. It is important to stay out of the 'boredom zone' because that is the space, we can easily find ourselves trying to fill up by going back to temporary gratifying activities that we are working to overcome. If you feel boredom, there are two things you can do. One is to feel the feelings that arise and go into some kind of meditation and do some breath work to move the energy. The other is to redirect the numbness that arises in boredom and do something that will help to elevate our mood and energy.

- *Clean a Closet / Bedroom / Garage / House / Car*
- *Go on a Hike / Go into the Water / Spend time in Nature*
- *Paint / Draw / Write / Do some form of Art*
- *Listen to Uplifting Music*
- *Read a Book!*
- *Listen to an Inspiring or Interesting podcast*
- *Call a close friend for support or simply to catch up*
- *Write out your goals for the next 6-12 months!*
- *Send 5-10 gratitude text messages to friends*
- *Lay down on your bed, close your eyes, and sleep if your body is tired*

The Dopamine Nutritional Protocol

The nutritional protocol is designed to help with the neurochemical withdrawal process and rebooting the brains neurotransmitter systems that have been burdened during the cycles of addiction. The biggest challenge people have in the withdrawal window is nutritional imbalances and deficiencies, for the most part. There are key vitamins, amino acids, minerals, and macro nutrients such as fatty acids that are critical for optimal brain function, blood sugar, hormone regulation, and neurotransmitter production. All of these factors are essential for cleansing the body of its chemical codependency from all forms of addictive substances and external dopamine reliance.

This is a sample blueprint that I would create for a client who is upgrading their health regime and looking to let go of addictive habits. The process of enhancing overall health is much the same as it is for overcoming addiction. In fact, it should be assumed that all pursuits of better health are really just attempts to overcome addictive habits that detour from good health in the first place.

This protocol can get more sophisticated, and I provide incredibly detailed nutritional programs in my other two books, The Holistic Health Mastery Program & The Inner Alchemy Youthening Program. You can review the recipe and supplementation sections of those books to go much deeper, but these basics will serve anyone who is recovering from addiction and beyond.

Morning Routine:
1 Liter of Spring Water + 1/4 teaspoon of Sea Salt
Morning Supplements
Green Vegetable Juice - 16-32 oz (Celery, Cucumber, Ginger, Green Apple +
1 table of chlorella, blue green algae, or spirulina)

Super Food Protein Smoothie - Sample Recipe
6-8 oz of Wild Blueberries
8-12 oz of Unpasteurized Coconut Water or Hemp, Almond, or Coconut Milk
1 TBL of Sprouted Sunflower, Almond, Coconut, or Brazil Nut Butter
1 TBL of High-Quality Protein Powder
1 TBL of Hemp Seeds (if more protein is desired)

Mid - Day Routine:
1 Liter of Spring Water (Can be broken up in 3-4 glasses over the afternoon)
1 Green Vegetable Juice, Herbal Tea Infusion, or Bone Broth
Light Meal (if desired) - Wild Caught Salmon - Organic Green Leafy Salad - Sweet Potato, etc.
2nd Round of Supplements that should be taken twice a day

Evening Routine

1 table of Apple Cider Vinegar diluted in shot glass of water 20 minutes prior to meal. (Increases stomach acid for added digestion)

*Nourishing and Satiating Meal - Specific to your metabolic type (fats-proteins-carbohydrates) - (See chapter **Mastering the Body: Optimizing Nutrition**)*

Take evening supplements 1 hour after consuming meal (let the food digest before drinking any liquids) + 1 Glass of Water.

Recommended Supplements

This list could be much more detailed and far more expanded. I left it simple because many people need to keep things simple in order to get started. If you want to go deeper, please review the back end of my book, The Inner Alchemy Youthening Program for a complete detailed supplement list with descriptions. Each of the following supplements below are for the dopamine reset process and will aid in helping the brain reboot its neurotransmitter set and aid in the detoxification process.

- Free Form Full Spectrum Amino Acids (Fermented Amino Acids preferably & contain all 8 essential amino acids)
- High Quality Magnesium
- High Quality - Full Spectrum CBD Sublingual Dropper
- Niacin - Flush Version for Niacin Flushing - Non-Flush Version for Vitamin B3 Support
- Full Spectrum B - Vitamins
- Vitamin B12 (Methylcarbylamine or Adenosyl cobalamin + Contains B9)
- L-Theanine (Matcha or Guayusa make for good coffee substitute because of its L-Theanine content)
- Tart Cherry Concentrate (highest source of natural melatonin - aids in REM sleep support)

The Dopamine Social Media Detox

This is an important consideration for redirecting the neuropathways of the brain due to the addictive nature of "smart" devices, global internet access, and social media platforms. Things are all things that we have grown accustomed too and resources we need to leverage in our techno-social world. The key to developing a healthy dynamic with technology and online platforms is to never become addicted to these things for personal amusement, entertainment, or for personal validation. That is the trap of the times we live in and these technologies have a far greater (and hidden) addictive nature to them than most other things. This is why we have to create a healthy space between our phones, our computers, and our social media habits in order to find out how addictive they can really become.

Consider this process as a temporary purge from social media influences on your brain. It's time to reacclimatize back into the felt experience of your immediate surroundings and your life as a whole. It's far too easy to distract ourselves by checking into the social media interface but this does not serve our brain, it actually worsens it to a minimal or even a significant degree. It is healthy to have a periodic cycle where you delete all social media apps from your phone and take a social media hiatus for days, onto weeks at a time as needed. When we simply delete the apps from our devices it can free up a tremendous amount of space in our mind and open up pockets of creativity you did not know where there. Even if you choose to use these platforms regularly, it is a good idea to make it a habit of deleting the primary apps and only using them when you are going to make a post or respond to a message. Otherwise, they take up space in our phones, in our minds, and are far too assessable that we can click the app anytime we want to distract ourselves from the present moment.

The Social Media Reset Protocol

The SM reset protocol is actually incredibly simple and straight forward. Ultimately what is recommended is to create a new attention-based relationship with social media platforms, checking our emails, scrolling on the internet, and reverting to checking our smart phones all together. By following the rest of the dopamine reset process, you will likely develop a new relationship with your digital devices and the applications you habitually check, out of pure habit but not necessarily with clear intention.

The simple idea is to schedule two distinct time windows in each day for checking your email and checking your social media accounts, including messages. This is a designated time for that activity and outside of those times, you simply do not check your phone or computer for emails or social media activity. You can pick the times, but it should be a 15-30 or maybe even 45–60-minute block of time, depending on how much time it actually requires of you to do what is needed to do. That is up to you, but you choose a time in the mid-morning preferable and then another time in the mid-later afternoon, as the day is concluding. This helps you get everything you need to get done in those windows, so you are not aimlessly wasting time, and you are being very intentional with how you spend your time on these platforms.

The second part of this, which is most important, is to delete your social media apps entirely off of your phone. I explained why this is important above and believe me, it will change how your brain respond to these applications when you have to reinstall them each time you choose to get back on it. It only takes a few seconds to reinstall it, no big deal at all. But that little gap in-between the thought of clicking the app out of habit, and having to install it, and re-login is a pattern interrupt that will help to create enough space between the thought of doing it and acting on it in the impulsive moment.

You may even consider completely removing the social media apps from your phone for an entire week. Doing a social media digital detox is incredibly healthy for the brain and for our emotional stability. If you feel like you have been staring too long at screens and your brain needs a digital dump, then you may want to consider getting off social media for a week, all together and simply give yourself a break from the virtual alternative reality, all together!

Final Thoughts

The addiction free lifestyle is a way of life, a way of being, and a path that can lead to incredible freedom. This is not a "diet", a short-term cleanse, or temporary approach to managing our addictions. This is an approach to living a life of inner clarity, self-discipline, optimal health, and personal power. This book has laid out the framework for overcoming addictions of all kinds and tapping into the subtle nature of how these addictions gain footing in our lives. Addiction, of course, is the single biggest challenge all human beings face, and serves as the initiation for immense growth, if we choose to accept the call towards recovery and integration that comes on the other end of the challenges we face along the way. This is not an easy path for anyone to walk. Recovering from the spirals of addiction and codependence is one of the hardest obstacles most of us must face in our lives, but it is also one of the most rewarding feelings anyone can experience, knowing they had assumed the courage, diligence, and persistence to see themselves through their stumbles along the path, and keep moving forward towards the finish line of becoming whole, healed, and complete within themselves.

There are multiple layers to the recovery process. It is not simply removing one layer by doing the dopamine reset - reboot - recovery process. This process happens in multiple instances and takes multiple forms as we go through our lives. This process serves as a simplified road map for moving through the layers of our own human experience, knowing that true healing occurs in waves, not just in a single instance. This book is meant to be a transformational manual that you can continue to refer back to over time, rereading sections that are most relevant in the moment, and provide golden nuggets of insight that you may have not seen in prior readings of them. As we evolve and grow, we begin to see things in a brand-new way. This book is meant to be a lifelong companion that sits by your bedside, is regularly visible on your countertop, or comes with you when you take space to be in nature.

The final words of encouragement I will leave you with here is to remain focused on who you choose to be, beyond the struggles and challenges in any given moment. Your vision for the future will powerfully aid you in going beyond the discomfort and temporary self-doubt of any challenging moment. When you feel those bouts of doubt, loss of confidence, instability, or general uncertainty, I want you to refer back to your goals, intentions, and purpose for pursuing an addiction free lifestyle. It is easy to lose focus and get knocked off center when we have lost track of our purpose. Make sure this does not happen to you. You can protect against this by following the steps in the dopamine reset process and taking the wisdom you received in this book and implementing it in your daily life.

Remember, one good habit leads to another. One positive action leads to another. One change in behavior will encourage the next. This is all about upgrading ourselves in any given moment, wherever there is an opportunity to grow, that is exactly where we lean into the process, and allow it to transform us, at the core. You have everything required to transform your life into the most incredible masterpiece you envision for yourself. Use your imagination in productive and inspiring ways. Let it be your guiding light towards a prosperous and truly fulfilling future. Everything is at your fingertips. All you have to do is make a decision that you will follow through until that future becomes your present moment. Let go of what does not serve and support that future, and you will be astonished by how fast the universe conspires to make that your new reality.

Blessings on the Journey,
Ronnie Landis